CRICKET BALL
About 1 cup
Use for cereal,
rice, pasta

TAKEAWAY COFFEE CUP
About 250 ml
Use for milk, yogurt,
soups

C000133188

TENNIS BALL
About ⅔ cup
Use for bread, rolls,
potatoes, small
serves of starch

DECK OF CARDS
About 85–110 grams
Use for serves of
beef, chicken,
pork, salmon

2 GOLF BALLS
About ½ cup
Use for beans,
hot cereals

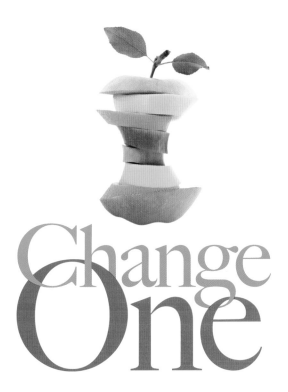

Change
One

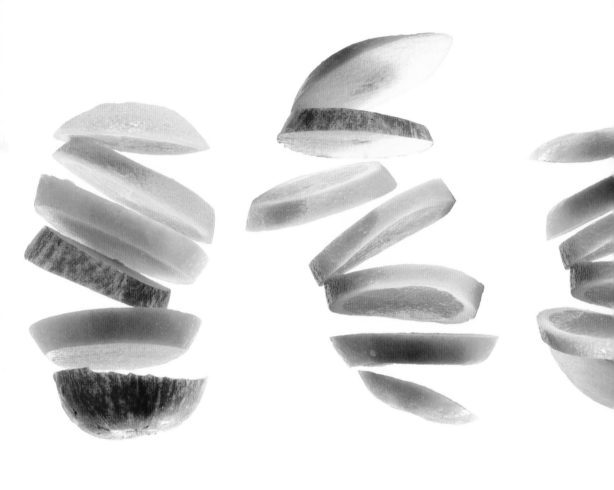

Change One

One

the DIET and FITNESS PLAN

Reader's Digest

Contributors

Most health books are conceived and written by just one person. *ChangeOne, the diet and fitness plan* has taken a different approach. As it has expanded and grown, *ChangeOne* has drawn on a team of doctors, writers, food experts, fitness experts and editors. For this updated edition, we'd like to thank the following people for their expertise and hard work.

Suzie Ferrie, an Advanced Accredited Practising Dietitian (AdvAPD) based in Sydney, Australia. Involved in both patient care and research, with diverse interests that include researching metabolism in health and illness, proteins and probiotics, Suzie has worked as a nutrition consultant on more than 10 books.

John Hastings, Peter Jaret and Mindy Hermann, the founding voices of the *ChangeOne* program. John has worked as a journalist covering medicine, nutrition and fitness for more than 20 years. Peter is the author of the Reader's Digest book *Heart Healthy for Life* and has also received an American Medical Association award for medical reporting. Mindy is a registered dietitian, and a speaker and consultant on weight loss and nutrition. She has co-authored the Reader's Digest book *Live Longer Live Better,* and was the nutrition writer for the American Medical Association *Family Health Cookbook.*

Selene Yeager, a trainer, triathlete and health-and-fitness entrepreneur, who developed the *ChangeOne* 10-minute-a-day exercise routines that you'll find inside.

Thanks also to **John Foreyt,** director of the Behavioural Medicine Research Center at Baylor College of Medicine, Texas, who originally shaped the *ChangeOne* approach.

The Editors

Note to our readers

This publication is designed to provide useful information to the reader on the subjects of weight loss, healthy eating and exercise. It should not be substituted for the advice of a doctor or used to alter any medical therapy or programs prescribed for you by your doctor. Make sure you consult your doctor before proceeding with any weight loss or exercise regime. The mention of specific products in this book does not constitute an endorsement by the author or the publisher. The author and the publisher disclaim any liability or loss, personal, financial or otherwise, which may be claimed or incurred, directly or indirectly, resulting from the use and/or application of the content of this publication.

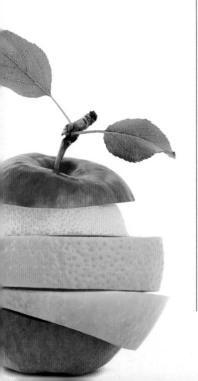

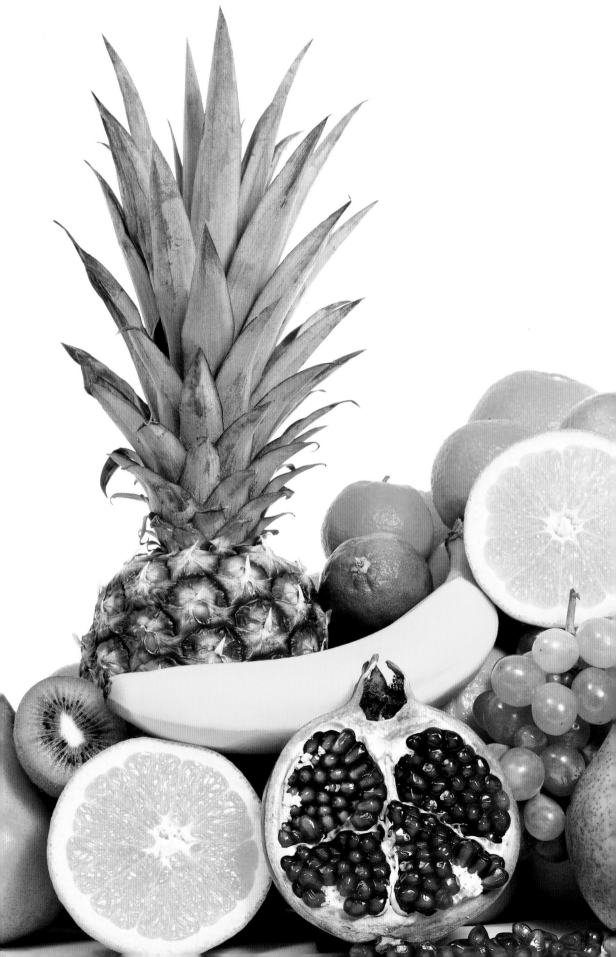

Contents

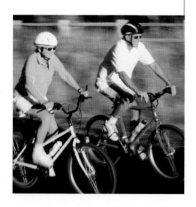
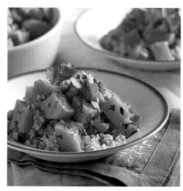
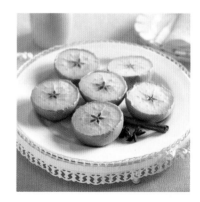

Part 3
ChangeOne Resources

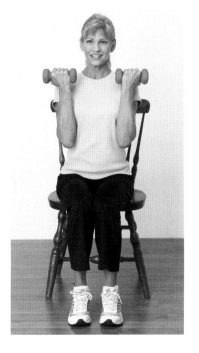
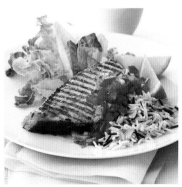
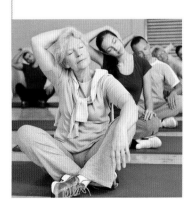

A program that works

How many diet plans have you tried? High protein? High carbohydrates? Low fat? Only eat grapefruit, or cabbage? You know the feeling. For a few weeks the latest fad seems to be working. You lose a few kilos, feel better about yourself and life in general, and then, bang – the weight comes back like a boomerang, and with a vengeance. Now you're left with two problems: you still have those kilos to lose and you feel like a failure.

That's why we created *ChangeOne, the diet and fitness plan.* You will lose weight without giving up the foods you love to eat. And you'll be stronger, in body and mind. By using advice from America's top nutritionists and dietitians and specially adapting it to Australia and New Zealand, we have come up with this completely original eating and fitness plan that takes the weight off...and keeps it off. In only 12 weeks – with just one simple change each week – you will win the weight-loss battle. *ChangeOne* is easy. It's different. And thanks to our testing, we know it works.

There's so much more at stake than looking good. Nearly two-thirds of the adult population in Australia and New Zealand is overweight, and around half of that group is clinically obese. That percentage in Australia alone has doubled since 1980. Obesity is now a national crisis in both countries, seriously affecting people's life expectancy and quality of life. Preventable diseases are now appearing in young people as well as the middle-aged and the elderly as a direct result of obesity. For instance, an increasing number of children are developing type 2 diabetes. It has been estimated that nearly two-thirds of cases of type 2 diabetes in men, and three-quarters in women, could have been avoided if being overweight were not an issue.

But that shouldn't be a surprise to us. Eating has become a national pastime in Australia and New Zealand. In shopping centres everywhere, restaurants and retailers have turned shopping and eating into a full-time hobby. On the road, fast-food outlets and takeaway places are legion. Shopping for food can be fattening, too. In many supermarkets, chocolate bars are just waiting for you at the checkout.

Lose weight *without* giving up the foods you love.

So what's the answer? A commitment to regaining control of what we eat, which is what *ChangeOne* will do for you. In this book you'll learn to:

- Put the focus back on how much you eat, rather than on what you eat. For all the talk about carbs, protein and fat, the thing that matters most is balancing how many kilojoules you eat in a day with how many kilojoules you burn in a day.
- Make permanent changes to how you eat and live. This is a program meant for life, not just 12 weeks.
- Feel confident that the advice we offer is based on thorough, sound scientific research.
- Enjoy the fact that *ChangeOne* is an easy, commonsense weight-loss program that actually works.

This new edition of *ChangeOne* will help yet more people transform their lives through healthier eating and movement. Read the 'success stories' in this book, and you'll see the response has been a resounding, 'Yes! It works!'

ChangeOne is one of the only weight-loss programs around that carefully meshes an eating program with exercise and lifestyle advice. Diet alone isn't enough to keep weight off. To make lasting changes, you need a well-rounded approach, one that bolsters your self-confidence and gets you a lot more active and happy.

While the first edition of *ChangeOne* featured loads of exercise advice and programs, it was based on conventional wisdom about fitness and movement. In this updated edition, we've exploded much of the popular thinking about fitness and come up with an approach that's a whole lot easier, more sensible and more intuitively appealing. You'll love our 10-minute-a-day strength and stretching plan, and you'll nod your head in agreement when we explain why how much time you spend outdoors is a top indicator of how healthy your lifestyle is.

Put it all together, and in only 12 weeks, you will get the training and practice you need to help win the weight-loss battle *permanently*. *ChangeOne* is easy. It's different. And it works. Using the ideas in this book, you can take charge of your life today, and you can succeed!

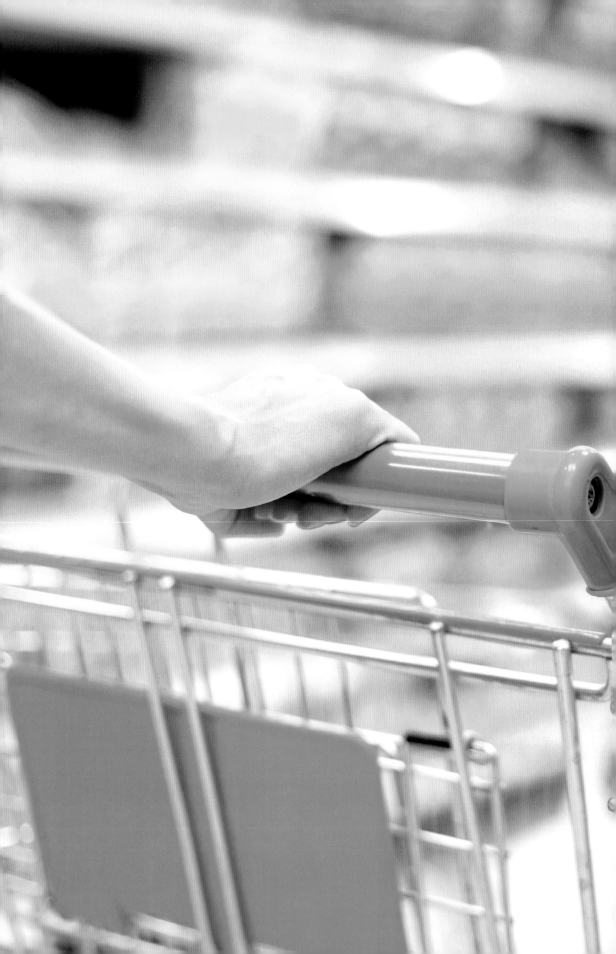

PART 1
DIET

ChangeOne
Quick-start guide

ChangeOne eating

The central theme of our 12–week program is that all foods are allowed in appropriate amounts. Most people will eat about 5500 kilojoules a day on this plan. Larger or more active people can add roughly 1500 kilojoules through extra serves of grain or protein each day. Here's an overview of the first four weeks.

Week 1: Breakfast

Around 1250 kilojoules

Eat a healthy breakfast and love it, even if you don't normally eat anything.

The basic menu

- One grain or starch – roughly 1 cricket ball's worth of ready-to-eat cereal; a slice of toast; or a roll (tennis ball).
- One high-calcium dairy food – 1 cup (250 ml) low-fat milk; or 1 tub (150 g) low-fat yogurt.
- Fruit – one piece or an equivalent amount of melon or berries.

Variations: champagne brunches, smoked salmon and bagels, even a morning parfait are fine if done the *ChangeOne* way.

Week 2: Lunch

Around 1500 kilojoules

You'll learn to recognise a sensible lunch that fits your lifestyle and tastes.

The basic menu

- One grain or starch – 1 tennis ball's worth of potato or a bread roll; two slices of sandwich bread; or a serve of pasta or rice.
- One protein – a small hamburger; thin palm-size slice of reduced-fat cheese; or 3 CD-size pieces of cooked deli meat.
- Fruit – one piece or an equivalent amount of melon or berries.
- Vegetables – as much as you want.

Variations: soups, salads and wraps can all work fine with sensible serve sizes.

Week 3: Snacks

Up to 840 kilojoules

Yes, you can have your cake – twice a day, if you watch yourself.

- Savoury – 1 handful of crisps, savoury biscuits, nuts in the shell or popcorn
- Sweet – 1 palmful of M&Ms, jelly beans, malted milk balls, raisins, boiled lollies; or a fun-size chocolate bar.
- Baked – 2 small biscuits; 1 cupcake; or a 5 cm square brownie (½ business card).
- Frozen – 2 golf balls' worth of frozen yogurt, sorbet or reduced-fat ice-cream; ½ tennis ball's worth of regular ice-cream; or an icy pole or fruit ice confection.

Week 4: Dinner

Around 1900 kilojoules

A full day's worth of dieting begins this week, and you'll never look back.

The basic menu

- One protein – 1 tennis ball's worth of prawns, scallops or crab; 1 deck of card's worth of chicken fillet, beef or salmon; or a serve of white fish the size of a chequebook.
- One grain or starch – 1 tennis ball's worth of rice, pasta, noodles or bread.
- Vegetables – as much as you want.

Variations: casseroles, Chinese buffets, grilled kebabs, stir-fries, barbecues.

The key principles

1. Make one change at a time. You can't become a new person overnight; lasting change requires a measured approach.
2. The secret of weight loss is understanding serve sizes, not maths. If you don't want to count kilojoules for the rest of your life, don't diet that way.
3. All foods are allowed. Let your meals be a source of healthy enjoyment and never skimp on flavour or pleasure.
4. Eating for a healthy weight is the same as eating for health. Think of *ChangeOne* as a way of life, and this will be the last time you *have* to lose weight.

ChangeOne living

While the first four weeks cover meals, the next eight weeks offer essential health lessons. Each week takes on an aspect of daily life that influences how you eat.

Week 5: Eating out

We'll ask you to go out for meals at least twice this week (yes, you *have* to visit restaurants) to practise ordering, and eating, only what you want.

Week 6: Weekends & celebrations

Plan to get together with family or friends, and not only will you be able to enjoy yourself, you'll learn to gracefully say 'no' when your mum or aunt turns into a food pusher.

Week 7: Fixing your kitchen

Take a hard look inside your refrigerator and pantry. Is the food you see going to help you lose weight or undermine your efforts?

Week 8: How am I doing?

Everybody take a deep breath. You're two months into the program so it's time to stop and assess your progress and clear any blockages.

Week 9: Stress relief

Stress has a way of sneaking up on you and eating often serves as a coping mechanism. We'll help you to identify and relieve those hidden pressures.

Week 10: Superfoods

Yes, eat the foods you love on *ChangeOne*. But you might wish to incorporate these foods that provide particularly good weight-loss benefits.

Week 11: Keeping on track

If the kilos start to return, they won't do it all at once. Your goal is to devise your own 'First Alert' program that will help you contain the gain.

Week 12: *ChangeOne*...for life!

You made it! So don't let boredom ruin the new you. Here's how you can make great food an ongoing source of pleasure – and maintain your weight loss.

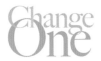
Welcome to *ChangeOne*

You've opened this book for one simple reason: you want to lose weight. Maybe a little, maybe a lot. Maybe you'd like to improve the reflection looking back at you from the mirror. Maybe you're hoping to fit more easily into an old pair of trousers or jeans. Or perhaps you simply want to be healthier and feel better.

Whatever your goal, *ChangeOne* will help you lose weight – and keep it off.

That may sound like a big promise. But there's really no mystery to dieting, despite the bewildering number of plans out there. Want to know a little secret? They all work. You can lose weight on almost any diet because only one thing matters in the weight-loss game: consume fewer kilojoules than you burn. All diets, even the seemingly crazy ones, restrict your kilojoules and that's why you lose weight. Eat sensible amounts of food and the weight will melt away.

Honest, sensible weight loss

So you won't find any silly gimmicks in *ChangeOne*. We're not going to make you become a vegetarian, a strict carnivore, a caveman or a goddess. But we're radically different in one crucial way. *ChangeOne* asks you to approach dieting one meal at a time, one week at a time. (*ChangeOne* means just that – one change at a time.) We won't overwhelm you on day one. Most diets ask you to throw out the way you eat overnight and adopt a new plan. The biggest problem with that kind of approach is that people will eventually go back to their old ways and gain back the weight they lost.

Imagine a psychologist who expects depressed patients to be happy after one visit. Or a language teacher who announces on the first day of class that students will be able to speak fluent French the next day. It sounds laughable because making a significant change takes time; new skills require practice. Yet instant change is what most diets ask for, which could explain why so many people end up regaining the weight they've worked so hard to lose.

ChangeOne slows dieting down so you can experiment and learn. But don't worry, the weight will start coming off right away.

In the first week, you'll make just one change to your diet: overhaul your breakfast, following one of the five suggested *ChangeOne* breakfast menus. Don't worry: we've counted the kilojoules for you. All you'll have to do is learn to recognise reasonable serves.

In the second week, while you stick with your new habit of eating a healthy, low-kilojoule breakfast, you'll move on to lunch. Again, we offer a variety of simple menu choices. All you do is choose one each day during the week.

In the third week, you'll focus on snacks. What do snacks have to do with dieting? Plenty. Snacks will keep you from

The *ChangeOne* team

To put *ChangeOne* to the test, the team that made the original book in the USA recruited volunteers from around America – and now a group in Australia is taking the *ChangeOne* challenge – people just like you who wanted to lose weight to look and feel better. When people were offered the chance to try the program, the response was overwhelming, and the results were just as positive. Over the 12 weeks, the volunteers lost an average of 8 kg. Just as important, they honed skills and strategies that have helped them to keep the weight off. Throughout this book, you'll hear first-hand how they shaped the *ChangeOne* plan to work for them.

getting too hungry and strengthen your will-power. We offer you satisfying choices that will help, not derail, your diet.

In the fourth week, with breakfast, lunch and snacks up and running, you'll move on to what's typically the biggest meal of the day: dinner. You'll find a tantalising variety of great-tasting dinner menus and tried-and-true strategies for keeping serve sizes under control.

Voilà. By the end of the fourth week, you will have reworked your diet, reduced kilojoules and fat, and discovered new ways to enjoy good nutrition and great-tasting food. And you'll be watching the weight melt away.

This measured approach makes it easy to experiment with each meal, allowing you to incorporate food that you enjoy into your diet. By focusing on one meal at a time, you'll discover more about the way you eat. You may find that eating a reasonable breakfast and lunch is easy, but at dinner you go overboard. Or maybe snacks are your biggest stumbling block. You'll also gain confidence as you succeed in getting each meal under control. Then in the following eight weeks you'll tackle the big issues dieters face, such

continued on page 19

Dieting as a tennis match

Reading the health pages of newspapers and magazines could make you feel as if you're at Wimbledon. One day you'll read that carbohydrates are terrible and fat is fine; the next day you'll hear the opposite. What's the real answer? Well, it may be years – even decades – before the scientific debate over low-carbohydrate and high-carbohydrate diets is resolved.

But maybe it doesn't matter. Consider a study that tested two very different diets. The first was low in carbohydrates and very high in fat (15 per cent of kilojoules came from carbs, 53 per cent from fat and 32 per cent from protein).

Ultimately, the protein vs carbs debate is missing the point.

The second diet was high in carbohydrates and low in fat (45 per cent of kilojoules came from carbs, 26 per cent from fat and 20 per cent from protein). The only thing they had in common was that each totalled 4200 kilojoules a day. When the two groups of volunteers stepped onto the scales after six weeks, guess what? On average, all of them had lost nearly the same amount of weight and body fat.

High fat, low fat, high protein, low protein – in the end, none of it made a whit of difference on the scales. What mattered was kilojoule intake. The key to losing weight is as basic as that.

Ready, steady...lose

Yes, you want to lose weight. But before you start, it's worth checking to make sure you've got what it takes to succeed. To test your readiness, answer these 10 questions by circling the appropriate number in the right-hand column.

1. Which term best describes your attitude towards losing weight?

Enthusiastic	4
Positive	3
Lukewarm	2
Resigned	1

2. How much weight do you want to lose?

4.5–9 kg	4
9.5–18 kg	3
18.5–27 kg	2
28 kg or more	1

3. How would you rate your chances of reaching your goal?

Excellent	4
Very good	3
So-so	2
Poor	1

4. How do you feel about being physically active?

Enjoy it	3
Don't really mind it	2
Hate it	1

5. Which of the following statements best describes you?

Once I make up my mind to do something, I do it	3
My intentions are good, but my will-power is sometimes weak	2
I tend to get discouraged easily	1

6. How important is losing weight to your health?

Very important	3
Somewhat important	2
Not very important at all	1

7. How well do you deal with stresses and strains in your life?

Very effectively	3
So-so	2
I get frazzled easily	1

8. How much time do you spend in front of the TV on a typical day?

Less than an hour	4
One to two hours	3
Three to four hours	2
Four or more hours	1

9. Which of these statements best describes your knowledge about losing weight and keeping it off:

I know what it takes	4
I'm pretty sure I know	3
I'm confused by conflicting advice and diet plans	2
I have no idea where to start	1

10. Think about the people closest to you. How are they likely to react to your decision to diet?

Very enthusiastically	4
Somewhat positively	3
Sceptically	2
Negatively	1

Turn to the next page to add up your score.

Quiz score

Now add up your score. If you had a total of 22 or more, you're ready, but a lower score is no cause for alarm. Many dieters feel grim about their chances early on. Look for the ones or twos in your responses, then read the answers below to boost your readiness.

1. Enthusiasm doesn't guarantee success, but it does help. If yours needs a tune-up, draw a line down the middle of a piece of paper. In the left-hand column, write all the benefits you expect to get from losing weight. In the right column, jot down all the obstacles you anticipate. Finally, begin thinking about ways you could get around those obstacles in order to achieve the benefits you've listed.

2. Experts say your first goal should be about 10 per cent of your current weight. With a reasonable goal, you're less likely to get discouraged before you reach the finishing line. It may not seem like much, but people who lose 10 per cent look better, feel more confident and energetic, and are ready to set their next goal.

3. Despite discouraging words to the contrary, many people do lose weight and keep it off. Researchers at two American universities have been keeping track, in the National Weight Control Registry, of people who succeed at weight loss. We'll share many of the strategies that spell success for these successful slimmers.

4. Not everyone likes to get hot and sweaty. But you'll stand a better chance of succeeding if you become more active – walking, swimming or playing football with the kids, riding a bicycle round the neighbourhood, gardening, taking the stairs instead of the lift.

5. A lot of frustrated dieters want to put the blame on will-power failures. The surprising truth is that you don't need a rock-solid will to lose weight. You need strategies that will spare you from having to rely on will-power all the time. You'll find them here: ways to ward off hunger; ways to navigate restaurants; and ways to satisfy your sweet tooth on fewer kilojoules.

6. Better health is a bonus for *everyone* who sheds excess weight. Carrying around too much weight increases your risk of diabetes, heart disease and some cancers. The changes in *ChangeOne* are designed to help you not only to lose weight but also to become healthier.

7. Too much stress can undermine even the most determined dieter's plans. All of us face stresses and strains in our lives. What matters is how you deal with them. In *ChangeOne* we'll introduce you to effective ways to take the sting out of stress – techniques that will help you get through even the rockiest times.

8. The more television people watch, studies show, the more they're likely to weigh. Ask yourself this: would you be willing to give up just half an hour of TV three times a week to lose weight and feel a whole lot better? If so, you've just jumpstarted your chances of success.

9. Feeling a little unsure of the facts? Don't worry. In *ChangeOne,* we do more than just tell you what to do. We explain why, based on the solid research. The more you know about gaining and losing weight, the better your chances of meeting your goal.

10. The support of family and friends makes a big difference when you're trying to make a change for the better. But they may not be as supportive as you'd like. If that's true for you, remember that you are the only person whose opinion matters. You can do this on your own.

continued from page 16
as how to eat prudently at restaurants, manage stress and transform your kitchen into a place for healthy eating. Best of all, you'll learn skills that will help you eat sanely for the rest of your life. Losing weight is something you want to do only once. With *ChangeOne*, you'll take the time to get it right.

The numbers behind *ChangeOne*

The meals and menus you'll find in the following pages are more than just delicious. They've been designed to offer maximum nutrition with a sensible number of kilojoules. That's important. When you're cutting back on kilojoules, you certainly don't want to cut back on vitamins, minerals, fibre and the other health benefits of good food. The beauty of *ChangeOne* is that you don't have to weigh every gram or calculate every kilojoule. We've done that for you. The *ChangeOne* meal plans are designed to meet the following daily guidelines.

- **Kilojoules:** from 5500 to 7000
- **Kilojoules from fat:** approximately 30 per cent
- **Saturated and hydrogenated fats:** no more than 10 per cent
- **Fibre:** at least 25 grams
- **Calcium:** approximately 1000 milligrams
- **Fruits and vegetables:** 2 serves of fruit and at least 5 serves of vegetables a day

The kilojoule target of 5500 to 7000 a day is the one used in most diet programs run by experts in the field of weight loss. Not everyone needs the same number of kilojoules, of course. A large person uses up more kilojoules than a small one, and a very active person uses more than someone who doesn't get around much. As you'll discover, *ChangeOne* is designed to

What you'll find inside

On the following pages, you'll find regular features packed with dozens of helpful tips and plenty of advice based on the latest weight-loss research.

ChangeOne Menu

Meals and recipes that will help you to cut kilojoules without sacrificing flavour or the pleasures of eating. And our photos are accurate – the serve sizes you see pictured reflect what you'll be eating.

Help!

Troubleshooting tips to help you to overcome many of the most common obstacles along the way to successful weight loss.

Success Stories

Insights from people who have used the *ChangeOne* approach to shed weight and keep it off.

Fast Track

Optional strategies to help you to speed your progress.

The key is to
eat enough
so you do *not*
feel hungry.

let you set your own kilojoule target and adjust it along the way to suit your needs.

You'll also notice that *ChangeOne* meals don't cut fat to unrealistically low levels. In fact, you may be surprised to find that some of our meal plans contain slightly more than the 30 per cent of kilojoules from fat that is generally recommended. The latest research shows that diets with a decent amount of fat – the healthy kinds, of course – are more successful than diets that restrict fat to an absurd minimum. Another key to success is foods that are higher in fibre, which help people feel fuller longer. We've made sure the meals we offer include both fats and fibre, as well as all the other nutrients you need.

ChangeOne is designed to help you to slim down gradually, from half a kilo to 1.5 kilograms a week. People who lose weight at a steady, moderate pace like this are the most likely to keep it off. But many dieters are impatient to slim down. If you are one of them, *ChangeOne* offers 'Fast Track' features with suggestions to help you drop kilos faster.

Sound simple? We hope so. Taking the mystery and frustration out of weight loss is the goal of the *ChangeOne* diet and fitness plan.

Getting started

The basic *ChangeOne* meal plans you'll find in this book contain about 5500 kilojoules a day. That's a reasonable goal for many people who want to lose weight. But if you're very active or weigh more than about 85 kilograms, you may want to set your target at 7000 kilojoules. People who are physically active burn more kilojoules minute by minute than people who are sedentary. People who are heavy burn more kilojoules than lighter people, because they use more energy carrying around the extra weight.

What's the ideal target for you? Here's what we recommend.

Aim for 5500 kilojoules if:

■ You're a woman who usually does less than half an hour's worth of physical activity (including walking and other everyday activities) most days.

■ You're a fairly inactive man who weighs less than 85 kilograms.

Aim for 7000 kilojoules if:

- You get at least half an hour's worth of vigorous exercise most days of the week.
- You weigh more than 85 kilograms.

Keep in mind that you can always adjust your kilojoule target up or down during the program. If you aren't losing weight as quickly as you'd like, you can reduce your kilojoule level. (We don't recommend going below 5500 kilojoules a day, however, because a diet that is skimpy is likely to fall short on vitamins, minerals and other nutrients you need.) If you feel too hungry on most days, you can increase it. The key is to *not* feel hungry. Researchers have found that dieters quickly adjust to a lower kilojoule level, so if after a few weeks you're still starving, eat a little more. Once you reach your weight goal, we'll help you find a kilojoule target that balances the energy you take in with the energy you burn.

Real rewards

Most people on a diet want to see changes on the scales. That's natural. We recommend that you weigh yourself once a week, preferably every Monday (it will help you stay honest over the weekend). Use the same scales, and choose the same time of day. Keep a log of your weight.

But remember, logging weight loss on the scales is only one way to measure your progress, and not necessarily the best way. If you're losing fat and adding muscle, for instance, your weight may remain the same but you'll look and feel a lot better (and your waistline is likely to slim down). One of our *ChangeOne* volunteers actually stopped lifting weights when the numbers on the scales weren't dropping as fast as he would have liked. But he looked great, and the strength training had a lot to do with that. We convinced him to start exercising again and to pay less attention to the scales and more to the way he looked and felt.

That's good advice for anyone beginning a diet. Keep an eye on your image in the mirror, your clothes size, your energy and the notches on your belt, and you'll enjoy all the rewards of slimming down.

The 7000 Club

If you decide to base your food intake on 7000 kilojoules a day instead of the 5500 *ChangeOne* plan, don't worry about counting every extra kilojoule. Here's all you have to do.

- At breakfast, double your serve of cereal, toast, bagel or bread roll.
- At lunch or dinner, double your serve of protein (that is, your meat, chicken, fish or tofu serve). Or, at dinner, double your serve of starch or grain.

The *ChangeOne* plan is designed to help you slim down gradually, from half a kilo to 1.5 kilograms per week.

The *ChangeOne* approach to eating is based on sensible, proven principles that transcend fads and trends. The *ChangeOne* approach to exercise is equally sensible and equally honest. And in the spirit of honesty, it needs to be acknowledged: while it is possible to lose weight through dietary changes alone, for long-lasting health and weight loss, exercise is essential. Research proves it, and common sense acknowledges it.

Look at it this way: How many hours of your day are spent sitting or lying down? For many adults today, it is as high as 23 out of 24 hours! Often, our daily routine moves us from one resting spot to the next – bed to TV to kitchen table to car to work desk, and then nine hours later, through the same routine in reverse. But we weren't built for such sedentary living. From prehistoric times to just a few decades ago, the typical person spent much of his day on his feet, doing energy-burning, heart-enhancing labour. It is no coincidence that the beginning of the obesity epidemic in Australia and New Zealand coincides almost perfectly with the emergence of modern conveniences that have removed the need to exert ourselves.

Society's answer to the sedentary lifestyle has been the billion-dollar fitness industry. But it hasn't helped us much. For one thing, the exercise establishment makes things too complicated, with all its jargon and measurements and quotas and programs and costly gear. Put simply, the fitness industry is guilty of imposing a fitness approach that is essentially meant for athletes on everyday people like us.

The *ChangeOne* approach to exercise and fitness is much simpler than that, and doesn't require any expertise. It is based on the premise that healthy movement should happen all the time, not in 30-minute work-outs a few times a week. And you can forget about having to buy expensive gear, too. All you need is your

Water, water...

What can you quench your thirst with? Here's the *ChangeOne* approach to drink.

- Coffee or tea is fine. If you take either with milk or sugar, choose skim or a non-dairy (low-kilojoule) whitener, and use an artificial sweetener.
- Drink plain water, and lots of it. Soda water and mineral water are also acceptable choices. They quench your thirst – and reduce appetite – with no additional kilojoules.
- Avoid regular soft drink, with all its sugar and empty kilojoules.
- Fruit juice is healthy, but adds lots of kilojoules without fibre, so you're better off eating whole fruit and drinking a glass of water.
- One glass of wine or beer per day is acceptable. They add more than 419 kilojoules to your day's total kilojoule intake, but there's a debate about whether those kilojoules will slow your overall weight loss.

optimism and willingness to succeed. Specifically, we define healthy exercise as these simple goals.

- Walking for relaxation and energy, each and every day.
- Stretching and strengthening a few muscles, each and every day.
- Getting outdoors as often as you can.
- Living with a high-energy, upbeat attitude, and letting it influence your daily choices.

Notice that there are no wardrobe changes, no gyms, no big-time commitments, no special gear involved with any of that, so you're not expected to reach into your pocket and spend yet more money on fitness gear that won't often see the light of day. Rather, the *ChangeOne* approach to fitness says exercise can and should be embedded in all that you do. Live the high-energy way, and you'll burn more kilojoules, strengthen your heart and help keep the weight off – for good, not just the short-term.

You'll find great advice and directions in Part 2, starting on page 234, to help you shift from sedentary to active living, one small step at a time.

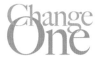

WEEK 1

Breakfast

How does this sound? This week you'll start *ChangeOne* by eating breakfast every morning.

Maybe you don't eat breakfast. Plenty of hopeful dieters skip the first meal of the day. What better way to make my weight-loss diet work, the thinking goes, than not eating? People reckon they'll end up taking in fewer kilojoules that way.

In fact, it works the other way round. People who miss breakfast often end up consuming more kilojoules during the day. Those who start the day with a healthy meal, meanwhile, are more likely to stick to healthy eating throughout the day

In this chapter, you'll find several great breakfasts, along with simple ways to adapt them to your own tastes. Every day this week, help yourself to whichever *ChangeOne* breakfast strikes your fancy. Experiment – and don't worry if you try something that doesn't fill you up. The rest of the day you can eat the way you normally do. That's all there is to taking your first step towards losing weight – and keeping it off.

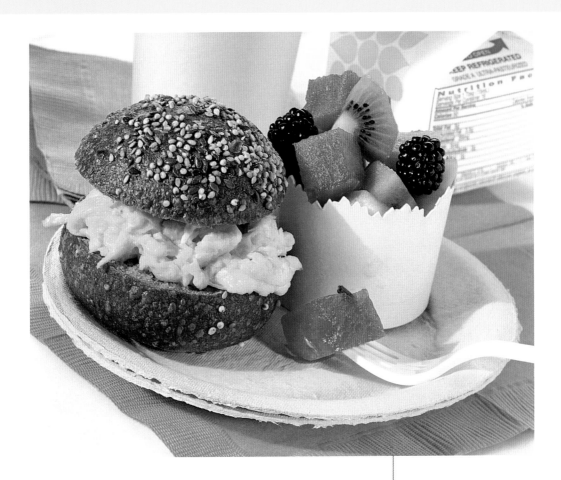

Egg on a roll

1 egg, scrambled, poached or hard-boiled

1 small wholemeal roll, about 50 g (tennis ball)

½ cup (115 g) fresh fruit salad (2 golf balls)

⅔ cup (160 ml) skim or reduced-fat milk

1366 kJ, 326 kcal, 20 g protein, 8 g fat (2 g sat fat), 217 mg cholesterol,
45 g carbohydrate (22 g sugars), 5 g fibre, 421 mg sodium

Instead of	Try
Egg	½ cup (100 g) low-fat cottage cheese 60 g wafer-thin ham
Wholemeal roll	1 English muffin 1 small pita bread 1 slice wholemeal toast
Fruit salad	⅔ cup (160 ml) orange juice 1 orange 1 banana 1 apple

Time-saver

This is a breakfast you can make at home to eat straight away or take with you. Or ask a café or sandwich bar to make it for you. If you're making scrambled egg at home, remember you only need to use a small amount of butter – about ½ teaspoon should be enough.

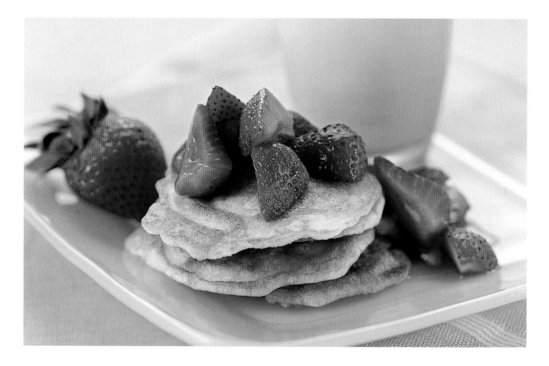

Pancakes with berries

4 pancakes

1/2 tablespoon maple syrup
(1 syrup bottle cap)

1/2 cup (85 g) strawberries, sliced
(2 golf balls)

3/4 cup (190 ml) reduced-fat milk

1276 kJ, 305 kcal, 15 g protein, 10 g fat (3 g sat fat),
65 mg cholesterol, 39 g carbohydrate (25 g sugars),
3 g fibre, 413 mg sodium

PANCAKES

Makes 16 pancakes to serve 4
1/2 **cup (75 g) self-raising flour**
1 1/2 **teaspoons caster sugar**
1/4 **teaspoon bicarbonate of soda**
3/4 **cup (190 ml) buttermilk**
1 **tablespoon vegetable oil**
1 **medium egg**
1/2 **teaspoon pure vanilla essence**

1. Whisk the flour, sugar and bicarbonate of soda in a bowl. Make a well in the centre. In another bowl, whisk the buttermilk, oil, egg and vanilla essence until blended. Pour into the well in the flour and whisk to combine. Allow batter to stand for 5 minutes.

2. Meanwhile, coat a large non-stick frying pan with cooking spray and set over medium heat until hot but not smoking.

3. For each pancake, pour 1 tablespoon batter into the pan. Cook for 3 minutes or until bubbles appear on the surface and begin to burst. Turn and cook for 1 to 2 minutes or until the other side is golden.

4. Make 4 pancakes for yourself. If not cooking for others, you can cover the extra batter and keep in the fridge for the next day. Or cook all the pancakes, wrap the extra in foil and keep in the fridge for a day or the freezer for a week. Reheat wrapped pancakes in a 180ºC oven for 10 minutes.

Instead of	Try
4 pancakes	1 slice French toast or 1 slice cinnamon toast (standard bread slice)
Maple syrup	fresh fruit coulis

Why breakfast is the key

If you usually skip breakfast, you may need a little convincing to get you started. Many of the volunteers who tested *ChangeOne* weren't breakfast eaters either. What they discovered was that starting the day with a healthy meal was the single most important change they made. 'I was amazed, really amazed', one *ChangeOne* volunteer told us. 'Starting to eat breakfast changed the way I ate all day long. It really made the difference.'

Don't just take our word for it. In an experiment conducted at Vanderbilt University in Nashville, Tennessee, researchers recruited overweight women who usually skipped breakfast. All the women were put on a 5000-kilojoules-a-day diet. One group divided kilojoules between just two meals: lunch and dinner. The second group ate those meals plus breakfast. Twelve weeks on, the breakfast eaters had lost 7.7 kilograms; the women who skipped breakfast had shed 5.9 kilograms.

Wait a minute, you might say. Weren't both groups consuming the same number of kilojoules? No, the researchers concluded. The women who ate breakfast were more likely to stick to the 5000-kilojoule diet. Those who went hungry until lunch were more likely to cheat a little.

If you skip breakfast, this study showed, you're likely to eat more, not less, than if you start the day with a meal.

> Four out of five successful dieters eat breakfast every day of the week.

Breakfast serves

To help you to assess serve sizes, we use both standard measurements and the *ChangeOne* serve-size guide. In the breakfast serves below, members of the 7000 Club can double the starch or grain serve.

Type of food	Example	Amount	*ChangeOne* guide
One starch or grain	Cornflakes	1 cup (25 g)	Cricket ball
	Porridge	½ cup (115 g)	2 golf balls
	Toast	1 slice	
	Bread roll	Small (50 g)	Tennis ball
One dairy or high-calcium food	Low-fat milk	1 cup (250 ml)	Takeaway coffee cup
	Low-fat yogurt	1 tub (150 g)	
One piece of fruit	Orange, apple	1	1 fist
	Berries, cut fruit	½ cup (115 g)	Cupped handful
Optional	Butter, jam	1 teaspoon	Thumb tip
	Nuts	1 tablespoon	Thumb

The reason is pretty obvious when you think about it. The longer you go without eating, the hungrier you get. And the hungrier you get, the more likely you are to devour anything you can get your hands on. When you start the day with breakfast, you begin by taming the hungry beast inside and make it easier to keep cravings in check.

You'll also be starting your day with an easy success: of the three meals, a healthy, sensible breakfast is the simplest to achieve. That will help you stay on track for the day. Psychologists say that levels of two brain chemicals that give us a sense of control – cortisol and adrenaline – peak very soon after we get up. The confidence they provide may make it easier to stick to our good intentions, such as a healthier diet. These chemicals ebb later in the morning, so it can be tougher to say no to the biscuits someone brings into the office – especially if you're feeling extra hungry because you skipped breakfast.

Still not convinced? Here's a compelling argument: most successful slimmers eat breakfast. Since 1994 researchers at two universities in the US have been gathering data on people who manage to lose 14 kilograms or more and keep the weight off for at least one year. The project, called the National Weight Control Registry, is designed to learn – from the people who know best – what it takes to lose weight permanently. And guess what? Four out of five say they eat breakfast every day.

Help!

'I'm just not hungry in the morning. Do I really have to force myself to eat something if I'm not hungry?'

Give it a try. One reason you're not hungry may be that you're not used to eating so early. So try this: start off with a few bites of something that sounds appealing – toast, say, or a muesli bar – for five mornings in a row. After two or three mornings, you might start to notice your early-morning appetite increasing. Also, schedule dinner a little earlier than usual if you can and eat only enough to feel satisfied without being stuffed. This will increase the chances of your appetite waking up when you do. If you're still struggling, eat just one item from a *ChangeOne* breakfast – a piece of fruit, for instance – and save the rest for a midmorning mini meal.

Making the change

Choose a *ChangeOne* breakfast each day this week. Mix and match the meals any way you like. The important thing is to start your day with a good breakfast and then go on with life – and the rest of your day's regular meals. Don't worry that you'll end up consuming more kilojoules than usual. Like a lot of breakfast converts, you're likely to feel less hungry midmorning and at lunch time.

Don't let the morning rush at your house get in the way. Putting breakfast together doesn't have to require more time than it takes to fill a bowl with

Change One Fast Track

Hoping to drop a size before your next school reunion? Determined to cut a slimmer figure in your swimsuit next summer? To speed your progress, choose one or more of these Fast Track changes this week.

Eat breakfast twice

Instead of having your usual lunch, make your midday meal another *ChangeOne* breakfast. Eating breakfast twice during the day isn't our idea. Several major cereal manufacturers have claimed it to be a novel weight-loss method.

Help yourself to a bowl of their flakes for breakfast and lunch, they promise, and you can have a full dinner and still shed weight. It works, especially if high-kilojoule lunches are your downfall.

Be more active

Add 15 minutes of extra physical activity to your schedule every day this week. Walking is fine: a quick circuit of the office complex, or up and down a few flights of stairs if they're handy.

Aim for 15 minutes of activity every day when you would otherwise have been inactive. And here's why. If you weigh 82 kg, for instance, you burn about 9.2 kilojoules a minute sitting in a meeting or parked in front of the TV. If you get up and take a walk, you more than double that number, to 20 kilojoules. Quicken your pace to a brisk walk and your metabolism burns up 30 kilojoules a minute.

The benefits can add up fast. Sitting still you burn just 139 kilojoules every 15 minutes, but brisk walking burns 454 kilojoules in the same period.

Keep a food diary

People who are asked to keep close track of what they eat during the day, researchers found, almost always begin to lose weight – even if they don't deliberately go on a slimming diet. There are several reasons for this.

When you're keeping a food diary, you become more aware of what you eat. And when you know you have to write down every nibble, you think twice before you eat a Danish pastry at your midmorning coffee break or a piece of chocolate cake for afternoon tea.

Keeping a food diary also reveals eating patterns you may not have been aware of – the fact that you snack more than you imagined, for instance, or that you are most inclined to eat late in the day. Those insights can help you shape the best strategy for losing weight. You'll find a handy Daily Food Diary form and instructions on page 345. Track your eating in it every day this week.

Speed up the program

Although our volunteers like the week-by-week pace of *ChangeOne*, you could do the first four weeks' assignments in less time to speed your weight loss. For example, give yourself three days for breakfast, four days for lunch, three days for snacks and four days for dinner.

That would get you through the first changes at a quicker pace and have you dieting from breakfast to bedtime in two weeks, instead of the four we recommend. The trade-off is that you won't have as much time to experiment with meals to find the foods that satisfy you, and you could miss out on the opportunity to discover – and solve – problems in your eating patterns. But if your goal is to look stunning for your beach holiday and you don't have a lot of time...

cereal, scatter a little fruit over it and pour on the milk.
If you're really in a hurry:

- Set the table for breakfast before going to bed. You'll save time, and the breakfast table will be an instant reminder for you when you get up.
- Take care of one or two morning tasks the night before. Instead of deciding what to wear after you get up, for example, select the next day's outfit before you go to bed.
- Prepare a fruit salad on Sunday so that you can quickly serve yourself some the first few mornings of the week.
- Set your alarm clock for 10 minutes earlier than usual.

If all else fails, keep a box of muesli bars and plenty of fresh fruit to hand for an easy-to-pack breakfast.

Behind the *ChangeOne* breakfast menu

Each *ChangeOne* breakfast is designed to supply around 1250 kilojoules or less. That's enough energy to power your morning and still get you started on losing weight.

What's more, each *ChangeOne* breakfast includes at least one food that's rich in fibre. There are several good reasons for this. The biggest shortfall in most people's diets is fibre: we should get about 30 grams a day to be at our healthiest; we average around 15.

Fibre defends us from several common health problems. It's also a key player in a healthy weight-loss diet. Because it's filling, fibre makes a meal feel more satisfying on fewer kilojoules. One type – soluble fibre – absorbs water to form gels that slow down digestion, so fibre-rich foods stay with you longer than other foods, keeping hunger at bay. (For more on fibre-rich foods, see 'More good reasons to fill up on fibre' on page 36.)

To test the hunger-taming effects of fibre-rich foods, scientists at the University of Sydney compared two seemingly similar breakfasts: a bowl of bran flakes, which are high in fibre, and a bowl of cornflakes, which are not. Volunteers in the bran cereal group reported feeling less hungry later in the morning than

continued on page 33

Help!

'What if I can't find a tub of yogurt with only 340 kilojoules? Or a muesli bar that has 500 kilojoules? How exact do I have to be?'

Don't get too hung up on exact kilojoule counts. If you can come within 40 to 80 kilojoules of the recommended amount in the target food, you'll be fine. Remember, the *ChangeOne* program is more about recognising healthy foods and eating reasonable serves than it is about counting kilojoules.

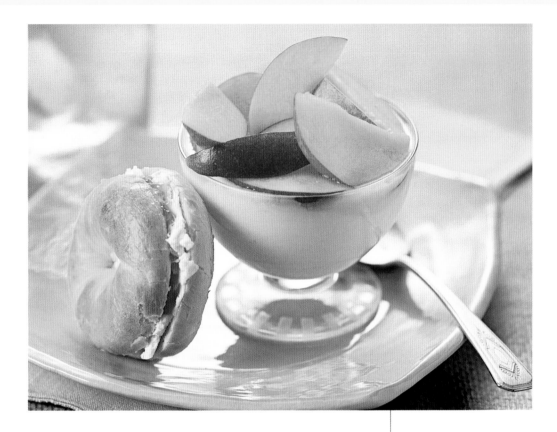

Bagel delight

½ ordinary-size bagel, or 1 mini bagel, split in half

2 teaspoons reduced-fat cream cheese (2 thumb tips)
  or 1 tablespoon yogurt cheese (see below) (whole thumb)
  or 2 tablespoons reduced-fat sour cream

1 teaspoon jam (thumb tip)

1 peach, sliced

1 tub (150 g) sugar-free or natural non-fat yogurt
  (tennis ball)

1151 kJ, 275 kcal, 16 g protein, 2 g fat (1 g sat fat), 10 mg cholesterol,
47 g carbohydrate (26 g sugars), 4 g fibre, 363 mg sodium

Time-saver
*Cut bagels in half when
you bring them home
from the supermarket,
then freeze them in a
resealable plastic bag.*

HOW TO MAKE YOGURT CHEESE

Line a plastic coffee filter, or a small sieve, with a filter paper,
and rest the filter on a bowl or measuring jug. Pour in 200 g
fat-free or low-fat natural yogurt (use a yogurt that does not
contain gelatine). Cover and refrigerate for at least one hour.
The liquid in the yogurt will drip through the filter paper,
allowing the yogurt to thicken into a spreadable 'cheese'.

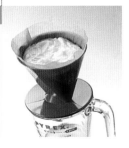

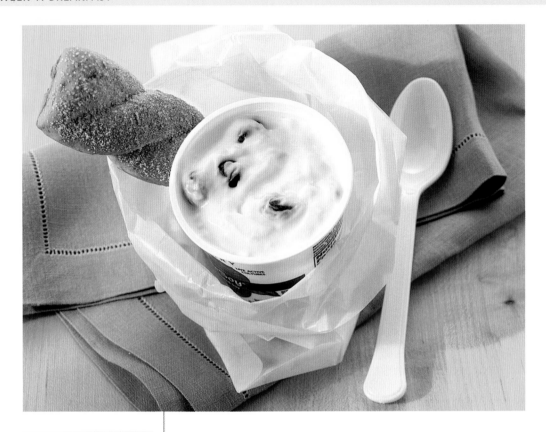

Time-saver

Pack a breakfast in a bag the night before so you can grab it and go in the morning.

HEALTH TIP

Fresh fruit is low in kilojoules but high in fibre: ½ cup (75 g) blueberries has 170 kilojoules and 2 g of fibre. Or use other fruit: an apple has 195 kilojoules and 1.8 g fibre; an orange 250 kilojoules and 2.7 g fibre; 3 plums 130 kilojoules and 1.4 g fibre; 1 cup (150 g) strawberries 170 kilojoules and 2 g fibre.

Breakfast on the go

1 muesli bar, 500 to 670 kilojoules

½ cup (75 g) blueberries (2 golf balls)

1 tub (150 g) natural or sugar-free, non-fat or low-fat yogurt

1114 kJ, 266 kcal, 12 g protein, 4 g fat (<1 g sat fat), 8 mg cholesterol, 45 g carbohydrate (29 g sugars), 4 g fibre, 202 mg sodium

ABOUT MUESLI BARS

Muesli bars are not always as healthy and innocent as you might think – some brands contain a lot of fat and sugar. Those at about 500 to 670 kilojoules may be a bit harder to find than their heavyweight cousins, but with a bit of careful label reading you'll find flavours you like. Look for a bar with at least 1 gram of fibre. But if you have a favourite that contains no fibre, go ahead and enjoy it – there's fibre in the fruit you eat with it.

continued from page 30
those who ate cornflakes. Similarly, researchers at the New York Obesity Research Center at St Luke's-Roosevelt Hospital pitted a sugary, low-fibre breakfast cereal against porridge, a high-fibre cereal. When volunteers ate the sweetened flakes, they tended to eat as much at lunch as if they'd had nothing but a glass of water at breakfast. When they sat down to a bowl of porridge, they felt fuller for longer and ate up to 40 per cent less for lunch.

A fruity choice

ChangeOne breakfasts also include at least one serve of fruit. Fruit, like whole grains, is a terrific source of fibre. One apple has 1.8 grams of fibre, which is 10 per cent of the recommended daily amount. Also, most people who hit the recommended goal of seven serves of fruits and vegetables a day get at least one of those at breakfast.

When we say fruit, we mean fruit you can chew. Fruit juices are fine now and then, but many are surprisingly high in kilojoules, especially if they've been sweetened (when they'll be called a drink or cocktail). A 250 ml glass of cranberry juice drink contains a hefty 590 kilojoules. Even apple juice has around the same number of kilojoules as cola. What's more, most fruit juices don't have nearly as much fibre as the fruit they're made from. Compare 150 ml of these juices with their whole fruit:

Orange juice
Kilojoules: 225
Vitamin C: 59 mg
Fibre: 0.2 g

An orange
Kilojoules: 250
Vitamin C: 86 mg
Fibre: 2.7 g

Apple juice
Kilojoules: 240
Vitamin C: 21 mg
Fibre: negligible

An apple
Kilojoules: 195
Vitamin C: 6 mg
Fibre: 1.8 g

Grapefruit juice
Kilojoules: 210
Vitamin C: 47 mg
Fibre: negligible

A grapefruit
Kilojoules: 200
Vitamin C: 58 mg
Fibre: 2.1 g

ChangeOne encourages you to help yourself to fruit not only at breakfast but for snacking, too. We stop short of saying you can eat as much fruit as you want because most

continued on page 36

Set the breakfast table the night before for easier mornings.

33

The cereal story

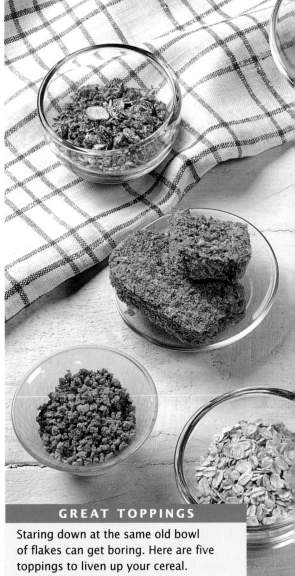

A good bowl of cereal, cold or hot, is one of the best breakfast choices you can make, as long as you select wisely. Try to find cereals with lots of dietary fibre – at least 3 grams per serve. And check the ingredients for whole grains like oats or wheat. Pictured on the right are several familiar breakfast cereals in serves that contain about 420 kilojoules.

A PERFECT BOWL OF CEREAL

²/₃ cup (25 g) bran flakes (tennis ball)
2 tablespoons raisins or sultanas
(2 thumbs)
1 cup (250 ml) skim or reduced-fat milk
2 teaspoons chopped nuts or sunflower seeds (optional, adds 125 kilojoules)
(2 thumb tips)

1135 kJ, 271 kcal, 15 g protein, 1 g fat (<1 g sat fat),
10 mg cholesterol, 51 g carbohydrate (37 g sugars),
5 g fibre, 386 mg sodium

MAKE YOUR OWN MUESLI

You can create your own signature breakfast cereal by mixing oats with your favourite dried fruit and seeds. Here's a muesli that will last for days.

■ 1⅓ cups (125 g) porridge oats
■ 60 g ready-to-eat dried apricots, chopped
■ 60 g banana chips
■ 2 tablespoons (25 g) pumpkin or sunflower seeds

Mix and store in an airtight container. This will make enough for 10 serves.

GREAT TOPPINGS

Staring down at the same old bowl of flakes can get boring. Here are five toppings to liven up your cereal.

■ 1 tablespoon unsweetened desiccated coconut (210 kilojoules)
■ 1 tablespoon chopped banana chips (125 kilojoules)
■ 2 teaspoons chopped almonds (210 kilojoules)
■ 2 teaspoons sunflower seeds (245 kilojoules)
■ 1 teaspoon mixed cinnamon and sugar (85 kilojoules)

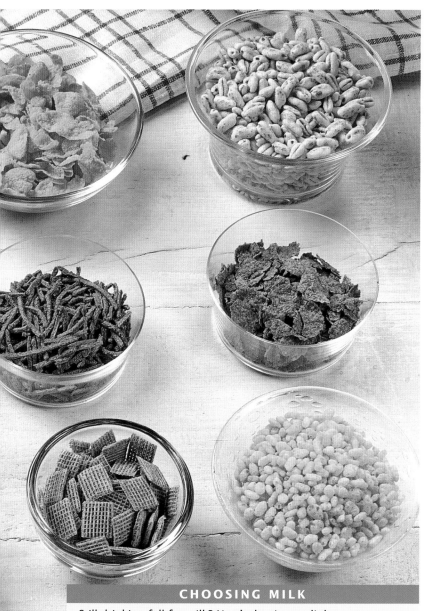

CHOOSING MILK

Still drinking full-fat milk? Now's the time to lighten up.
Take it one change at a time: step down from full-fat to
reduced-fat, then from reduced-fat to skim. It won't take
long before lower-fat milk tastes as good as what you were
drinking before. Here's what you'll save in artery-clogging
saturated fat and kilojoules in each ½ cup (125 ml).

Type of milk	Saturated fat	Kilojoules
Full-fat	4.9 g	345
Reduced-fat	2.3 g	244
Skim	0.1–0.4 g	175
Soy beverage	0.4 g	170

HOT CEREALS

If it's cold outside,
there's nothing like
a steaming bowl of
hot cereal to warm
you up. Porridge is
the classic, but you
can choose from
many others.

■ Instant oat cereal
■ Weet-Bix with hot
   milk
■ Wheat bran cereal
   with hot milk

continued from page 33

fruit contains a fair amount of sugar, which adds kilojoules to your diet. But frankly, we've never met anyone who got fat eating too many mangoes. If the choice is between a pastry or chocolate bar and a piece of fruit, reach for the fruit.

Weight loss secrets from the dairy

Something else you'll find in *ChangeOne* breakfasts: most meal plans include low-fat milk or yogurt. Low-fat dairy products are a terrific low-kilojoule source of calcium, which you need for a key trio of health reasons: calcium helps to keep bones strong, it reins in blood pressure, and research studies suggest that calcium may lower the risk of colon cancer.

continued on page 38

More good reasons to fill up on fibre

With all the attention being given to carbohydrates, protein and fat, it's easy to forget fibre. But when you're dieting, fibre could well be the part of food most worthy of focus.

Fibre, which is the indigestible part of food, gives whole grains, fruits and vegetables their snap, crunch and crispiness. And since your body can't digest fibre, it passes through without adding any kilojoules.

The research tells the story. A recent two-year study indicated that people who ate the most fibre were least likely to gain weight and body fat over time. In another study, researchers followed nearly 3000 men and women over 10 years. Those who regularly ate fibre-rich foods ended up weighing nearly 5 kg less, on average, than those with low fibre intakes.

Chances are they scored in other ways, too. Fibre-rich foods have been shown to lower LDL cholesterol, the bad stuff. University of Toronto researchers showed that a diet that gets more than one-third of its kilojoules from fibre-rich foods like fruit, vegetables and nuts can lower LDL cholesterol by 33 per cent. Volunteers on a high-fibre diet saw their LDL numbers drop within the first week.

Fibre eaters are also less likely to develop diabetes as adults. In two major studies conducted by scientists at the Harvard School of Public Health, people who ate the most fibre from whole grains had the lowest risk of type 2 diabetes: high-fibre grains were shown to cut their risk of contracting the disease by 30 per cent.

And here's one more reason to reach for whole grains, fruits and vegetables: many studies show a lower risk of several kinds of cancer among people who include lots of fibre in their diet. By eating a healthier diet based on plant foods, most of us could cut our cancer risk by at least one-third, experts say.

Fibre is the perfect diet food: no kilojoules and very filling.

Change One Success Stories

Winning the battle against temptation

When Debra Outlaw first started on *ChangeOne*, she knew immediately that it was different from other diets.

'I never had to go through the awful "consuming hungries" that I had experienced on other plans. When you phase in major changes over four weeks, it gives your system plenty of time to adjust to the new kilojoule levels for each meal.'

Now 53 kilos lighter, she is much healthier and more in control of her eating than ever before. 'Staying with the plan consistently is key', she says. 'With dedication and perseverance, every temptation does not become a war.'

Debra found that one of the most helpful changes she made to her routine was to eat breakfast. 'I had always skipped breakfast unless we were going out to eat', she says. 'I didn't realise how it affected my energy level. One Sunday morning I was late for church and had to go without breakfast. By the time I finished helping out, I was so weak! I now have a full appreciation for breakfast and enjoy it so much.'

Debra also tried not to look for excuses to eat. 'If the plan was a good plan, and I knew that it was, then it would serve me well for every meal, every day', she says. 'I could not see special events as a time for indulging. I had to focus on the joy and celebration and not the food. I could no longer use stress as an excuse to eat, either.'

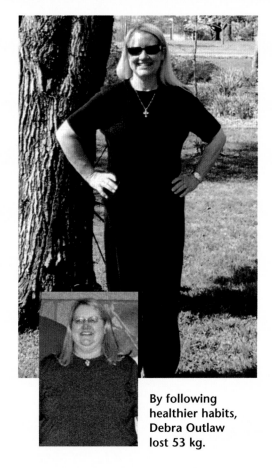

By following healthier habits, Debra Outlaw lost 53 kg.

For Debra, the trick is faithfully following her new healthy habits. 'If you truly want to develop new habits, you need to be consistent', she says. 'People tell me they could never stick to the plan every day, as though that would be such a burden. I think it's just the opposite. When you go on and off the plan, losing weight seems much harder. Temptations really do lose their power with consistency.'

continued from page 36

Calcium also turns out to have a surprising weight-loss benefit. The evidence first showed up in a study to test whether the blood pressure of men could be lowered by adding 300 grams of low-fat yogurt to their daily diet. The readings dropped and, as an added bonus, the men also lost weight – 5 kilograms in a year, on average.

Another study showed that dieters who ate three to four serves of low-fat dairy products daily lost 70 per cent more weight in six months than people on the same diet who were not eating dairy foods. And those in the dairy group lost more fat around their middles.

The magic ingredient in dairy products seems to be calcium. One two-year study found that university-age women who ate a low-calcium diet gained weight; women who got plenty of calcium maintained a steady weight, or even lost a bit.

Why? Experts have found that getting too little calcium triggers the release of a hormone called calcitriol, which tells the body to store rather than burn fat. When calcium levels are high, calcitriol levels stay low, and the body burns fat instead of storing it. Calcium's not quite the whole story, as subjects who took a calcium supplement pill in the diet studies didn't lose quite as much weight as people who got the mineral in their meals. However, this may suggest that something else in dairy products may help spur weight loss.

But what if you're lactose-intolerant? Many people have an intolerance to milk because they don't have enough of the lactase enzyme, vital for digesting milk sugars. Consuming too much dairy food can then cause uncomfortable wind or diarrhoea. But the amount of lactose in different dairy foods varies enormously, and you may find that even with low lactase you are able to digest small amounts of milk, yogurt or hard cheeses without discomfort. It is worth experimenting to find out how much you can tolerate: start by adding small amounts of yogurt or cheese to your diet and increase gradually.

Pop a pill?

When you're trying to cut back on kilojoules, you may be worried you are also cutting back on the vitamins and minerals that are essential for good health. Advice to dieters often includes a recommendation to take a daily multivitamin to ensure adequate intakes of these valuable nutrients, but you should discuss this option with your doctor before deciding to go ahead with it.

Recent research has raised concerns that nutrients taken in supplement form do not work the same way they do when consumed naturally in foods. And a balanced, well-planned diet should meet your needs for vitamins and minerals, even during weight loss. However, if you feel that your intake of vitamins and minerals is insufficient, then a multivitamin once a day might be something to think about.

Of course, you don't have to drink milk or eat other dairy products to be healthy or lose weight. You can substitute low-fat soy or rice beverage and get your calcium in other ways – from a supplement or in calcium-fortified foods, for example. The *ChangeOne* menu includes several foods with added calcium to help you to reach the recommended level. Other non-dairy sources rich in calcium include tofu, almonds, sesame seeds, calcium-fortified orange juice and canned fish (such as salmon) that are eaten with their bones.

Changes ahead: lunch

This week, while you focus on breakfast, keep an eye on what you eat for lunch. Don't change your lunch menu; we'll get to that next week. Eat the way you usually do for the rest of the day. Just note where you have lunch and what you eat. Be aware of the choices you have: eat out? at your desk? in a pub? And be alert to how you feel. Do you jam lunch into the middle of a frantic day, or is it a relaxed time? On at least one day – each day of the week if you have time – write down what you eat for lunch and estimate the serve sizes.

More breakfast choices

Can't find something you like from among the breakfasts suggested in this chapter? Starting on page 309, you'll find more quick and delicious *ChangeOne* breakfast ideas.

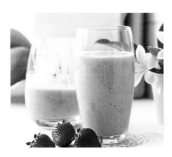

Tropical smoothie
page 309

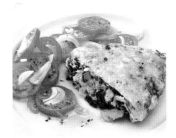

Vegetable frittata
page 310

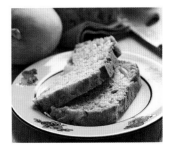

Peach and yogurt loaf
page 311

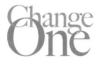
WEEK 2

Lunch

Contrary to what you've heard, the single biggest problem any slimmer faces in the battle of the bulge isn't what they eat, it's how much. We now annually consume more food per person, on average, than we did 15 or 20 years ago. How is that possible? Take a look at lunch.

Double cheeseburgers with two rashers of bacon, extra-large soft drinks, super-size chips – runaway inflation has hit the lunch counter.

This week sanity prevails. You'll eat delicious lunches that satisfy without having to resort to excess.

For many people lunch presents the biggest challenge of the day. We grab our midday meals in the middle of crowded schedules, work, errands and distractions. And because lunch is the meal we're least likely to eat at home, we typically have less control over what's on the menu.

But that's all the more reason for you to learn ways to make lunch a great-tasting, sensible meal. With some advance planning, and by using the lunches in this chapter and on pages 312 to 317, you'll be able to keep your kilojoules in line and still enjoy your midday meal.

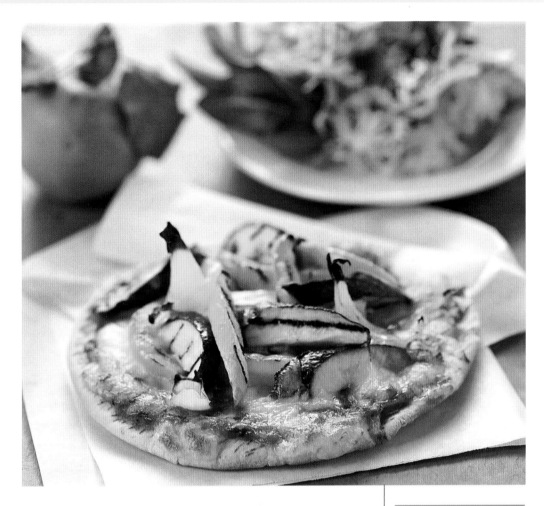

Pizza and salad

Pita pizza:

1 mini pita bread (60 g)
1 tablespoon tomato sauce (1 thumb)
¼ cup (25 g) reduced-fat mozzarella, grated (surface of palm)
Grilled vegetables

1 green salad with 1 tablespoon fat-free dressing
(1 salad-dressing cap)
or 2 teaspoons vinaigrette (2 thumb tips)

1 apple

To prepare pizza:
Spread sauce on the pita bread, sprinkle with cheese, top
with grilled vegetables and bake at 180°C for 5 minutes or
until cheese bubbles. For ham or pepperoni pizza, use half
the amount of cheese and top with 2 thin slices of meat.

1424 kJ, 340 kcal, 14 g protein, 6 g fat (3 g sat fat), 19 mg cholesterol,
57 g carbohydrate (28 g sugars), 6 g fibre, 978 mg sodium

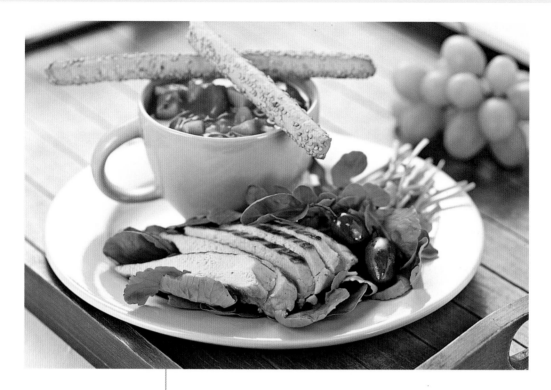

Soup and salad

1 cup (250 ml) fresh vegetable soup (takeaway coffee cup)

2 breadsticks, small

1 green salad (unlimited) topped with:

55 g grilled chicken (half your palm)
2 tablespoons olives (two thumbs)
  or 1 tablespoon chopped nuts (1 salad-dressing cap)
  or 1 tablespoon grated cheese (1 salad-dressing cap)
1 tablespoon fat-free dressing (1 salad-dressing cap)
  or 2 teaspoons vinaigrette (2 thumb tips)

1586 kJ, 379 kcal, 24 g protein, 14 g fat (4 g sat fat), 62 mg cholesterol, 38 g carbohydrate (7 g sugars), 4 g fibre, 777 mg sodium

ABOUT SOUP

Soup is great for staving off hunger. Researchers at an American university found that chicken and rice soup was more filling than the same amount of chicken and rice with a glass of water. Why? Soup is satisfying because it brings out all the flavours of its ingredients. Also, soup may linger in your stomach, which will keep you feeling full.

Instead of	Try
Vegetable soup	Gazpacho (230 kJ)
(1 cup/250 ml, 460 kJ)	Mushroom (630 kJ)
	Spinach (630 kJ)
	Carrot and coriander (440 kJ)
	Lentil (1050 kJ)
	Minestrone (565 kJ)
	Tomato (455 kJ)

Don't let lunch send you off course

Let's face it: food purveyors have our number. Super-size it! Two for the price of one! Twenty-five per cent extra free!

We're conditioned to look for a bargain, and more food for less money sounds about as good as it gets. 'For only a little bit more I can get large fries and a large cola with that double hamburger with bacon? Yes, please.'

But consider the numbers. A double hamburger with cheese and bacon provides a massive 2520 kilojoules. Add on the large fries and get another 2100 kilojoules. With a small drink – or what passes for small these days – you're up to about 5500 kilojoules. That's the basic *ChangeOne* kilojoule target for a whole day, all in one meal!

Of course, most slimmers know better than to order a double hamburger with cheese and bacon. But even healthy-sounding lunch selections can hide a surprising number of kilojoules. 'I always thought chicken was the healthiest choice', one of our volunteers told us. Then she learned that at one leading restaurant chain, a single serve of crispy chicken with dips packs 2310 kilojoules. An individual-size pizza? Throw on lots of high-fat toppings like sausage, salami or cheese and the kilojoules can exceed 3360. The same is true of innocent-sounding veggie burgers and seemingly healthy salads smothered with high-fat dressings.

Lunch serves

These meal plans use both standard measurements and the *ChangeOne* serve-size guide. Here's what a standard serve looks like.

Type of food	Example	Amount	*ChangeOne* guide
One starch or grain	Potato	Medium	Tennis ball
	Bread roll	Medium	Tennis ball
	Rice, pasta, noodles	⅔–1 cup (140 g)	Tennis ball
One protein	Cheese, grated	¼ cup (25 g)	Covers surface of palm
	Lean hamburger	55 g	1 cm thick coaster
	Cooked ham	85 g	3 CDs
One fruit	Orange, apple	1	1 fist
	Berries, cut fruit	½ cup (75 g)	Cupped handful
Vegetables		Unlimited	

You get the point? Unless you know what to select – and make sure that you can get it – you could find yourself having to choose between going hungry or going overboard on kilojoules.

Check-in

Over the past week you began to take control of breakfast. If you weren't a breakfast eater before, you've become one. If you were already sitting down to the breakfast table, you've started helping yourself to healthier choices or more sensible serves. Don't fret if you missed a day or two. Don't worry if you ended up grabbing a Danish pastry one morning on the way into work. The important thing is not to fall into the trap of thinking you failed just because you had a mishap or two. What matters is that you're finding time to sit down first thing in the morning to a breakfast that starts your new healthy diet off on the right track.

If you're not quite there yet, consider taking another week to get breakfast under control. With the confidence that comes with making just one change for the better, you'll find it easier to move on to the next. If you feel happy with breakfast, you're ready to move on to lunch.

Making the change

This week, while you keep up the good work at breakfast, help yourself to your choice of the *ChangeOne* lunches pictured in this chapter. *ChangeOne* lunches contain about 1500 kilojoules. That includes everything – food and drink. Compare that with the kilojoules in most fast-food and pub meals and you'll see why sticking to the *ChangeOne* menu will speed your weight loss.

The meal plans you'll find here include lunches you can make at home, lunches you can pack, lunches you can order at a good sandwich shop that's willing to do it your way, and even a fast-food meal that will work for you. Mix and match them any way you like. If you prefer to have pretty much the same lunch every day, that's fine. If variety is the spice of your life, help yourself. What matters is sticking as closely as you can to the *ChangeOne* lunch meal plan every day this coming week.

As much as possible, decide in advance what and where you're going to eat. In one step you're in control. No more searching the vending machine for something, anything, that looks halfway healthy. No more raiding that bag of tortilla chips or devouring a chocolate bar because you're famished and it's the only edible item in your desk drawer.

Instead, consider some other options.

If you eat most of your lunches out: Make a list of the *ChangeOne* lunches that you'll be able to order at your favourite lunch spot or company cafeteria. Try to choose a

continued on page 47

Change One Fast Track

If you're anxious to speed your progress, choose one or two of the following Fast Track changes and you're likely to see kilos melt away faster.

Turn off the TV

At least three times this week, turn off the television and walk for half an hour when you would otherwise have sat in front of the TV. It doesn't take a genius to figure out that sitting around watching television is bad for anyone's waistline. Yet even researchers have been surprised by the link between TV viewing and tubbiness.

Many recent studies indicate a link between television viewing and higher risk of obesity. An American study found that women watching three hours of television a day have an average body mass index (BMI) 1.8 points higher than those watching for just one hour. For a 170 cm woman, that's an extra 5.4 kg. (To calculate your BMI, go to page 343.)

Hate to miss your favourite shows? Record the ones you really want to see. By fast-forwarding through the advertisements you'll save at least eight minutes per half-hour show – extra minutes you can grab to do something active and keep off the couch.

Put down your fork

When you eat too fast, you deny your body the time it needs to signal that you're full. It takes about 20 minutes from the time you start eating for your stomach and brain to coordinate on these so-called satiety signals.

This week, lay down your knife and fork after each bite. Take notice of what happens when you slow down. Savour what you're eating. And try another tactic: the minute you feel satisfied, get up from the table. Stop eating, even if there's still food on your plate.

Pour it on

This week carry a bottle of water with you and take a swig whenever you feel thirsty. That way you'll be less tempted to grab a sugary, kilojoule-filled drink. And drink one glass of water with lunch and dinner. When you include a glass of water with your meal, you get some kilojoule-free help on quenching your hunger along with your thirst.

Use the 50 per cent solution

Lunch serves, like dinner, are often larger than most of us want or need. No matter when you eat the biggest meal of your day, giant serves can really pile on the kilojoules. This week downsize your main courses. Serve up half of what you normally would eat. After you're done take a few minutes to relax and savour the meal. If you're still hungry, help yourself to half of what's left over. Otherwise, get up from the table.

Create a diversion

Identify one time of the day when you're eating for no other reason than because that's when you typically eat. This would not be a regular mealtime, but perhaps a midmorning coffee break, afternoon snack or late-evening splurge.

Now instead of eating at that time, do something else – something that really appeals to you. Read the paper, take a brief stroll, pursue a hobby, call a friend – anything that gets you through that period. You may find that the reason you ate at that time was habit, not hunger. Develop a new habit – one that doesn't involve food – and you could cut more than 420 kilojoules a day.

Chef's salad

Green salad topped with:

25 g reduced-sodium roast chicken or turkey breast (1 CD)
25 g reduced-sodium cooked ham (1 CD)
25 g reduced-sodium cheese (1 CD)
1 tablespoon fat-free dressing (1 salad-dressing cap)
  or 2 teaspoons Italian dressing (2 thumb tips)

1 medium wholegrain roll (55 g) (tennis ball)

½ cup (85 g) diced melon (cupped handful)

1214 kJ, 290 kcal, 24 g protein, 10 g fat (4 g sat fat), 50 mg cholesterol, 27 g carbohydrate (12 g sugars), 4 g fibre, 571 mg sodium

TIPS FOR TOPPING YOUR SALAD

Combine any three of these to top your salad. Serve size for each is 25 g (the size of a CD, or as indicated), slightly less for cheese, unless otherwise noted.

- Turkey breast
- Chicken breast
- Lean roast beef
- Shredded chicken
- Cooked ham

- Canned tuna (in water)
- Cheddar
- Gruyère
- Edam
- Grated parmesan
  (surface of your palm)

- Tofu cubes (1 thumb)
- Kidney or other beans, 2 tablespoons (2 thumbs)
- Chopped nuts, 1 tablespoon (1 thumb)

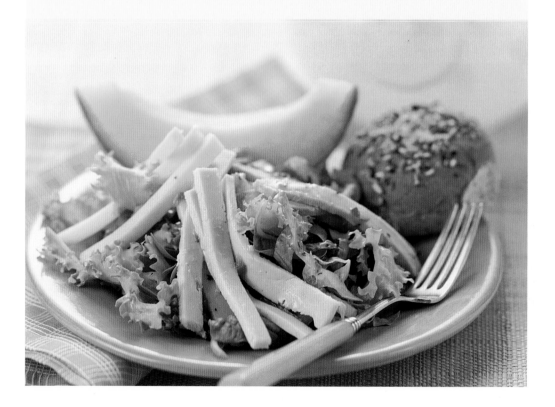

continued from page 44

place that will do it your way, including keeping serve sizes under control. When in doubt, check the serve sizes in this chapter for a rough idea of what a *ChangeOne* lunch should look like, and keep the handy visual equivalents in mind. Before you dig into lunch, make sure that what's on your plate matches up. At some lunch places, you may eat just half of what you're served. If possible, ask for a take-away container when giving your order, and enjoy the extra tomorrow. Think of it as two meals for the price of one. Now that's a bargain.

If you usually eat at home: Choose the meals you think you'll like the best from the *ChangeOne* lunch suggestions. Or each day this week, try a different one. You may find that something you wouldn't normally eat tastes great and really fills you up. Remember, there's little risk. If you feel ravenous by mid-afternoon, you can have a snack and your usual dinner later. Eventually you may want to stick to one or two particular meals (see 'Keep it simple', below). If you end up selecting a wide variety, consider writing each day's lunch menu on your calendar. When you begin to feel hungry as midday approaches, you'll know exactly what's coming.

If you plan to pack a lunch: Make up your shopping list and buy what you'll need at the beginning of the week. Don't forget lunch bags and storage containers. If your early mornings are a mad rush, do as much preparation as you can the night before – until you get in the swing of packing your lunch, it's easy to rush out the door empty-handed. Write 'Lunch?' on a Post-it and stick it on the refrigerator or front door to make sure you won't forget.

Keep it simple

Many people prefer not to have to decide every day what they're going to eat. They find it comforting to open up the lunch box to the same cheddar and pickle sandwich with an apple and an oat and raisin biscuit. And talk about being in control: if you eat the same lunch every day, you never have to wonder about how many kilojoules you're consuming.

Help!

'I don't have a refrigerator at work to store my packed lunch. Should I worry about food going off?'

It depends. If your packed lunch includes meat, fish, eggs or dairy products (apart from hard cheeses), here are some simple ways to keep it cold and safe.

- Freeze a small plastic bottle of water or carton of fruit juice to use as a sandwich chiller (pack on top of your sandwich), then as a drink after it defrosts.
- Use a refreezable ice pack.
- Buy an insulated lunch box.
- Peel eggshells of hard-boiled eggs only when you're ready to eat them.

Some slimming experts even recommend the eating of monotonous meals. In one study volunteers who were offered a four-course meal consumed 44 per cent more kilojoules than those offered just one course.

Still, not everyone wants to sit down to the same thing every day. And there's a virtue to variety. By trying out several *ChangeOne* lunch options, you'll find the ones that work best for you. All that really matters is arriving at a plan for lunch that you can stick with.

Behind the *ChangeOne* lunch menu

Some of the choices found on the *ChangeOne* lunch menu may surprise you. Like avocado slices. Peanut butter. Cheese. Nuts. None of these would make its way into a low-fat diet. Yet we've included them in *ChangeOne* for a good reason. The latest evidence shows that you don't have to cut way back on fat to lose weight. New data shows that most people shed weight more successfully on diets containing moderate amounts of fat than they do on very low-fat regimens.

Surprised? No wonder. For years nutritionists have told us to cut back on fat. All fat. Too much fat on the menu makes people fat, they said. Gram for gram, fat contains twice as many kilojoules as protein or carbohydrates. And just as bad, it puts our hearts and arteries at risk by increasing cholesterol. Or so they said.

And we listened. Over the past three decades, the total number of kilojoules from fat in the average diet has fallen considerably and is still falling.

But now, in a stunning reversal, the experts are offering very different advice. Some fats are actually good for our hearts, they say. What's more, slashing fat from your diet, rather than helping you to lose weight, may actually make it harder to maintain a healthy weight. Very low-fat diets could even be unhealthy.

Good fat, bad fat

The truth is, experts have long known that there are various kinds of fat. The two main categories are saturated fat and unsaturated fat. Saturated fat comes mainly from animals,

continued on page 51

Change One Quiz

Ready for lunch?

Thinking over the food choices you made last week will help you to find the best ways to master the midday meal this week. Complete these nine questions by circling the number to the right of the appropriate answer.

1. Last week how often did you know in the morning what you'd have for lunch?

Never	1
A few days	2
Most days	3
Every day	4

2. How often did you know at least where you would have lunch?

Never	1
A few days	2
Most days	3
Every day	4

3. How often did you grab whatever happened to be handy?

Most days	1
Several days	2
Rarely or never	3

4. Which phrase best describes the choices available to you at lunch?

Very little choice	1
Some choice – same three or four things	2
Ample choice – varied and interesting	3

5. How would you rate your typical lunch?

Not very healthy	1
Healthy enough	2
Very healthy	3

6. How many serves of vegetables did you typically eat at lunch? (Chips don't count.)

None	1
1	2
2 or more	3

7. What was your usual choice for a sandwich bread?

White or French roll	1
Wholemeal, rye or other dark brown bread	2
Multi-grain or other wholegrain bread	3

8. How often did you eat lunch at home this past week or bring lunch to work?

Never	1
1–2 times	2
3–4 times	3
5–7 times	4

9. What was your usual drink at lunch?

Regular soft drink	1
Sweetened fruit drink	2
Milk	3
Sugar-free soft drink or water	4

Turn to next page to total your score.

Quiz score

Add up the numbers you've circled in the right-hand column.

   A score of 24–30: You're already well on your way to eating a good lunch.

   A score of 19–23: A few simple strategies could help to make the switch to a *ChangeOne* lunch easier.

   A score of 9–18: Okay, you've got serious work to do. By improving your lunches, you can take a giant step towards trimming kilojoules and slimming your waistline. Put ticks beside questions that scored a 1 or 2. Then look for the corresponding answers in the key below for tips that will help you this coming week.

1, 2, 3. If you have no idea where you'll have lunch – or what you'll choose – you're at risk of eating whatever's handy when lunch time rolls around. That could spell trouble for your diet. On pages 44 and 47 you'll find tips on how to master lunch by planning ahead.

   Of course not all of us always know ahead of time where we'll eat lunch. If that sounds like you, then it's time to keep a very close watch on serve sizes, wherever the lunch hour finds you.

4. Not much choice available? Your best option may be to bring lunch with you. You'll find several tasty packable lunches in the *ChangeOne* menus. If you're pressed for time in the morning, put your lunch together the night before.

5. Is your lunch falling short on good nutrition? Most of what's available at fast-food restaurants and other lunch cafés is high in fat and sugar and low in fibre and nutrients. If your typical lunch rarely sees a green vegetable, it needs work. If there's a big juicy cheeseburger on your plate – well, you already know there's work to do. If the lunch venues available don't offer much choice, your best bet is to pack your lunch.

6. What, no vegetables? You're missing out on one of the best healthy slimming foods around. Follow the *ChangeOne* menu this week and you'll get at least one serve at lunch, usually two.

7. White bread? You'll get more nutrients – and feel fuller for longer – when you eat breads that are made from wholemeal or rye flour. You'll get even more fibre, as well as healthful vitamins and minerals, from breads that contain whole grains like oats.

8. Not the lunch box type? Don't dismiss the idea out of hand. This week give it a try for a day or two. There's no better way to control exactly what and how much you eat. Many people find that packing a lunch relieves them of the pressure of having to choose the food they'll have when they're hungry.

9. Sugary soft drinks pack a load of kilojoules (about 545 in a 330 ml can). Some experts place much of the blame for the country's growing weight problems on the popularity of sugary drinks.

   That's an awful lot of kilojoules from foods that don't supply much else in the way of nutrition. Switch to a sugar-free drink or have a glass of still or sparkling water, and you'll shave 545 kilojoules from your diet, just like that. A small glass of fruit juice will provide vitamin C, which will facilitate the absorption of iron from your meal. For a longer drink, why not mix fruit juice and sparkling water?

   Skim or reduced-fat milk, a great source of calcium, is another smart beverage choice. Yes, milk supplies kilojoules. But it's also loaded with protein and calcium, which is essential for healthy bones. And, as you discovered last week, there's new evidence that it also helps to speed weight loss by encouraging your body to burn more fat.

continued from page 48

either in the form of meat or the fat in cheese, milk and other dairy foods. Unsaturated fat comes mainly from plants and fish. One of the biggest sources in our diets is vegetable oils such as corn, sunflower, olive and peanut.

The real culprit, when it comes to heart disease, is saturated fat. Because of its chemical composition, saturated fat causes the body to churn out additional artery-clogging LDL cholesterol.

Unsaturated fat, in contrast, has been shown to lower LDL. It can also raise HDL cholesterol, the friendly form that removes dangerous cholesterol from the body. The result: getting plenty of unsaturated fat protects your arteries from hardening. Global studies bear it out: the less saturated fat and more unsaturated fat people eat, the lower their risk of heart disease.

So why did so many nutritionists recommend cutting back on all fat? Because some of them thought the good fat/bad fat message was too complicated for people to understand. By telling people to cut back on all fat, the thinking went, saturated fat levels would fall. And with the country's waistline expanding, cutting back on total fat didn't seem like such a bad idea. Now it does.

Carbohydrates aren't so simple

When we listened to that flawed advice and dutifully cut back on fat, we replaced it largely with carbohydrates, mostly the processed kind found in white bread, biscuits, sugar and confectionery. That's bad news for two reasons.

First, it turns out that a high-carbohydrate, low-fat diet of this kind increases levels of triglycerides, a form of fat in the blood. Higher triglyceride levels are strongly linked to a greater danger of heart disease.

Second, a diet low in fat and high in processed carbohydrates may actually make it harder, rather than easier, to lose weight. Fat decreases the rate that the stomach empties, helping us to feel full for longer. And unlike slowly digested unprocessed foods, processed carbohydrates are quickly absorbed and send blood sugar levels spiking up rapidly. This sharp increase in blood sugar triggers a surge in insulin from the pancreas and the blood sugar level decreases again, leading to hunger pangs only an hour or so after eating, and the temptation

Plan on eating half of your restaurant lunch and taking home the rest.

Friendly hamburger

1 regular (55 g) lean hamburger (1 cm thick coaster) on bun with lettuce, salsa, tomato sauce or mustard, pickle

1 green salad topped with chopped vegetables (tomato, red cabbage, capsicum) (unlimited)

2 tablespoons fat-free dressing (2 salad-dressing caps)

1425 kJ, 340 kcal, 25 g protein, 8 g fat (3 g sat fat), 38 mg cholesterol, 38 g carbohydrate (8 g sugars), 7 g fibre, 452 mg sodium

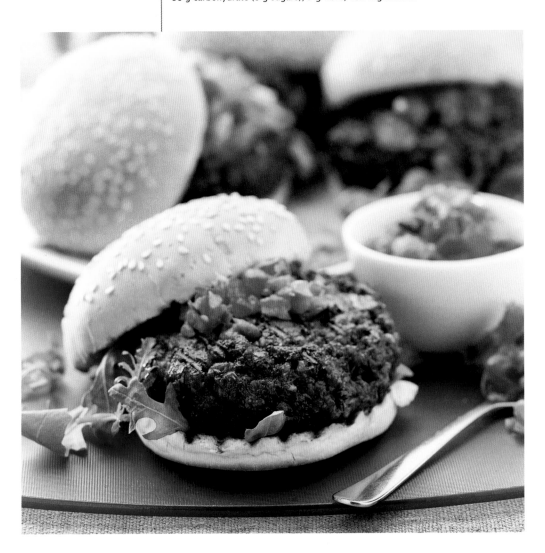

to grab another snack. That's a vicious cycle. The job of insulin is to help the sugar enter the muscles to fuel activity, and to promote storage of excess energy as fat. This works well when sugar is released gradually into the blood, and when you are getting enough exercise to use up excess sugar. Unfortunately, sudden blood sugar spikes, causing frequent surges of insulin, may be priming the body to store more fat, particularly if you are inactive.

There's still much left unresolved about carbohydrates, the role of insulin and the effect of blood sugar levels. But one thing is clear: cutting back on fat and filling up with processed carbohydrates like low-fat biscuits, rice crackers and sweets hasn't made us thinner. We're fatter than ever. And evidence is accumulating that a diet with moderate amounts of fat may make it easier to shed excess weight.

Eat fat, get slim

Consider the surprising results of an experiment conducted at Brigham and Women's Hospital in Boston, USA. Thirty overweight people followed a low-fat diet. In the same study, another group of 31 overweight people followed a diet with a moderate amount of fat – very much like the *ChangeOne* diet. Six months later volunteers in both groups had lost the same amount of weight. But after 18 months a tell-tale difference surfaced. By then, only 20 per cent of the people in the low-fat group were still on their diet, compared with 54 per cent of those in the moderate-fat group. What's more, the moderate-fat slimmers, as a group, had lost more body fat and reduced their waistlines more than the low-fat dieters.

continued on page 56

Help!

'Last week I was so hungry by the middle of the morning that I felt almost light-headed. Is that normal?'

Well, the light-headed part is. Hunger can make you feel woozy. It can also make you feel distracted or grumpy. If you get that hungry, however – at any time of the day – it's time to eat something. If you're especially heavy or active, you may need more kilojoules. Your body is burning more to keep you moving.

We're not talking about devouring jam doughnuts. In a kilojoule-reduced diet like *ChangeOne*, it's important to make every kilojoule count for nourishment. Choose snacks that do what they're supposed to do: take the edge off hunger. Next week we'll take a closer look at snacks. For now, try one of the following if hunger threatens.

- A piece of fruit
- A handful of nuts (about 25 g)
- All the celery or carrot sticks you like
- A glass of tomato or vegetable juice
- A mug of clear chicken or miso soup
- A glass of skim or reduced-fat milk, or a small tub of low-fat yogurt

Don't be afraid to reach for a snack. One recent survey found that snacking wasn't the downfall of most failed slimmers; what got most into trouble was eating too much at one of the three big meals of the day. Tame your hunger and you'll stay in control.

Build a better sandwich

Believe it or not, a deli can be a dieter's best friend. The options are endless, and if you're vigilant, you can make a satisfying and sensible sandwich.

Whether you're ordering over the counter or making your own, keep an eye on what's in even the supposed lightweight choice – chicken or turkey, tuna, even meatless options. Make sure you don't overstuff a sandwich with 140–225 grams of meat – twice as much as it's smart to swallow in a meal – or smother it in mayonnaise (as much as 2940 kilojoules worth in a tuna sandwich).

What you get can be a day's worth of kilojoules between two slices of bread. Not only will that blow your diet, it will also slow down your progress.

What you want is what you see here. Check out these *ChangeOne* tips for building a better sandwich.

THE PERFECT DELI SANDWICH

Chicken with gruyère

2 slices wholemeal bread
55 g reduced-sodium chicken breast (2 CDs)
15 g gruyère (credit card)
Sliced tomato, seeded mustard

½ cup (55 g) shredded lettuce, carrot, cabbage, red onion (cupped handful)

½ cup (85 g) melon salad (cupped handful)

1507 kJ, 360 kcal, 25 g protein, 17 g fat (5 g sat fat),
69 mg cholesterol, 27 g carbohydrate (10 g sugars),
6 g fibre, 377 mg sodium

Bread
- Wholegrain roll (tennis ball)
- Rye bread, 2 slices
- Pumpernickel bread, 2 slices
- Flour tortilla (wrap), medium (dessert plate)
- French, ciabatta or sourdough bread (2 mobile phones)
- Soft finger roll, 7.5 cm (length of longest finger)

Meats or alternatives
- Cooked ham, 55 g (2 CDs)
- ½ cup (85 g) tuna salad (made with reduced-fat mayonnaise) (2 golf balls)
- Lean roast beef, 55 g (2 CDs)
- Corned beef, 35 g (2 CDs)

Cheese or alternatives
- Reduced-fat cheddar, 15 g (credit card)
- Additional meat or tuna, 25 g (CD or table tennis ball)
- 2 tablespoons peanut butter (2 thumbs)
- 2 tablespoons hummus (2 thumbs)

Vegetables
- Lettuce and tomato
- Grilled vegetables (unlimited)
- Spinach leaves (unlimited)
- Rocket or watercress (unlimited)
- Thinly sliced apple, 3 slices
- ¼ avocado, sliced

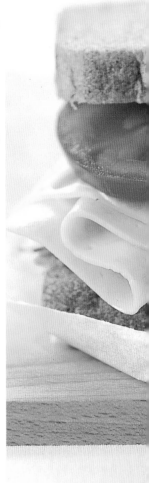

Deli delights

You can enjoy your deli favourites if you keep to a modest 55 g of filling (the equivalent of a couple of CDs). That said, here are popular cooked, cured and processed meats ranked from best to 'wurst' based on kilojoules and artery-clogging fat. There's no harm in enjoying them once in a while, but keep in mind that they're all higher in kilojoules than leaner fillings like smoked chicken and turkey breast.

- Prosciutto (all fat removed)
- Roast beef/pork
- Pastrami
- Corned beef

- Garlic sausage
- Liver sausage (liverwurst)
- Salami
- Chorizo

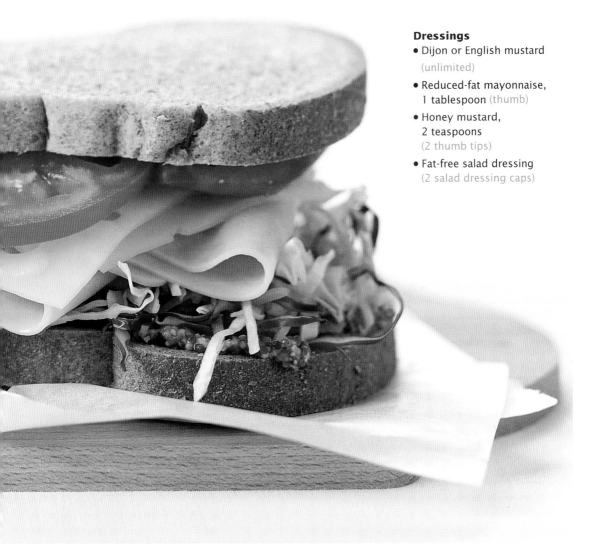

Dressings

- Dijon or English mustard (unlimited)
- Reduced-fat mayonnaise, 1 tablespoon (thumb)
- Honey mustard, 2 teaspoons (2 thumb tips)
- Fat-free salad dressing (2 salad dressing caps)

continued from page 53

Why? One reason, researchers say, is that a diet with moderate amounts of fat is simply more satisfying than a harsh low-fat regimen. It's a healthy diet people can live with. And that's the only kind of diet that really works over the long term. Another reason may be that people eating moderate amounts of fat are less likely to overdo simple carbohydrates, and keep their hunger in check more easily.

The new advice is the same whether you hope to protect your heart or shed excess weight. Replace saturated fat with unsaturated fat wherever you can – by switching from butter to olive oil, for instance, and by eating less meat and more fish. (Fish is abundant in polyunsaturated fats, particularly a form that contains omega-3 fatty acids, which have been shown to protect the heart.) Keep serve sizes under control so you don't overdo the kilojoules. And steer your diet away from simple carbohydrates like sugar and white bread and towards more complex carbohydrates like those in wholegrain breads and cereals. These recommendations are the basis of the *ChangeOne* menu because they are the surest strategy for slimming down and keeping weight off.

The perfect slimming food

Something else you'll notice about the *ChangeOne* lunch menu: it features plenty of vegetables. Every meal includes at least one serve, often two. No other food fills you up on fewer kilojoules while delivering more nutrients. Vegetables are rich not only in fibre but also in disease-fighting antioxidants and phytochemicals. They're mostly complex carbohydrates, the kind that keep blood sugar levels from soaring too fast and then plummeting too quickly. Vegetables are so good in so many ways that they're free on *ChangeOne* – with the exception of potatoes, which are high in simple carbohydrates.

And as any chef will tell you, nothing brightens up a plate like dark leafy greens, red or yellow capsicums, a ripe tomato or rich orange carrot slices. On the *ChangeOne* lunch menu, *continued on page 59*

A BIT ON THE SIDE

Faced with a choice among side salads, choose one of these – and keep in mind that pickles are freebies.

- Green salad topped with chopped vegetables (tomato, cucumber, broccoli, capsicum, etc) (unlimited) with 2 tablespoons sliced olives, a few of shakes of olive oil, and vinegar
- 'Clear' coleslaw made with vinegar and a touch of sugar rather than mayonnaise (cupped handful)
- Three-bean salad with low-fat dressing (cupped handful)
- Italian-style pickled vegetables (unlimited)
- Grilled vegetables (if not too oily) (unlimited)
- Sliced or diced tomato (unlimited)

Mexican wrap

1 flour tortilla (18–20 cm), filled with:

55 g grilled chicken (half your palm)
1 tablespoon canned refried beans or kidney beans (1 thumb)
1 tablespoon grated cheese (1 thumb)
1 tablespoon guacamole (1 thumb)
1 tablespoon salsa (1 thumb)
Shredded lettuce and diced tomato (unlimited)

1 orange

To prepare the wrap:

Place chicken, beans and cheese on tortilla. Microwave for 30 seconds or until the filling is warm. Add the remaining ingredients, roll up and eat.

1584 kJ, 379 kcal, 26 g protein, 14 g fat (6 g sat fat), 61 mg cholesterol, 36 g carbohydrate (15 g sugars), 8 g fibre, 570 mg sodium

Time-saver
Buy pre-grated cheese sold in a resealable plastic bag.

ABOUT TORTILLAS

Choose a small or medium-sized tortilla to keep kilojoules in check. A large flour tortilla contains as many kilojoules as four slices of bread.

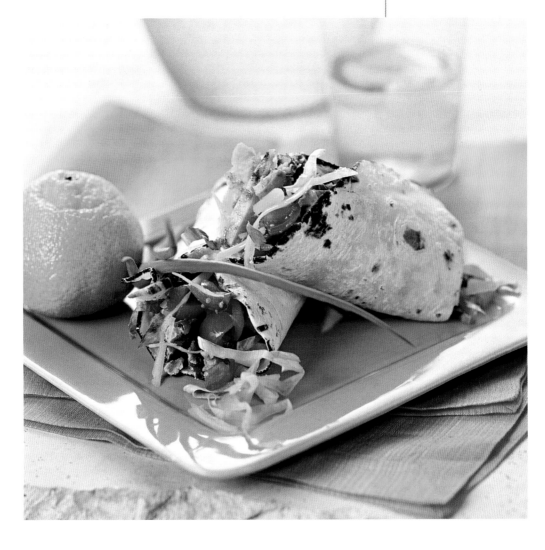

Change One Success Stories

Benefits far beyond just weight loss

When she decided to get healthy, Lyndel Walker felt pretty overwhelmed by the amount of weight she needed to lose.

'My husband's doctor had told him to try the Atkins Diet, but I just couldn't be convinced that the high-protein, high-cholesterol approach could be healthy in the long term', she says. Once she found out about *ChangeOne*, she 'knew that it could really help me do what I already knew I needed to do.'

With *ChangeOne*, Lyndel has already lost 48 kg and plans to lose another 13 kg.

Besides her weight loss, Lyndel lists other benefits from *ChangeOne*. 'I can now fit into airline seats, bend over to tie my shoes or paint my toenails, climb up into the kids' wooden cubby house without worrying about breaking it, and shop in the "regular" clothes sections. I have truly enjoyed being more physically active and just having a sharper mind and much more energy. Two of my grandchildren were visiting this summer from France, and I could go to the zoo, ride a bike, swim and just play so much better than in the past.'

Lyndel is thrilled about her family and friends' reactions to her weight loss, too. 'My husband never made me feel bad about my weight, but he has enjoyed being able to get his arms around me again', she says. 'My children know that it means I will have more years to be a grandmother to their children and are happy about that.'

She also hears many comments about the amazing changes in her appearance.

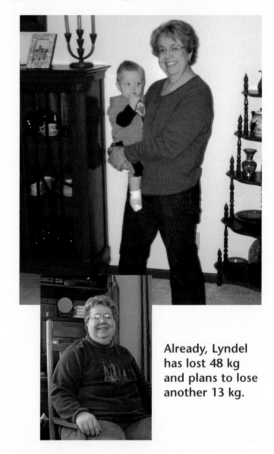

Already, Lyndel has lost 48 kg and plans to lose another 13 kg.

'When I see casual acquaintances that I haven't seen for quite a while, they seem to respond strangely to me, and then I realise they do not even recognise me.'

Lyndel advises anyone who's trying to lose a significant amount of weight to be patient, as the results may take a while to show. 'When I started, I knew that it would take at least a year to really get anywhere with my weight, but I also knew that it would take the rest of my life to stay at a reasonable weight', she says. '*ChangeOne* has helped me make changes that can last a lifetime.'

continued from page 56
you'll find many clever ways to add a serve or two of vegetables to your sandwiches and soups to make them more filling and more flavoursome without piling on kilojoules.

Changes ahead: snacks

While you're settling on your *ChangeOne* meals for breakfast and lunch, be aware of times during the day when you have a snack attack – and what you typically do about it. Don't feel that you have to change your snacks just yet. But be aware of how you feel, the choices you've given yourself, and what you usually do to satisfy your cravings. If you have time, keep track of all the snacks you eat, and about how much of each you eat. In the next chapter we'll take a closer look at hunger and the best way to satisfy it.

More lunch choices

Can't find something you like from the lunches suggested in this chapter? Starting on page 312, you'll find more quick and delicious *ChangeOne* lunch ideas.

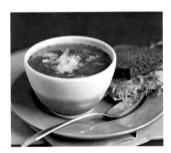

Hearty split pea soup
page 312

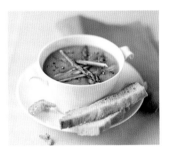

Cream of asparagus soup
page 313

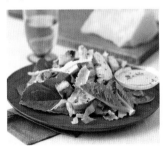

Grilled chicken caesar salad
page 315

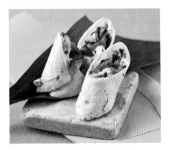

Roasted vegetable wraps with chive sauce
page 317

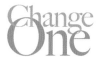

WEEK 3

Snacks

An entire chapter on snacks? In a book about losing weight? Are we serious? Of course we are.

Over the next few days, you'll learn how to use two snacks a day to take the edge off hunger and make losing weight *easier*.

We think you'll be surprised at what you learn. In fact, one of the dieters in our *ChangeOne* pilot group asked to repeat the snacks week. 'It wasn't until I filled in a food diary that I realised how often I snacked during the day', he explained. 'And it wasn't until we tackled snacks that I saw how often I ate something when I wasn't even all that hungry.' After two weeks of focusing on snacks, he really began to drop the weight.

You may too. For years nutritionists – and our mothers – told us not to eat between meals. Snacks seemed like they were the enemy. But now a new way of thinking about snacks has emerged. The two snacks a day recommended in *ChangeOne* will help you to stay on track. Eating something between meals, many experts say, can be one of a dieter's smartest strategies.

Nuts & seeds

Nuts and seeds are filled with proteins and healthy fats, which makes them nutritious but dense in kilojoules. They are also filling, so if you eat them slowly, it won't take many to reduce hunger. Here is a selection to eat to equal a 420-kilojoule snack (the size that *ChangeOne* recommends).

- Peanuts, in shells, 10 (handful)
- Pistachios, in shells, 30 (handful)
- Sunflower seeds, in shells, 25 g (palmful)
- Almonds, 16 to 20 (palmful)
- Pumpkin seeds, in shells (handful)
- Peanut butter, 1 tablespoon (thumb)

HEALTH TIP

Try to buy your nuts with their shell still on. Opening them takes time, so you're less likely to eat too many. And for many people, the cracking, splitting, picking and sorting are as satisfying as eating the nuts themselves.

ABOUT PEANUTS

Peanuts – actually a legume rather than a true nut – and peanut butter have become diet darlings of late. At Harvard University, a study showed that slimmers eating peanuts and peanut butter found it easier to stick to their diets. More good news: they're filling, they keep hunger at bay and they may also be good for your heart.

From top: pistachios, pumpkin seeds, peanuts, almonds (left), and sunflower seeds

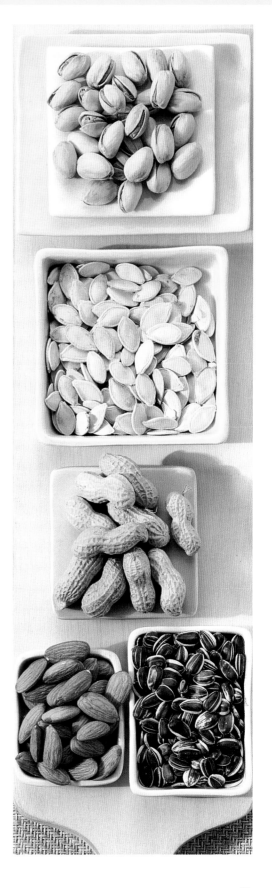

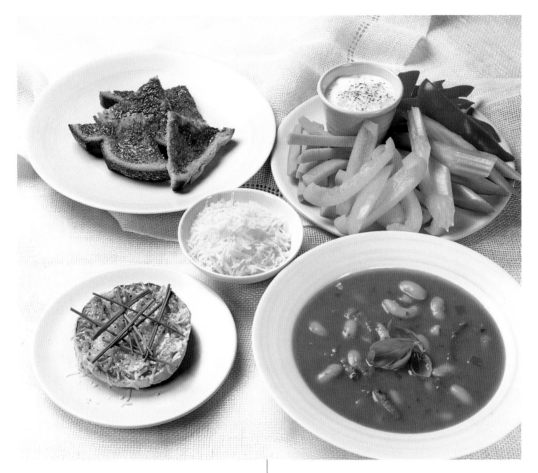

Savoury surprises

Break out of snacking boredom with change-of-pace foods like these. All provide 420 kilojoules or less.

- Soup: minestrone, vegetable, tomato, 1 cup (250 ml) (takeaway coffee cup)
- V-8 juice, 1 cup (250 ml) or more (drinking glass)
- Wholemeal toast, 1 small slice, spread sparingly with butter and yeast extract
- Reduced-fat, mature cheddar, 40 g (small matchbox)
- Peanut butter, 1 tablespoon (thumb), on a normal-size rice cake

Clockwise from top left: wholemeal toast with Vegemite, crudités, minestrone soup, muffin pizza and reduced-fat cheddar (centre)

- Muffin pizza: half an English muffin, topped with 1 tablespoon pasta sauce and 2 tablespoons grated cheese, then grilled until cheese bubbles
- Hard-boiled egg
- Rye crispbread, spread with 2 tablespoons reduced-fat hummus
- Breadsticks, 3, with 3 tablespoons tomato salsa
- Pumpernickel, spread with 30 g reduced-fat cottage cheese, plain or flavoured
- Crudités (unlimited), with 3 tablespoons tzatziki or another yogurt-based dip

Make snacks work for you

When we asked the *ChangeOne* volunteers to describe the single biggest fear they faced in dieting, many of them listed 'hunger'. That's not surprising. Dieters often think they have to resist hunger in order to lose weight. This week, we want you to pay close attention to hunger cues. And instead of resisting them, we want you to feed them – with a healthy snack. Here's why.

Hunger is an extremely powerful force. Getting enough fuel for our bodies is essential to survival. It is a matter of life and death, literally, so the body has a variety of internal signals that alert it when its energy stores are dipping low. Some come from the stomach. Some originate in the brain.

The longer we go without eating, the more powerful those signals become. It doesn't take long before they're so urgent that almost all we can think about is food. As hunger intensifies, will-power weakens. If you get hungry enough, you'll reach for anything.

That's where smart snacking comes in. Help yourself to something sensible when you feel hungry, and you'll help to ensure that hunger pangs don't destroy your determination to lose weight.

Concerned that snacking will make it harder to lose weight? Don't worry. Surprisingly, several large studies have found no link at all between the number of snacks people eat and how much they weigh. Even people who snack before bedtime – once considered a big diet taboo – don't seem to be any more likely to be overweight than people who don't.

Eating more often than just three times a day might even have advantages over the three-meals-a-day pattern when it comes to health. In a study at St Michael's Hospital at the University of Toronto, researchers tested two nutritionally identical diets. One group of volunteers ate their allotted food in three main meals. The others ate the same food in the same amounts but divided it into

17 snacks. Compared to the three-meals-a-day group, the snackers actually saw their cholesterol levels drop. The experts concluded that eating smaller meals more frequently kept blood sugar and insulin levels down, which in turn reduced the body's output of cholesterol. That's good, of course, and for anyone who wants to lose weight those results hint at even more good news: holding blood sugar and insulin levels steady can also keep hunger in check.

How we snack

Almost everyone has at least one snack a day. Half of the people in a survey conducted by Columbia University in New York snacked two to four times a day. Afternoons were their favourite snack time, when they were most likely to reach for something salty. The next favourite was before bedtime, when many people's taste buds yearn for something sweet, like chocolate or ice-cream.

Naturally, 17 snacks a day might be overdoing it a little. But one or two during the day – that's a proven key to dieting success. Just ask the successful slimmers who are part of the American National Weight Control Registry. A majority report that they eat five times a day: three small main meals and two snacks.

This week, help yourself to a snack when you feel hungry. But before you start reaching for the snacks, we're going to ask you to do one simple thing: make sure you're really hungry.

Learn to spot hunger cues

In this chapter, we've grouped snacks and desserts. One reason is that the same foods often serve either function (frozen yogurt, fruit, a piece of chocolate, a sweet biscuit), depending on when we eat them. Another is that most of us think of snacks and desserts as optional foods, a treat that's not part of our basic diet. On *ChangeOne* you can help yourself to sensible serves of snacks and desserts. All we ask is that you reach for them to satisfy genuine hunger.

Isn't that the reason most of us eat in the first place? Surprisingly, the answer is no. Weight loss experts say we typically eat for reasons that have nothing to do with genuine physical hunger. We take a box of buttered popcorn or a packet of chocolate-covered nuts to our seat in the movies simply because that's what we've always done. We eat because someone just brought a birthday cake into the office, and who can resist? Often we take up our knives and forks simply because it's meal time. Or because everyone else is eating.

continued on page 68

Change One Fast Track

To speed your progress, choose one or two of the following optional Fast Track changes this week.

Downsize your dishes

Serve sizes aren't the only things that have grown bigger in recent years. So have the plates and bowls on which they're served. If you have a tendency to pile your plate high and finish it all, try switching to smaller dishes.

Use a side plate instead of a dinner plate for your main dish. Ignore the giant pasta bowls and use a smaller cereal bowl to serve spaghetti. If the plates you already have won't do, buy an inexpensive set of 'downsized' plates and bowls for everyday use. Another clever way to make a little less food seem like more: use a dessert fork instead of a regular fork and a teaspoon for your soup and cereal.

Slim your sips

Plenty of people look to a cola for a pick-me-up in the mid-afternoon. If you're still reaching for soft drinks or other beverages sweetened with sugar, you're drinking a lot of kilojoules that aren't doing much to satisfy hunger.

Studies show that these drinks slip down without triggering satiety signals. If you drink a 330 g can of cola you'll consume 545 kilojoules or more before you know it. This week, switch to sugar-free versions of your favourite drinks. Or try something new and add a squeeze of fresh lemon or lime juice to a glass of sparkling mineral water.

Go for the gold

If you're a walker, increase your pace this week. On Day One, walk at your normal pace and keep track of how long it takes you to do your normal circuit. On Day Two, try shaving a minute off your time. Be aware of how you feel. A good brisk walk should leave you feeling winded but not gasping for air.

The quicker your pace, the more kilojoules you burn each minute. An 82 kg person burns about 25 kilojoules per minute walking at a leisurely 3.8 kilometres an hour. Walking at 5.5 kilometres an hour burns about 27 kilojoules per minute, while speeding up to 7.2 kilometres an hour (power-walking) burns about 33 kilojoules per minute. You'll also increase your fitness level, which will translate into more stamina and energy.

If you swim, jog, bicycle, exercise at a gym or do another kind of activity, nudge your workout a bit this week by putting in a little more time or pushing the intensity a little harder.

Skip the butter

Accustomed to smothering bread or rolls with butter? One small knob of butter – 8 mm x 2.5 cm – contains a massive 150 kilojoules and 4 g of fat, most of it saturated. If you smear a lot of butter on bread, you can easily total 500 kilojoules or more on butter alone.

This week, enjoy the unadulterated flavour of bread without all those extra fat-laden kilojoules. Choose wholegrain varieties of bread and rolls. The extra fibre they contain will slow digestion and make you feel fuller, and you'll get so much extra flavour that you may not even miss that butter. Or at least not terribly.

Savoury snacks

Do you have a craving for potato chips and other savoury chips and snacks? Then go ahead and have some – just not too many. The following lists show you gram weights and/or quantities of each snack food that equal 420 kilojoules or less.

Savoury chips

- Potato chips 20 g (cupped handful)
- Reduced-fat chips (such as rice chips), 22 g (cupped handful)
- Vegetable chips, 21 g (cupped handful)
- Thick-cut crisps (such as Pringles), about 10 (18 g)
- Reduced-fat Pringles, about 15 (22 g)
- Tortilla chips, about 12 (22 g)
- Prawn crackers, about 32 (30 g)
- Bagel chips, about 8 (20 g)

Savoury biscuits

- Rye crispbread (such as Ryvita), 3
- Ritz, 6
- Rice cakes, regular thick, 3
- Rice cakes, thin, 6
- Breadsticks, 4
- Pappadams, mini, 26 g (2 cupped handfuls)
- Multigrain crispbread, 3
- Pretzels, 26 g (about 1 handful)

Popcorn

- Popcorn, popped in a pot (about 3 handfuls)
- Microwave popcorn, butter flavour (about 1 handful)

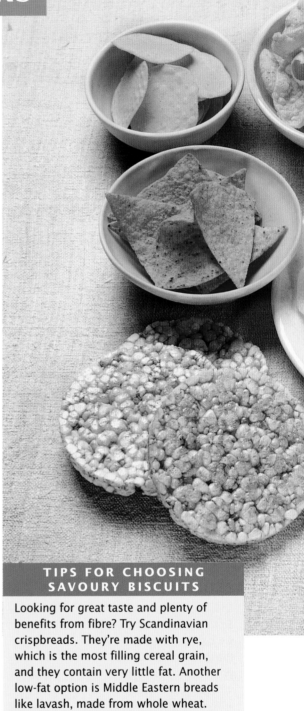

TIPS FOR CHOOSING SAVOURY BISCUITS

Looking for great taste and plenty of benefits from fibre? Try Scandinavian crispbreads. They're made with rye, which is the most filling cereal grain, and they contain very little fat. Another low-fat option is Middle Eastern breads like lavash, made from whole wheat. Enjoy both of these plain or topped with a little low-fat hummus, roasted capsicum dip, peanut butter or reduced-fat soft cheese.

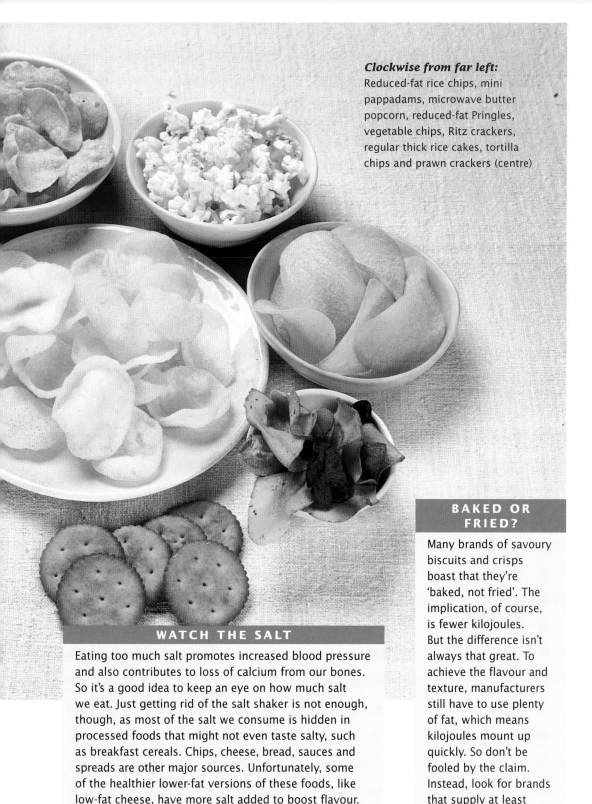

Clockwise from far left:
Reduced-fat rice chips, mini pappadams, microwave butter popcorn, reduced-fat Pringles, vegetable chips, Ritz crackers, regular thick rice cakes, tortilla chips and prawn crackers (centre)

WATCH THE SALT

Eating too much salt promotes increased blood pressure and also contributes to loss of calcium from our bones. So it's a good idea to keep an eye on how much salt we eat. Just getting rid of the salt shaker is not enough, though, as most of the salt we consume is hidden in processed foods that might not even taste salty, such as breakfast cereals. Chips, cheese, bread, sauces and spreads are other major sources. Unfortunately, some of the healthier lower-fat versions of these foods, like low-fat cheese, have more salt added to boost flavour. Check the label – if a food contains more than 400 mg sodium per serve, avoid it or use only small amounts.

BAKED OR FRIED?

Many brands of savoury biscuits and crisps boast that they're 'baked, not fried'. The implication, of course, is fewer kilojoules. But the difference isn't always that great. To achieve the flavour and texture, manufacturers still have to use plenty of fat, which means kilojoules mount up quickly. So don't be fooled by the claim. Instead, look for brands that supply at least 1 g fibre and less than 3 g fat per serve.

continued from page 64

The experts call these reasons for eating, environmental cues. Something in our surroundings triggers the urge to eat. You may not be hungry in the sense that your body is running short of fuel. In fact, you may have just finished a big, filling meal. But the sight or smell or memory of past occasions prompts the urge to eat and you help yourself, often without thinking.

Emotional eating

Environmental cues aren't the only reasons we eat when we're not really hungry. Many of us eat for emotional reasons, too. After all, food can be comforting. It's part of being sociable. Getting together over a meal with friends or family can be a pleasant way to relax and enjoy each other's company after a long and busy day. And of course, food simply tastes good.

The pleasure we get from food has a biochemical basis, researchers say. When we eat something delicious, the experience triggers the release of endorphins in the brain, the same 'feel-good' chemicals that have been associated with 'jogger's high'. Certain foods may have their own mood-enhancing effects. Carbohydrates are thought to increase the absorption of an amino acid called tryptophan, which in turn boosts levels of serotonin, another biochemical associated with mental wellbeing.

There are other reasons why eating is linked to emotions. If your parents comforted you or rewarded you with food, for instance, you may tend to reach for something to eat when you're feeling low or want to give yourself a reward for a job well done. If you get into the habit of eating something when you're feeling bored, you'll find yourself feeling hungry every time boredom strikes.

The same can be true for feeling lonely. 'I'd get home from work at the end of a long day, which was a hard time for me after being divorced', one *ChangeOne* volunteer recalled. 'I'd have dinner. And then, maybe because I was feeling lonely, I'd just go on eating and eating. Sweets. Biscuits. I wasn't hungry. Somehow it just seemed to make me feel better. Recognising that pattern made a big difference for me.'

The problem with environmental and emotional eating is obvious. If you eat when you're not genuinely hungry, you'll almost certainly consume more kilojoules than your body needs. There are healthier ways than overeating to deal with

Food provides comfort and consolation. Unfortunately, neither has anything to do with nutrition.

Change One Quiz

The hungry me

Tick only the boxes with the statements that apply to you. Tell yourself the truth; nobody but you needs to see your answers. Then, add up your score.

- ❐ When I go to the movies, I almost always get popcorn, chocolate or some other treat.
- ❐ When I'm very busy, I sometimes don't even notice that I'm hungry.
- ❐ On stressful days, I often find it relaxing to eat something.
- ❐ If I'm bored and there's food around, I'll eat it.
- ❐ It's no big deal for me to say no to treats if I'm not really hungry.
- ❐ There are certain foods I really crave, like chocolate or salty snacks.
- ❐ I like the feeling of being really hungry when I sit down to a meal.
- ❐ I have a tendency to eat everything on my plate even if I'm not really that hungry.

- ❐ If I'm feeling a little down or blue, eating something can really help.
- ❐ If there's a plateful of biscuits or potato chips in front of me, I won't be able to resist taking some.
- ❐ I have to be careful about having junk food around the house. If it's there, I'll eat it.
- ❐ My way of dealing with stress is to get up and do something.
- ❐ As long as I know I'll be sitting down to a meal soon, I can deal with feeling hungry.
- ❐ Dinner just doesn't seem to be dinner without dessert.
- ❐ I definitely don't like the feeling of being hungry.

Turn to next page to add up your score.

stress, boredom or loneliness. Simply distracting yourself by doing something else you enjoy – listening to music, phoning a friend, reading a book, watching a film, going for a walk or doing a crossword puzzle – often works. How do you know if environmental or emotional cues are controlling when and how much you eat? The first step is paying attention to what genuine hunger feels like.

Last week, you began to be more aware of times during the day when you felt hungry between meals – and what you did about it. Using what you learned then, do 'The hungry me' quiz on this page.

Quiz score

Add up the number of boxes you ticked according to colour.

❒ green _____
❒ red _____
❒ yellow _____

What your score means

❒ If you ticked mostly green boxes, at least you're not snacking because you're bored or stressed. This week, choose your snacks from among the recommended *ChangeOne* snacks and you'll keep kilojoules under control.

❒ If you ticked mostly red boxes, you tend to be an 'on cue' snacker. You reach for a snack not necessarily because you're hungry but because of cues in the environment around you. Recognising those cues – and asking yourself if you're really hungry – could help you to avoid taking in kilojoules you don't really want.

❒ If most of the boxes you ticked are yellow, you tend to be an 'emotional' snacker. You have the urge to eat something when you're feeling anxious, sad or lonely, or under stress. Many people do. Recognising what real hunger feels like – and finding ways other than eating to deal with your emotions – will help you to control kilojoules and also eat more healthily.

If your score was divided evenly among greens, reds and yellows, you're half way to becoming a smart snacker. The tips in this chapter will guide you the rest of the way there.

Knowing when you're genuinely hungry

One day early this week, try a simple experiment. If you typically have either a midmorning or midafternoon snack, skip it. Delay the next meal to about an hour later than usual. Then pay attention to how you feel. After you've gone four or five hours without eating anything, your body will begin to send out physical hunger cues. Some of these come from a part of the brain called the hypothalamus. When blood sugar levels fall, the hypothalamus senses an impending energy crisis and begins to issue 'feed me' orders by way of the central nervous system. Your tummy growls. Your thoughts focus on food. You may find yourself getting a bit irritable.

This physical hunger is different from the emotional or environmental kind, and it is not the same as a food craving. Food cravings focus on specific foods. You may crave chocolate when you're feeling lonely, or a fast-food hamburger when you're travelling in the car. Cravings are almost always responses to emotional or environmental cues.

Physical hunger isn't so specific. When your body needs more energy in the form of food, you don't focus on the taste of a particular food. You want any food that will fill you up.

Two key questions

As part of your hunger test this week, try another experiment. When you finally sit down to eat, make a point of slowing down and paying attention to how you feel as you eat. Notice what it feels like as your sensation of hunger gives way to the feeling that you're satisfied.

During the rest of this week, each time you feel the urge to have a snack between meals, pause for as long as it takes to ask yourself these two simple questions: Am I really hungry? Can I wait until my next meal to eat? If the answers are a resounding Yes! and No! help yourself to a snack. But if your answer is lukewarm, wait a bit. Get up and change what you're doing. Here are some options.

- Take a quick walk
- Drink a big glass of water
- Make a phone call
- Do a necessary chore such as dusting, tidying up or organising papers
- Wash your face or hands
- Brush your teeth
- Practise a relaxation technique like deep breathing
- Fill in three words on a crossword puzzle
- Flick through a magazine or newspaper

continued on page 75

Calcium choices

Not only does calcium build strong bones, new research shows that it also helps the body to burn fat. Try some of these calcium-rich, dairy-based snacks in 420 kilojoule serves.

- Low-fat or non-fat yogurt, natural or sugar-free and with fruit (200 g)
- Yogurt smoothie: in a blender, mix 115 g non-fat natural yogurt, ½ cup (125 ml) reduced-fat or skim milk and 255 g frozen unsweetened strawberries
- 1 cup (250 ml) reduced-fat or skim milk, plain or flavoured with syrup, or used to make a cup of cocoa
- Reduced-fat soft cheese (25 g) with celery sticks
- 1 cup (250 ml) sugar-free rice pudding or custard made with skim or reduced-fat milk

Sweet snacks

As long as you trust your will-power enough to stick to our serve sizes, then *ChangeOne* has some sweets for you. Here are 420 kilojoule helpings of some favourites.

Sweets

- M&M's, 30 (half a handful)
- Chocolate frog, plain, 1
- Smarties, 1 packet fun size
- Maltesers, 1 packet fun size
- Caramel-peanut chocolate bar, 1 fun size
- Chocolate and wafer bar, 10 g, 2
- 'Lite' chocolate bar, 1 regular
- Milky Way bar, 1 treat size
- Fudge, 1 regular
- Chocolate mint thins, 3
- Jelly beans, about 16 (30 g)
- Marshmallows, large, 5
- Fruit gums, 5
- Rolos, 4
- Boiled lollies, 4

Fruit

There's no denying that fruit is good for you, but the kilojoules in fruit can add up. We recommend buying medium-sized fruit when possible, but having a serve that's a little larger won't undo your *ChangeOne* plan.

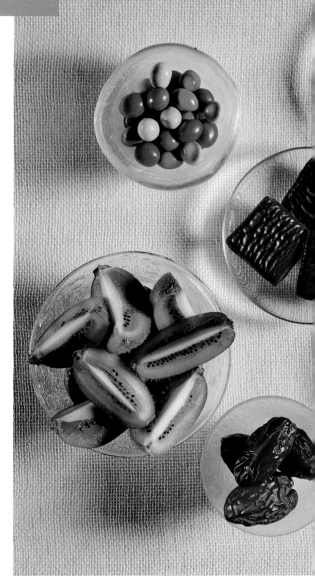

- Dried apricots, 6–8 (40 g) (half a handful)
- Sultanas, 3 tablespoons (three thumbs)
- Grapes, ¾ cup (20 g) (tennis ball)
- Apple, 1
- Orange, 1
- Banana, 1
- Melon balls, 1 cup (160 g) (cricket ball)
- Pineapple chunks, fresh, ½ cup (75 g) (2 golf balls)
- Fresh dates, 4
- Kiwifruit, 3
- Banana chips, 20 g (handful)

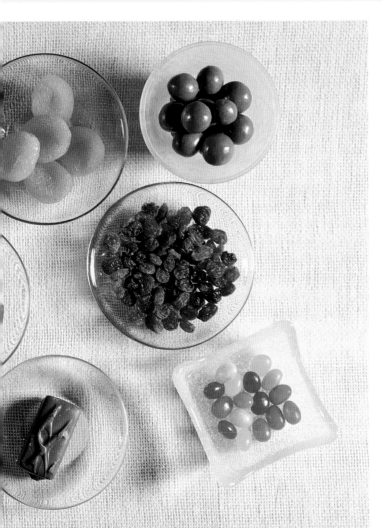

Clockwise from far left:
M&M's, dried apricots, Maltesers, sultanas, jelly beans, Milky Way bar, fresh dates, kiwifruit and chocolate mint thins (centre)

WHY CAN'T FRUIT BE UNLIMITED?

It's good and good for you, so why can't you eat as much fruit as you want? Because the natural sugar content of fruit gives it more kilojoules than are in most vegetables. *ChangeOne* suggests two serves of fruit, one at breakfast and one at lunch, plus the option of a third for a snack. Eating more than that is all to the good from the viewpoint of general nutrition, but keep in mind that the extra kilojoules could slow down your weight-loss efforts.

SWEET STRATEGIES

When nothing but lollies will do:

Minis are in. Buy the smallest pieces you can find. From the label, calculate how many pieces add up to 340 to 420 kilojoules. (You'll probably need a calculator to do this!) Eat them one by one, taking time between bites to savour them completely.

Hide and seek. Packets of fun- and bite-size lollies and bars are easy to find in supermarkets. A serve is one or two pieces. Put them in an out-of-the-way spot – say, high in a cupboard behind the wine glasses – and then go there only to take out what you'll eat for the day. If you have to pull out some wine glasses before you can get a treat, you'll have time to reconsider your need.

Buy high-quality lollies that you really like. When the flavour is intense or when you're eating a favourite, you'll be satisfied with less.

73

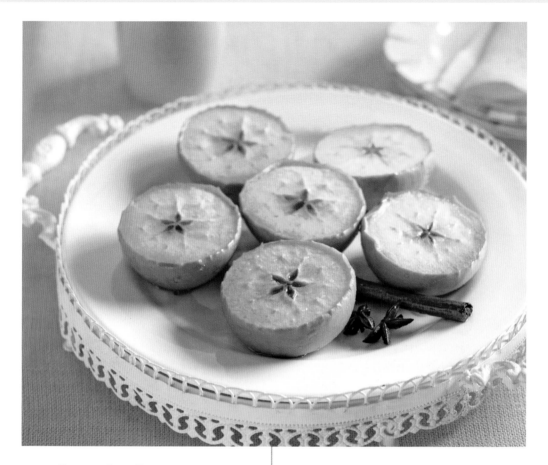

Baked desserts

Cakes, pies, baked custards and hot fruit puddings are deservedly popular. Here are serves of some favourites that provide about 420 kilojoules.

- **Plain sponge, 1 slice**
  (about ¹⁄₁₂ of the cake)
- **Fruit pie (apple, berry, etc)**
  (as thin as you can slice it and still see it, about 4 forkfuls)
- **Brownie, 5 cm square**
  (half a business card)
- **Chocolate gâteau, 1 slice about 1 cm thick** (lip-balm width)
- **Cupcake with icing, 1**
  (regular patty pan size)
- **Crème caramel, low-fat, 140 g**
  (small yogurt tub)

Baked apple

Halve a small Granny Smith apple and sprinkle it with cinnamon and sugar, plus a few star anise if you have some. Cover and microwave for 3 minutes or until soft.

Spiced pineapple

Sprinkle 2 slices of fresh pineapple (about 100 g) with 2 teaspoons soft brown sugar mixed with a pinch of ground ginger. Cover and microwave for 2 minutes, then top with 1 tablespoon reduced-fat sour cream.

Glazed bananas

Slice a small banana into 2.5 cm pieces. Sprinkle with ½ teaspoon soft brown sugar and dot with ½ teaspoon butter. Microwave for about 1 minute until bubbly.

continued from page 71
With any luck you'll be distracted enough that, if you weren't hungry, you'll forget about snacking. Food cravings typically disappear as quickly as they come, and hunger from environmental or emotional cues lasts only as long as the cues are right in front of you.

But if, after five minutes or so, you're still hungry, then it's time for a snack.

Reach for a snack that satisfies

Snacks seem to be everywhere these days. Vending machines are crammed with them. Supermarkets have entire aisles devoted to them. There are snacks at the check-out counter, as well as snacks at the movies, snacks at the service station and snacks at the newsagents.

And like so much else on the food landscape, many of these so-called snacks are oversized, fat-laden, kilojoule-laden extravaganzas. The biscuits on sale at deli counters these days are often the size of saucers. Family-size bags of potato chips or tortilla chips look big enough to feed hundreds. Even cookbooks have felt the pressure: in 1967 one cookbook's recipe for brownies made 36; in the latest edition, the exact same recipe makes 16 brownies. The fact is, even what passes for an individual-size serve these days can spell big trouble when you're trying to lose weight. A 200 gram bag of tortilla chips can easily contain almost 4200 kilojoules. Of course, you could stop eating when you start feeling satisfied. But who among us is able to do that with these nutritional booby traps?

Nibblers can take heart, however. We've put together a wide selection of good-tasting, low-kilojoule snacks that will tame your hunger without scuttling your diet. Of course you'll find carrot and celery sticks on the list,

continued on page 79

Help!

'My husband lost 2.5 kg in two weeks. I've barely lost anything. And we seem to be eating the same amount of food. What's going on?'

You're different people. Some people can eliminate one thing from their diet – sugary soft drinks, for instance – and begin losing weight immediately. Others have to watch everything they eat, and still their progress seems slow. There are many reasons. Some people's metabolic rate is higher than most, so they burn more kilojoules even when they're just sitting around. Some people do a lot of fidgeting during the day, which also burns kilojoules. One study found that fidgeters can burn more than 2100 kilojoules a day jiggling their legs or pacing about.

If you're feeling frustrated by the slow speed of your weight loss, consider making an additional Fast Track change. (You'll find Fast Track suggestions on page 65.) And don't give up. Remember the tortoise and the hare. Even with weight loss, slow starters can be the first ones across the finishing line.

Frozen treats

In summer, or at any time really, most people love a frozen dessert. Here are lots with fewer than 420 kilojoules. The trick is to indulge and enjoy yourself, without going over the top. Remember, they're a treat.

Iced treats

- Frozen yogurt, 60 g (1 scoop), 335 kilojoules
- Reduced-fat ice-cream, 60 g (1 scoop), 380 kilojoules
- Super premium chocolate ice-cream, 2 tablespoons (golf ball), 420 kilojoules
- Sorbet, 60 g (1 scoop), 250 kilojoules
- Fruit-flavoured icy pole, 78 ml, 210 kilojoules
- Home-made sorbet, see below (2 golf balls)

Frozen fruits

- Frozen grapes, ¾ cup (175 g) (tennis ball)
- Frozen banana, 1
- Frozen strawberries, 1 cup (250 g) (cricket ball)

Easy sorbet:

1. Freeze a can of fruit in heavy syrup.

2. Take out of the freezer 30 minutes ahead of serving time and place on the benchtop. Open the can at both ends and push out the contents into a food processor. Add ½ cup (125 ml) apple juice and process until smooth.

3. Serve soft, or refreeze.

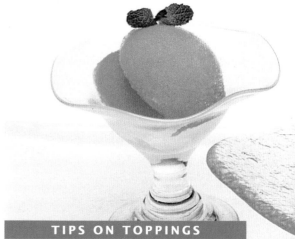

TIPS ON TOPPINGS

If you could have a tablespoon of topping on your ice-cream, what would you choose? Here are some favourites rated from lowest to highest in kilojoules per tablespoon. Remember that those over 210 kilojoules may have to stand in for your second snack of the day.

	kilojoules
Raisins	115
Crunchy cereal	120
Chocolate sauce	170
Chopped almonds	195
Butterscotch topping	220
Chocolate chips	220
Strawberry coulis	225
Hot fudge sauce	295
M&M's	300
Chocolate flakes	300

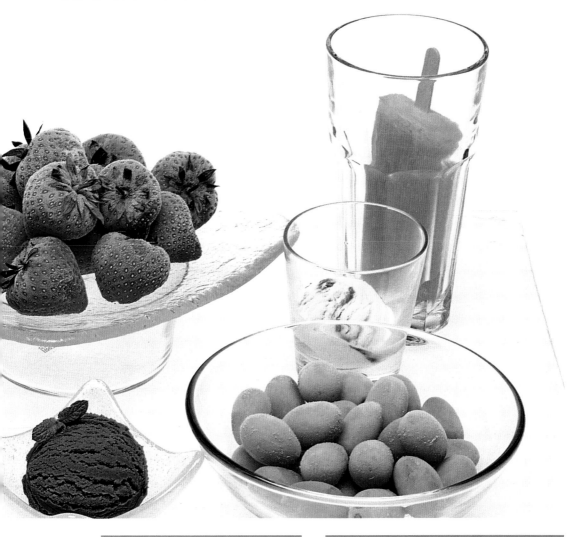

Clockwise from top left: home-made sorbet, frozen strawberries, orange and lemon icy pole, frozen yogurt, frozen grapes, super premium chocolate ice-cream

CHOOSING FLAVOURS

Frozen desserts in fruit flavours, for example strawberry and peach, are lowest in kilojoules because the fruit takes the place of higher-kilojoule, higher-fat ingredients such as full-fat milk and cream. The highest-kilojoule ice-creams are vanilla and those varieties with added bits such as toffee or nuts.

ABOUT FREEZING FRUIT

Fruit is easy to freeze and refreshing to eat. Start with your choice of ripe fruit – grapes, bananas, berries, melons, peaches, pineapple, plums, mangoes, nectarines – whatever you like. Cut whole fruit into bite-size pieces. Place on a baking tray and freeze until firm. Remove from the tray and place in a resealable plastic bag or container. Store in the freezer until needed.

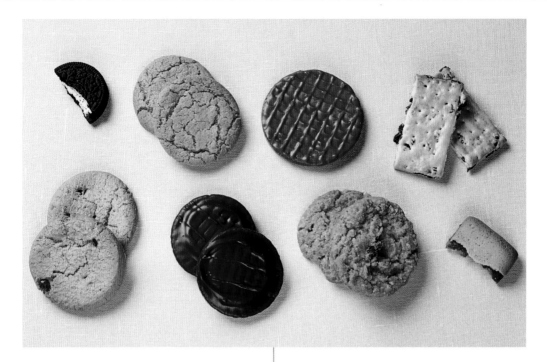

Biscuits

Biscuits and cookies are a special treat, whether home-made or bought. Here is a list of how many you can eat for a snack or sweet indulgence that will be 420 kilojoules or less.

- Butter crunch, 2
- Chocolate chip, 5 cm, 2
- Oat and raisin, 5 cm, 2
- Ginger nut, 5 cm, 2
- Rich tea, 2
- Jaffa cake, 2
- Fruit slice, 2
- Cream-filled plain or chocolate sandwich, 1½
- Fig rolls, 1½
- Biscotti, 1
- Digestive, plain or with milk chocolate, 1

Clockwise from top left: cream-filled chocolate sandwich, ginger nut, milk chocolate digestive, fruit slice, fig roll, oat and raisin cookie, Jaffa cake, chocolate chip cookie.

TIPS FOR BUYING BISCUITS

Don't rush to buy lower-fat versions of regular biscuits: they just don't taste as good, they tend to cost more and most shave off few, if any, kilojoules. And be careful of serve sizes when it comes to biscuits bought at the deli – not only are they huge in circumference, but they can be thicker than a normal biscuit. Often, one-third of a large biscuit is all you need; save the rest or share.

continued from page 75
simply because they make excellent munchies. But you'll also find some surprises, like Jaffa cakes, pistachios, tortilla chips and even chocolate buttons.

Behind *ChangeOne* snacks

Every *ChangeOne* snack contains about 420 kilojoules – enough to ease hunger pangs and still keep you within your kilojoule guidelines. We've chosen snacks that offer plenty of flavour. It may be obvious, but it's worth repeating: if something doesn't taste good, don't eat it. Why waste kilojoules on a low-fat biscuit that tastes like sawdust when you can help yourself to a handful of rich-tasting nuts or a piece of pita with sizzling salsa?

Beyond good taste, a snack worth its kilojoules should also be satisfying in other ways. If it's hot and humid, you want something cool and refreshing, like a real fruit sorbet. If you're inside on a cold, rainy day, you want something delicious, like hot chocolate, that will warm you up. A snack should also satisfy your hunger long enough to tide you over until the next meal. Research shows that snacks that take up a lot of volume per kilojoule – popcorn, or fruit and yogurt smoothies blended with ice, for instance – tend to make people feel fuller on fewer kilojoules.

Unlimited snacks

Some foods are so low in kilojoules that you can have as much as you want. Here are a few.
- Sugar-free icy pole
- Raw capsicum slices
- Cherry tomatoes
- Carrots and celery sticks
- Sugar-free fruit jelly

Snacks that pack a lot of nutrition also turn out to be more satisfying and filling than those with a lot of empty kilojoules. Remember the handful of nuts we mentioned? One recent study found that snacking on them may actually help people to keep their weight down. The reason: nuts are loaded with protein, vitamins and, yes, fat. With all that, it doesn't take many to satisfy your appetite. Munch on low-fat biscuits, which are made up mostly of simple carbohydrates, and you can go on eating and eating, hoping you'll find some flavour in the next bite, piling on kilojoules before you begin to feel satisfied. A few nuts, on the other hand, can give you that satisfaction.

Choosing a nutritious snack is important for another reason: when you're on a low-kilojoule diet, it's just good sense to make those kilojoules count. As we've said, a lot of us tend to think of snacks as a little something extra – a treat we allow ourselves that isn't really part of our slimming diet. We're kidding ourselves. In fact, treats are a surprisingly big part of what we eat during the day. According to one survey, about 20 per cent of our total kilojoules on average come from snacks – all the more reason to make sure those kilojoules deliver essential nutrients as well as good taste.

On *ChangeOne*, snacks will make up about 15 per cent of your total kilojoules. Naturally, since no one expects a snack to be a balanced meal in itself, we're including some less nutritious favourites just because they taste good. After all, it's not about never eating sweets, biscuits and other treats again. It's more about eating them less often and in reasonable serves, and enjoying them more.

Fitting a snack into your *ChangeOne* program

You can choose two snacks, or a snack and a dessert, or two desserts during the day. You can also dish up slightly larger serves of food at your meals, especially if you find yourself getting too hungry. As often as possible, try to make sure that one selection comes from the calcium choices on page 71. You already know the evidence linking calcium to weight loss. And getting enough calcium is important for strong bones.

Use snacks this week to help you to manage your hunger. If you get ravenous in the morning, eat something. If your appetite roars to life in the afternoon, grab a snack. Before you do, remember to take the hunger test. Ask yourself: Am I really hungry? Can I wait until my next meal?

Eight tips for controlling hunger cues

1. Instead of buying snacks at the movies, a match or some other event, chew a stick of sugar-free gum. Soon you'll associate the taste of gum, rather than high-kilojoule food, with that setting.
2. At parties, stand as far away as you can from the bowls of snacks.
3. On car trips, plan ahead and take a few *ChangeOne* snacks. If you have a tendency to munch in the car, bring just a single serve, not the whole box. Put the rest in the boot.
4. Buy snacks in small packs. If you buy the giant size to economise, divide it into single-serve-size sealable plastic bags or containers as soon as you get home.
5. Put the healthiest snacks where you'll see them first when you open a kitchen cupboard or the fridge. Hide the others behind them.
6. Don't snack in your office. (And don't keep bags of potato chips in your desk drawer.) Go somewhere else – kitchen, cafeteria, coffee area or outside. That way you won't associate your office with food.
7. At home, enjoy your snacks in the kitchen and nowhere else.
8. Don't eat to relax. Relax, then eat. Stress is such a big factor in diet that we've devoted a whole chapter to it. Look ahead to Week 9, which begins on page 182, for stress-busting tips.

ChangeOne Success Stories
Feeling better about herself

When Teresa Williamson first read about *ChangeOne*, she was intrigued by its simple and sensible approach. She gave the diet a try and has lost 34 kilograms and 96 centimetres.

'I feel so much better about myself and more self-confident because of the weight loss itself and the fact that I have done it on my own', she says.

Teresa's weight loss is not the only benefit she's gotten from *ChangeOne*. 'I feel good physically. I'm not out of breath all the time anymore from physical exertion', she says. 'I have also had a noticeable improvement in my asthma. I used to use an inhaler regularly, but now I seldom use it, because my body is not having to work as hard.' She adds, 'I can shop in the regular-size clothing section, something that I haven't done in many years. That is very exciting!'

Teresa loves the commonsense approach of *ChangeOne*. 'I know that I'm not doing any harm to my body by going on this diet. Diet pills can cause harm, as can fad diets. There are no special meals that must be bought – just good food from the supermarket. That means for me that if I continue throughout my life to follow *ChangeOne* principles, I should easily be able to maintain weight loss once I achieve my goal weight.'

The *ChangeOne* serve guides have helped Teresa keep her servings in check. 'Also, knowing that I should eat breakfast, a snack, lunch, a snack and dinner helps me tremendously. Now, I

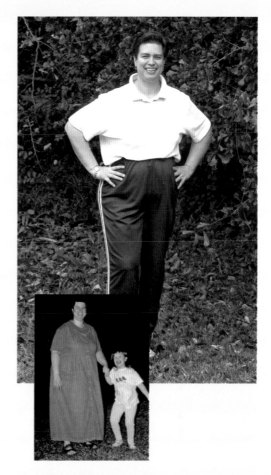

Teresa Williamson lost 34 kg and 96 cm on the *ChangeOne* plan.

eat because I'm hungry, whereas before, I ate whenever and whatever I wanted to.'

Teresa's friends and family are amazed by her progress. 'My sister-in-law told me that I am just melting away!' she says. 'People are always commenting on how good I look now and how much slimmer I look! My husband is proud of me and is constantly telling me that I am doing great and look good.'

Can't find something you like from among the snacks suggested in this chapter? Starting on page 326, you'll find more quick and delicious *ChangeOne* snack ideas.

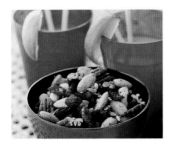

Curry-spiced fruits, nuts and seeds
page 326

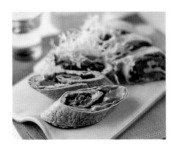

Roasted capsicum pinwheels
page 326

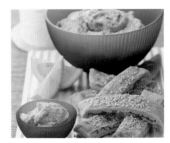

Sesame pita crisps
page 327

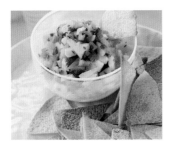

Tortilla chips
page 327

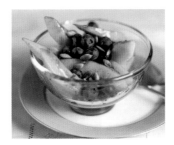

Melon salad with raspberry vinaigrette
page 328

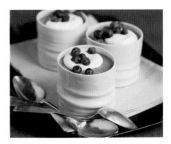

Blueberry mousse
page 329

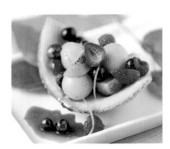

Fruit boats with orange and balsamic glaze
page 330

Changes ahead: dinner

This week, while you focus on snacking, start paying attention to what you have for dinner. Don't change what you eat. Just notice what it is. Also be aware of how much time you spend eating dinner. Record how many nights you eat in and how many nights you eat out at restaurants or friends' houses. If you have time, keep a food diary of your dinners for the week, listing the foods in them and approximately how much you ate. (You'll find an easy-to-use form on page 345.) Pay attention to the way you experience hunger and fullness, too. Those sensations can be a useful guide when it comes to eating sensible-size serves.

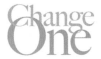

Dinner

Pull up a chair, it's dinner time.

For most of us dinner comes at the end of a long day of work or errands. It's the time when we relax and reward ourselves. If you've been following *ChangeOne* week by week, this chapter will complete a month of determination and healthy changes. Well done! You've taken control of breakfast, lunch and snacks.

This week we want you to enjoy tasty meals each evening, and to slow down and enjoy the company. By doing so, you'll actually eat less.

Dinners are typically the biggest meal of the day, as well as the source of the most kilojoules. That's why taking charge of dinner can have the biggest payoff when it comes to losing weight. Many of our *ChangeOne* volunteers saw their weight loss accelerate when they got dinner into shape. By being sensible about serves, and using the meals in this chapter and on pages 318 to 325 as a guide, you'll discover that you, too, can enjoy delicious dinners and keep melting the weight away.

Slow down, relax and enjoy dinner

On the following pages you'll find a tantalising selection of *ChangeOne* dinner suggestions, with plenty of ways to tailor them to your own tastes. We've made the menus as varied as possible to take advantage of the extraordinary culinary diversity available to us – from Chinese stir-fries to Italian pasta dishes to beefburgers on a bun. Of all the meals of the day, after all, dinner is the one that most reflects our family history, culture and special tastes.

(If you eat a lot of dinners out, you may want to glance at the next chapter, in which we take a look at strategies you can use to eat smart at restaurants. But first, take a few minutes to look over the dinner meal plans on these pages. They'll give you a good idea of what a *ChangeOne* dinner contains and what sensible serve sizes look like.)

When you sit down to dinner this week, there's one simple change you'll want to make, no matter what's on the table: slow down and savour the meal. Too often these days we're doing a mad dash from here to there, devouring meals without really taking the time to taste what's in front of us.

Dinner serves

These meal plans give weights as well as size indicators from the *ChangeOne* serve-size guide.

Type of food	Example	Amount	*ChangeOne* serve
One starch	Rice, pasta, noodles	140 g	Tennis ball
or one grain	Bread roll	Medium	Tennis ball
One protein	Chicken, beef	115 g	Deck of cards
	Tofu	85–115 g	Deck of cards
	White fish	170 g	Chequebook
	Oily fish such as salmon or mackerel	85 g	Deck of cards
Vegetables	Any vegetable, except potato	Unlimited	

And eating too quickly is one reason so many of us find ourselves struggling with weight.

So this week, give dinner your attention. Set aside enough time to be sure that you don't feel rushed. You may not be able to treat yourself to a leisurely dinner every night, but if you can guarantee that you enjoy an unhurried dinner at least three times during the coming week, you'll begin to see why savouring a meal is one of the simplest and smartest slimming strategies.

Here's why: research shows that just as the body sends hunger signals to the brain, it also communicates when it's had enough food. Those cues, called satiety signals, are the body's way of balancing kilojoules we consume with kilojoules we burn. They work effectively as long as we take time to notice them.

If you've ever got up from a Christmas dinner feeling as if you're as stuffed as the turkey, you'll know how easy it is to eat more than you need – sometimes a lot more. Studies show that it takes up to 20 minutes after food reaches your stomach for satiety signals to kick in.

Hence the problem with fast food, and fast eating in general, regardless of what's on the menu. Gulp down food in a big hurry and you don't give your body time to tell you, 'Stop, I've had enough!' You can end up consuming far more kilojoules than you need or even want.

'I realise now I was like a feeding machine', one of our volunteers told us. 'Hand to mouth, hand to mouth – I never paused. I just ploughed through whatever was in front of me. I never stopped to think about what it tasted like. Or how I felt. The change that made the biggest difference for me was learning to put my fork down every few bites and just stop for a minute.' As she learned, a leisurely meal gives your body and brain time to catch up with your fork. Slow down and you'll feel satisfied on far fewer kilojoules than if you rushed through dinner.

Making the change

Given how busy life is for many of us, taking time for dinner isn't always easy. You may have to rearrange your schedule a little. You may need to watch that episode of your favourite program later. You may have to reorganise an appointment or two.

> It takes up to 20 minutes after food reaches your stomach for satiety signals to kick in.

Even so, give it a try. Make it a goal that everyone in your house who plans to eat dinner sits down together. You'll find it's worth the effort, not only for the opportunity to relax and savour the meal but also for the new chance to spend time with your friends and family. If you're used to an eat-and-run approach to dinner, you can rediscover its pleasures – and make yourself a smarter eater – with these seven simple changes.

1. Arrange your schedule so you have at least 30 quiet minutes for dinner.

2. When you have dinner at home, always have it in your dining area. That way you won't associate food with other parts of the house – the sofa in front of the television, for instance.

3. If the menu allows, divide your meal into courses – for instance, a main dish and vegetables, salad and dessert. Choose the order that works best for you.

4. Make the meal the focus of dinner time. Turn off the television. Put away the newspaper. Let the answering machine take your calls. A little quiet music is fine, as long as it doesn't distract you from the meal.

5. Serve a glass (250 ml) of water with the meal. Between each bite, put down your fork and take a small sip of water. Sipping water forces you to slow down. Water with dinner also makes a meal more filling without adding kilojoules. Many people also find that it helps them to clear their palate and more fully experience the flavours in a meal.

6. Pay attention to how the food tastes. Notice how the flavours complement or contrast with one another. Take small bites and let them linger in your mouth so that the full flavour is released.

7. After a course, take a minute or two to relax, chat and savour what you've just eaten. It may sound paradoxical, but lingering over dinner could be an important key to maintaining a healthy weight.

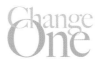

Change One Check-in

Last week you added snacks to your *ChangeOne* menu. You'll find that low-joule snacks help you to manage hunger and stay in control of what you eat. Still mastering the art of snacking? Struggling with breakfast or lunch? Then by all means take another week to get them under control. If you find you are too rushed in the morning to put together a proper *ChangeOne* breakfast, look back at Week 1 for some time-saving tips. If you're having trouble controlling serve sizes when you go out to lunch, try packing a lunch a few times this week. Still grabbing a chocolate bar from the vending machine when you suffer a mid-afternoon snack attack? Select a smarter snack from the *ChangeOne* suggestions in Week 3 or from the additional ideas on pages 326 to 330. And plan ahead to make sure a snack is handy when hunger strikes.

Change One Fast Track

In a hurry to see more weight come off? Choose one or two of the following Fast Track changes to help to speed your progress.

Early to bed

Surprisingly, insomnia or even regularly falling short on sleep by an hour or two may keep you from reaching your goal. Some researchers suspect that overtired people unwittingly compensate for their lack of energy by eating more.

Being short of sleep can also make people more susceptible to stress, and thus more likely to overeat. Whatever the reason, weight-loss experts recommend trying to get seven or eight hours of sleep every night.

If you've been burning the candle at both ends lately, say goodnight to late nights this week. If you find yourself repeatedly waking up in the night no matter when you go to bed – especially if you're a heavy snorer – talk to your doctor. You could have sleep apnoea, a common problem that can be treated easily. Being overweight is a common risk factor for this condition.

Have some fun

This weekend set aside time to do something enjoyable that also involves moving around. Walking, tennis, gardening, cycling, swimming – anything that takes your fancy, as long as it's active. Make it a family outing, if you like. Invite a friend. Or choose something you want to do just for yourself. Set aside at least an hour for activity.

Open your diary

Keep a food diary, again or for the first time. We've recommended it before, and we're recommending it again for one simple reason: research shows it's the single best way to jumpstart your diet. Now that you're adding dinner to the other *ChangeOne* meals, keeping a record of what you eat will help you to see how far you've come in changing your diet. It's also a great way to spot trouble: certain times of the day when you eat more than you'd like, or situations that trigger hunger cues. You'll find a sample food diary form on page 345.

Chew on this

Buy some packs of sugarless gum and place them everywhere: your kitchen, your desk, your car, your handbag, your briefcase. When you're tempted to reach for a snack, take a piece of gum instead. You may find that the act of chewing relieves your snacking impulses. Also, try chewing a stick of gum while you're cooking meals – there's no way you can sample things with gum in your mouth.

Get moving

Cutting back on kilojoules is the quickest way to start losing weight. But studies show that the best way to keep the weight off is to increase the number of kilojoules you burn by becoming more active. Exercise will also help you to replace fat with muscle, and that will make you look and feel trimmer.

If you aren't as active as you'd like to be, read the section on fitness – which begins on page 234 – and then get moving. This fitness plan offers a simple and easy way to ease yourself into a more active lifestyle that will have a significant impact on your ability to lose weight, and keep it off.

Knowing when
enough is enough

Paying attention to satiety signals is just one more way to make sure that you keep serve sizes under control. And in the end, serve size is really the key to the success of any slimming diet. Some dieters discover that once they learn to stop eating when they're no longer hungry – before they're too full – they automatically eat reasonable serves.

Learning the art of knowing when you're satisfied takes time, though. And it doesn't work for everyone. So practise memorising those serve sizes. The easiest way to get a sense of what several grams of different foods look like is to prepare meals at home as often as you can this week, and to use our suggestions of everyday objects for comparison and to judge serve sizes.

To follow the recipes in *ChangeOne* you won't need anything more exotic than kitchen scales, a measuring jug and standard measuring spoons. Kitchen scales that can be adjusted to zero after you place a bowl or plate on top make it quick and easy to weigh out the correct serve of pasta, for instance. Alternatively, you can divide up a 500 gram packet of pasta into six equal serves. A variety of individual serve-size storage containers will also come in handy. (For more on helpful shopping strategies, take a look at page 340.)

> Vegetables are so low in kilojoules, you can think of them as 'free' foods.

Behind the *ChangeOne* dinner menu

Each of the suggested *ChangeOne* dinner menus contains about 1900 kilojoules (some have a bit more). By following *ChangeOne* breakfast, lunch, snack and dinner recommendations, you'll consume roughly between 5500 and 7000 kilojoules a day – a level, as we said before, that guarantees you'll lose weight at a reasonable, healthy pace.

How can *ChangeOne* dinners be so thrifty with kilojoules? A big reason is that each dinner includes at least two serves of vegetables. Vegetables are so low in kilojoules – 90 grams of cooked spinach contains only 55 kilojoules, for instance,

continued on page 96

Grilled kebabs

What could be more delicious than marinated seafood, meat or tofu threaded onto skewers with colourful vegetables and then grilled to perfection?

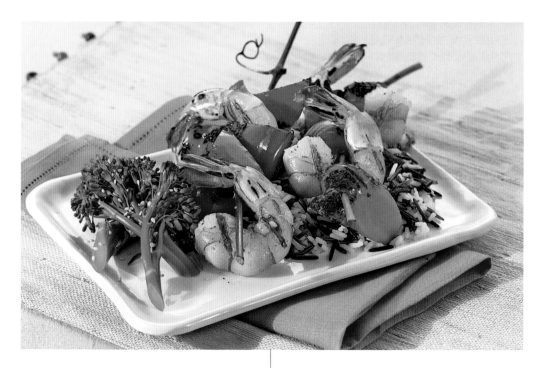

Prawn kebab feast

2 skewers prawn and capsicum kebabs

Sesame broccoli (cupped handful)

Wild and white rice (cricket ball)

1746 kJ, 417 kcal, 35 g protein, 10 g fat (1 g sat fat),
<1 mg cholesterol, 46 g carbohydrate (3 g sugars),
6 g fibre, 616 mg sodium

PRAWN AND CAPSICUM KEBABS

Serves 4
**450 g raw king or tiger prawns,
 marinated for at least 1 hour
1 green and 1 red capsicum, cut into
 2.5 cm squares
2 teaspoons olive oil
8 skewers**

1. Microwave the capsicums for 1 minute or until soft.

2. Thread the prawns and capsicum pieces onto skewers. Brush with olive oil.

3. Grill for 5 to 7 minutes or until the prawns are cooked (turning pink).

Serve bonus (extra food, few extra kilojoules): Add extra capsicums and other vegetables to make 3 or 4 more skewers, and help yourself to an extra one.

WILD AND WHITE RICE

Serves 4
**225 g mixed basmati and wild rice
Pinch of salt**

1. Bring a large saucepan of water to the boil. Add the rice and salt. Bring back to the boil and stir well, then lower the heat so the water is simmering. Cook for about 20 minutes or until the rice is tender.

2. Drain well, then allow to stand for 2 minutes before serving.

SESAME BROCCOLI

Serves 4

350 g broccoli florets
4 tablespoons salt-reduced chicken stock
2 teaspoons sesame oil
1 ½ tablespoons sesame seeds

1. Place a medium-sized non-stick frying pan on medium heat until warm.

2. Add the broccoli and stock, and cook for 7 to 10 minutes or until the florets are just tender. Remove from the heat.

3. Drizzle with the sesame oil and sprinkle with the sesame seeds.

Serve bonus: Add extra broccoli and stock.

Instead of prawns

- Firm-fleshed fish, such as tuna or salmon, 115 g (palm of hand)
- Skinned chicken breast, 115 g, cut into strips (palm of hand)
- Skinned chicken thigh, 85 g, cut into chunks (palm of hand)
- Lean steak, 85 g (palm of hand)
- Lean lamb, 85 g (palm of hand)
- Extra-firm tofu, 85 g (palm of hand)

Instead of capsicums

- Eggplant, in 2.5 cm cubes, sprinkled with salt, rinsed after 15 minutes and sprayed with cooking spray
- Button or open-cap mushrooms
- Cherry tomatoes
- Pickling onions*
- Red onion, in wedges*
- Garlic cloves
- Zucchinis, in 5 mm slices
- Carrots, in 2.5 cm pieces*

* Microwave for a couple of minutes to soften before grilling.

TIPS FOR GRILLING KEBABS

Let your imagination run riot with kebabs. The combinations of seafood, meat, poultry and vegetables are virtually endless. If you're grilling for a crowd, make all-vegetable and all-meat kebabs so it will be easier to time the cooking.

- Brush kebabs with fresh marinade during cooking for more intense flavour (but remember not to use the marinade you soaked them in). If you're using a sweetened marinade, move kebabs away from direct heat to prevent the sugar from burning.
- Turn kebabs over so that both sides cook evenly.
- Cover the ends of wooden skewers with foil to prevent burning, or invest in a set of metal skewers.

ABOUT MARINADES

Marinating imparts great flavour without many kilojoules. It also may fend off the formation of cancer-promoting compounds that form on meat and other animal proteins grilled at high temperatures. It's best to make your own marinades from ingredients such as oil, vinegar, lemon juice, yogurt, herbs and spices. If you buy a ready-made mixture, check that the kilojoule count and fat content are not exorbitant.

- To marinate, place your kebab ingredients in a bowl or resealable plastic bag. Add about 4 tablespoons of your favourite marinade – teriyaki, lemon-pepper, lime-ginger – and mix well. Refrigerate for at least an hour.
- Discard the marinade after removing marinated items.

Speedy stir-fry

There's no cooking method that's faster, healthier or easier than stir-frying.
You'll love blending vegetables with tofu (or with poultry, meat, fish or nuts)
for a fast stir-fry, and then creating sauces in the pan as you go.

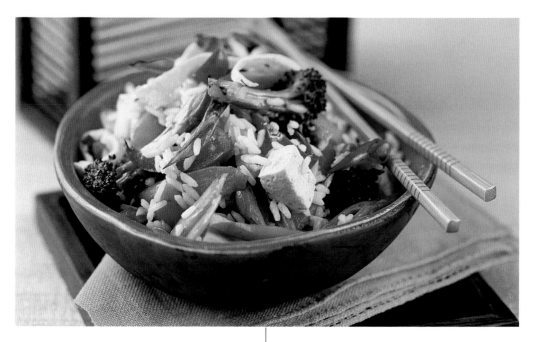

Colourful stir-fry

Fried rice with tofu and vegetables
(3 cricket balls)

1799 kJ, 430 kcal, 20 g protein, 8 g fat (1 g sat fat),
55 mg cholesterol, 58 g carbohydrate (17 g sugars),
3 g fibre, 360 mg sodium

FRIED RICE WITH TOFU AND VEGETABLES

Serves 4

1 cup (250 ml) dry white wine or
  salt-reduced chicken stock
30 ml salt-reduced soy sauce
2 tablespoons clear honey
1 tablespoon peeled and grated
  fresh ginger
350 g extra-firm tofu, diced
1 cup (200 g) long-grain white or
  brown rice
2 cloves garlic, finely chopped
5 spring onions (scallions), cut into
  5 cm pieces

500 g vegetables cut into bite-size pieces,
  such as 200 g broccoli, 100 g snowpeas,
  1 carrot and 1 red capsicum, or 1 packet
  (500 g) frozen mixed Asian vegetables,
  slightly thawed
freshly ground black pepper to taste
1 large egg, lightly beaten

1. Combine the wine or stock, 1 tablespoon
soy sauce, the honey and 1 teaspoon
ginger in a sealable plastic bag. Add the
tofu, push out the excess air, close and
shake gently to coat. Marinate in the fridge
for 1 hour, turning occasionally.

2. Cook the rice according to the packet
directions; keep warm. Lightly coat a wok
or large deep frying pan with non-stick
cooking spray and place over high heat
until hot.

3. Stir-fry the garlic and remaining ginger
until fragrant, about 1 minute. Add the
mixed vegetables, half the spring onions,
the rice, the remaining soy sauce and

pepper. Stir-fry until the mixed vegetables are heated through, about 4 minutes. Push the ingredients to one side of the wok and pour in the egg. Cook until almost set, cutting the egg into strips with a spatula.

4. Pour the marinade into a small saucepan and boil over high heat for 2 minutes. Add the tofu and marinade to the wok. Stir-fry until the tofu is heated through, about 4 minutes. Sprinkle with the remaining spring onions and serve.

Serve bonus: Use more spring onions and mixed vegetables.

Instead of tofu

You can use one of the following in the above recipe for about the same number of kilojoules.
- Salmon fillet, 265 g
- Pork fillet, 280 g
- Skinless chicken breast, 350 g
- Beef fillet, 225 g
- Boneless leg of lamb, 225 g
- Cashews, ½ cup (70 g)

ABOUT WOKS

If you don't have a wok, is it worth getting one? Yes. A wok is perfectly designed for low-kilojoule cooking, using little oil, and cooking vegetables and meat so quickly that they stay tasty and keep their flavour and nutrients. A wok is not just for Asian cooking. Use it anytime you need to sauté something quickly. When shopping for a wok, you'll have a number of choices.

- **Non-stick, flat bottom** Our favourite because it fits on top of any stove and washing-up is easy. However, it doesn't conduct heat as well as a traditional steel wok.

- **Traditional carbon steel** The traditional wok from Chinatown conducts heat extremely well, and the concave design makes it simple to keep the food cooking evenly. However, it requires regular seasoning with oil. A pre-seasoned carbon steel wok is easier to keep clean. For both types, wash and dry thoroughly after each use, then wipe with a little vegetable oil to avoid rust.

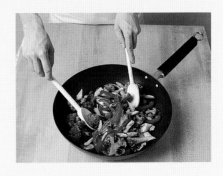

TIPS FOR STIR-FRYING

Most of us associate stir-frying with Chinese cooking, but this low-fat cooking method can be used to create healthy meals with flavours from round the world. Use this dinner menu's Asian-themed stir-fry recipe to create other international delights.

Cuisine	Instead of broccoli, snowpeas	Instead of soy sauce, ginger
Mexican	Assorted capsicums, sweetcorn	Squeeze of lime juice, fresh coriander
Italian	Green beans, tomatoes	1 tablespoon olive oil, fresh basil
Thai	Unchanged	2 tablespoons each lime juice and peanut butter
Greek	Eggplant, assorted capsicums	2 tablespoons each lemon juice and olives

93

Succulent stew

Every culture in the world has a recipe for slow-cooking chunks of meat with lots of vegetables. A traditional beef stew can take pride of place.

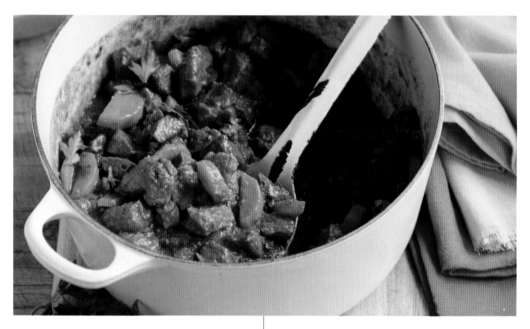

Beef stew dinner

Beef stew (2 cricket balls)

Egg noodles (1 cricket ball)

2050 kJ, 489 kcal, 48 g protein, 14 g fat (5 g sat fat),
120 mg cholesterol, 41 g carbohydrate (4 g sugars),
3 g fibre, 351 mg sodium

BEEF STEW

Serves 8
2 tablespoons vegetable oil
1.5 kg stewing beef, cut into 3 cm cubes
1 large onion, chopped
2 tablespoons plain flour
1½ cups (375 ml) beef stock
1 can chopped tomatoes, about 400 g
2 carrots, halved and sliced
freshly ground black pepper
fresh flat-leaf parsley leaves, to serve

1. Heat half the oil in a large heavy-based saucepan over high heat. Brown the beef in several batches, stirring often, for 3–4 minutes per batch; the meat will at first stick to the pan, until it begins to sear, so add a little more oil between batches if necessary. Set the beef aside.

2. Reduce the heat to medium. Fry the onion in the remaining oil for 5 minutes, or until soft and golden, stirring frequently to prevent burning. Sprinkle over the flour and stir for 30 seconds. Gradually stir in the stock, scraping the base of the pan to stop lumps forming.

3. Stir in the tomatoes and return the beef to the pan. Cover and bring to the boil, then reduce the heat as low as possible, so the liquid is only just simmering. Cook, covered, for 1 hour, stirring occasionally.

4. Add the carrots, cover and cook for 45 minutes, stirring occasionally. Remove the lid and cook, uncovered, for a further 10 minutes, or until the sauce is thickened and reduced slightly – you might need to increase the heat a little to keep the liquid at a simmer. Season with freshly ground black pepper and sprinkle with parsley.

Serve bonus: Increase stock and vegetables.

EGG NOODLES

Serves 4
200 g egg noodles
pinch of salt

1. In a large saucepan, bring 12 cups (3 litres) of water to the boil. Add the noodles and salt and cook according to packet instructions, until al dente.
2. Drain the noodles in a colander, shaking so that all water drains out. Refrigerate any extra.

Instead of egg noodles

If you'd prefer to use pasta made without eggs, here are a few suggestions.
■ Plain noodles, fettuccine or tagliatelle
■ Farfalle (bow-ties)
■ Penne (short, straight quills)
■ Fusilli (spirals)
■ Rigatoni (short, ridged tubes)
■ Rice sticks (flat Chinese noodles)
■ Soba (Japanese buckwheat noodles)
■ Chinese wheat noodles

ABOUT STEWING BEEF

Beef for stewing – chuck, blade, round, brisket and flank – is from flavoursome, less expensive, tougher cuts that become tender when cooked slowly in liquid. All are similar in kilojoules and nutrients. Cooking slowly in moist heat breaks down the tough connective tissue. Generally, the longer the cooking time, the more tender the result. It's best to buy a whole piece of beef and cut it up yourself, discarding any excess fat.

TIPS ON ROOT VEGETABLES

Carrots, parsnips, turnips, onions and potatoes store well and all supply fibre and an assortment of vitamins and minerals. Root vegetables such as these are well suited to stewing, or cut into 2.5 cm chunks and try these other ways of preparing them.
■ **Roast.** Toss with a bit of olive oil and roast in a tin for 30–45 minutes at 230ºC, until soft and caramelised.
■ **Mash.** Boil for 3–5 minutes or until soft. Mash or purée with milk or stock, a pinch of salt, freshly ground black pepper and a small knob of butter.
■ **Simmer.** Place in a pot with enough stock to cover and simmer, covered, about 15 minutes or until the liquid is absorbed and the vegetables are soft.

ABOUT STOCK

Stock is a must-have ingredient for healthy, slimline cooking. It adds lots of flavour and moisture, with very few kilojoules.
■ Home-made stock, made by simmering bones (chicken, beef, veal or fish) or seafood shells with vegetables and herbs in water to cover, has a rich flavour. Bought chilled fresh stock is an alternative, although it is quite expensive and often very salty.
■ The best aromatic vegetables for stock include carrots, onions, leeks, celery and garlic. Avoid cabbage, broccoli and other members of the cabbage family, as they can make stock bitter, and strong-tasting parsnips, swede and brussels sprouts, which tend to dominate.
■ If you don't have time to make stock, or have none in the refrigerator or freezer, you can use stock made from bouillon powder or paste or good-quality stock cubes.

continued from page 89

and 80 grams of cooked sliced carrots just 85 kilojoules – that you can think of them as 'free' foods and help yourself to as much as you want.

One exception is vegetables that are creamed or sautéed in butter or oil. Another is fried vegetables. In these cases check serve sizes. Weight for weight, the fat in butter, cream and oil has more than twice as many kilojoules as either protein or carbohydrates. So even small amounts can drive up the total. A teaspoon of butter (about 5 grams) packs 143 kilojoules; a teaspoon of oil contains 168 kilojoules.

With those numbers in mind, the *ChangeOne* menus on these pages have been chosen in part because they're relatively low in fat. But we've been careful to include some fats, especially the unsaturated kinds that can improve cholesterol levels. Fat adds flavour and enjoyment to food. Diets with a moderate amount of fat offer much more variety and flexibility than strict low-fat diets. As long as you keep serve sizes under control, you can eat any kind of food you enjoy, even if it contains fat.

Remember, new research findings show that when you're trying to lose weight, diets with moderate amounts of fat work the best. Several recent studies have shown that slimmers are more likely to stick to low-joule diets if those diets get 25 per cent to 35 per cent of their kilojoules from fat. Very low-fat diets, in contrast, are so difficult to follow that most people give up and go back to their old ways of eating. Of course, it's wise to eliminate fatty foods that you don't really like or want. It's smart, too, to replace saturated fat with unsaturated fat. You can do this easily by using olive oil instead of butter, for instance, and choosing a reduced-fat mayonnaise. But don't become too preoccupied with fat. Managing serve sizes is a much smarter way to keep kilojoules under control.

Help!

'I often don't get home from work until late – which means I eat dinner just before going to bed. I've heard eating before bedtime causes food to turn straight to fat. Is that true?'

Worry not. As long as you have sensible serves at dinner, what you eat won't magically appear on your thighs tomorrow. Despite what some fad diets tell you, the timing of meals makes virtually no difference to whether the kilojoules are burned up or stored as fat. It's the number of kilojoules in a meal that matters, not what time you eat.

Of course, many people don't like the feeling of going to bed on a full stomach. If you're one of them, try moving your dinner time back an hour. Choose meals that take a little less time to prepare. Do as much advance preparation as you can, either the day before or over the preceding weekend. After you eat, take a walk. Many people find that walking helps them to digest a meal and encourages sounder sleep.

About high-protein and low-GI diets

We've all heard the buzz about high-protein diets. It's easy to see why they've proved so popular. Any diet that invites you to live on steak and eggs is going to attract attention.

But most doctors remain sceptical about high-protein diets. It's not that these regimens don't help people to lose weight. They do. A study conducted by scientists at Arizona State University in the US showed that young women who ate a meal high in protein burned more kilojoules during the next few hours than women who ate a high-carbohydrate, low-fat meal. The reason, researchers surmise, is that protein needs more energy to digest than carbohydrates do. That extra energy consumption showed up in slightly raised body temperatures for the women consuming high-protein meals.

Another study found that volunteers said they felt more satisfied after eating a meal with 29 per cent of its kilojoules from protein than after a meal with only 9 per cent of its kilojoules from protein. They also burned more kilojoules to digest the higher-protein meal. But keep this in mind: you'll burn a lot more kilojoules by taking a 15 minute walk after dinner than you will consuming extra protein.

Many high-protein foods, like meat, are also high in saturated fat, which can be rough on your arteries. More importantly, when you're controlling kilojoules, over-loading your diet with protein raises the risk that you'll come up short on other nutrients, such as the essential vitamins, minerals and fibre in vegetables.

The glycemic index (GI) is a measure-ment of how quickly foods are converted into blood sugar by your digestive system. The approach is simple: Foods that convert quickly into blood sugar (in other words, high-GI foods, primarily dietary sugars and simple carbohydrates) are bad for you; slow-to-digest, low-GI foods are good for you.

There is some validity to this premise as well, and indeed, most high-protein diets are low-GI, since protein is very low-GI

What if I'm losing weight too fast?

It sounds crazy, but it's dangerous to lose weight too quickly. Experts recommend losing no more than 1.4 to 1.5 kilograms a week.

Why? Because losing weight faster than that means you're burning off muscle as well as fat. Losing muscle tissue can lower your basal metabolic rate – the rate at which your body burns fuel – because muscle tissue requires more energy for maintenance than does fat. The less muscle you have, the fewer kilojoules you'll burn, and the harder it is to lose weight.

If you've lost more than 1.4 kilo-grams a week on average – more than 4 kilograms in three weeks – it's time to slow down. Add 850 to 1250 kilojoules to your diet by eating an extra snack or two each day, or increasing serve sizes slightly. And to make sure you don't lose muscle tissue, increase your exercise.

ChangeOne Success Stories

Living a healthy life together

Moderation is the key to a full life for Betsy and John Larimer. Since they decided to decrease serving sizes at the dinner table, they not only feel healthier, they've also dropped a few clothing sizes.

'In our house, we monitor the portions of everything we eat', Betsy says. Shortly after they were married, she gained what she liked to call 'wedding weight', and John was diagnosed with rising blood pressure and high blood cholesterol levels.

'When John's cholesterol skyrocketed, I knew it was time to start eating properly', Betsy says. 'We needed a new way of life, not a temporary diet or a quick fix. We read *ChangeOne* and learned how to make weekly improvements in our eating habits and lifestyles. In just three months, I lost 5.5 kilograms, and John lost almost 8. At first, eating healthy wasn't easy, but as our weight dropped, we were motivated to stick with it.'

To reduce kilojoules, fat and sodium, the couple trimmed their dinner portions in half. 'We found that we didn't need the large quantities of food we were accustomed to eating', says Betsy. 'I began asking our butcher to cut salmon and steak into sensible sizes for us, and at the deli, I ordered reduced-fat cheese and lean luncheon meats sliced thinly.

'We learned to eat slowly, taking time to enjoy our food, and soon we recognised when we felt satisfied as opposed to feeling stuffed. Eventually, John and I could differentiate between being truly

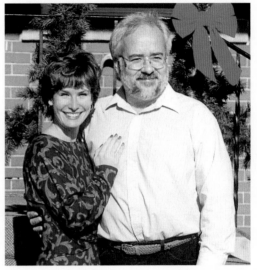

John Larimer lost almost 8 kg in three months on *ChangeOne*. His wife, Betsy, lost 5.5 kg in that time.

hungry and merely craving food as an emotional response.

'We limited our visits to restaurants, knowing that we could prepare healthy food ourselves', Betsy explains. 'Salads became a regular staple. The fibre filled us up, helping to limit our portions at dinner. We also ate nutritious breakfasts, lunches and snacks.

'My husband and I continue to eat well, motivating each other along the way', she confirms. 'Checking in on one another during the day is easy, since I'm an administrative assistant at the same company where John works as an engineer. Eating healthy can be tough at times, but we know that the benefits are immeasurable.'

food. One study showed that people on low-GI diets burned 335 kilojoules more per day that dieters on a low-fat diet. Plus, they reported feeling more energetic and less depressed and hungry. However, the glycemic index of a food can change based on what is being eaten with it.

Bottom line: There is truth in many of the popular weight-loss theories. But why put all your weight-loss hopes in one theory, since your goal is a lifetime of healthy weight – and good health as well. *ChangeOne,* by pairing plenty of protein with good fats and complex carbohydrates, is sensible, easy to track and provides all the protein and low-GI food you need to get the benefits. And there's evidence that this combination of nutrients keeps people feeling so good that they don't want to overeat!

The watchword is moderation. It's still the best advice around. Protein, carbohydrates and fat – you need them all. Tipping your diet too far in one direction or another forces you to cut back on the variety of foods you eat, which makes it harder to stick to a diet.

Goal-setting: it's finally time

Chances are you had in mind the weight you wanted to lose when you started *ChangeOne.* That's great. In fact, this week we want you to put your goal in writing – and sign your name to it.

Now it might seem puzzling that we have waited until the fourth week of the program to get to the topic of goals. But there are two reasons we waited.

The first is that it is impossible to set a reasonable goal when you are just embarking on a new skill. If you never played golf, for example, how can you

continued on page 106

Help!

'I've been putting in lots of time being active, and I haven't seen any results on the scales. What's wrong?'

Nothing. By being as active as you can, you're doing the right thing. The frustrating fact is that it takes a lot of exercise to lose even a small amount of weight. The average weight loss most people can expect from exercise alone is about 150 g a week.

So why bother? Try these three very good reasons.

1. Physical activity does burn kilojoules – and those extra kilojoules will help you to lose weight over time.

2. You'll be much more likely to keep the weight off. Almost all the successful dieters in the American National Weight Control Registry say that a big part of their success comes from exercise. On average they burn an extra 10,500 kilojoules a week doing physical activities.

3. Being physically active has been shown to improve people's mental outlook and boost self-confidence, two changes that can make it much easier to stick to a diet.

Don't stop exercising because you're not losing weight. Stay active and take another look at your diet. Make sure you're not consuming a lot of empty kilojoules in the form of sweetened drinks, including sports drinks and sugary tea and coffee. Readjust serve sizes to make sure yours are still within the *ChangeOne* guidelines.

Pasta perfect

Who doesn't love the taste and texture of spaghetti and noodles? Our advice: skip the ready-made tomato sauce and experiment for fun and flavour.

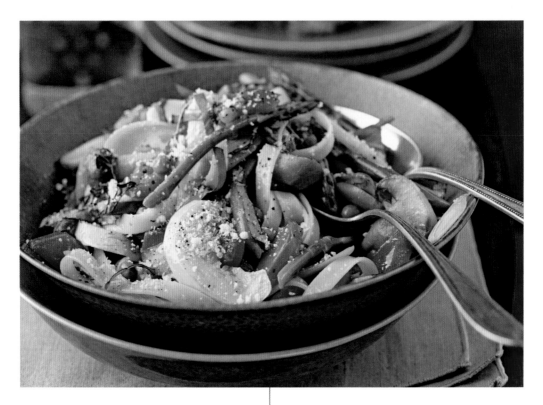

Pasta primavera dinner

Pasta primavera (2 cricket balls)

Italian salad (2 cricket balls)

1873 kJ, 448 kcal, 19 g protein, 20 g fat (3 g sat fat),
5 mg cholesterol, 48 g carbohydrate (8 g sugars),
10 g fibre, 456 mg sodium

PASTA PRIMAVERA

Serves 4

2 tablespoons olive oil
4 roma tomatoes, coarsely chopped
**1 medium carrot, peeled and cut into
  thin slices**
2 cloves garlic, thinly sliced
1 cup (75 g) sliced mushrooms
**¾ cup (185 ml) salt-reduced chicken
  or vegetable stock**
**500 g asparagus, trimmed, blanched
  in boiling water**

1 cup (150 g) frozen peas, thawed
**1 medium yellow zucchini cut into
  1.25 cm-thick slices**
¼ cup finely chopped basil
¼ cup (20 g) grated parmesan
200 g fettuccine

1. Heat oil in a medium non-stick saucepan over medium heat. Add tomato, carrot and garlic. Cook 10 minutes. Add mushroom and stock. Cook 10 minutes. Add asparagus, peas and zucchini. Cook until all the vegetables are tender, about 2 minutes. Add basil and parmesan. Cover; set aside.

2. While sauce is cooking, cook pasta in a large saucepan of lightly salted boiling water until al dente, following packet instructions. Drain. Place in a serving bowl. Add vegetable sauce and toss to combine.

Serve bonus: Increase all vegetables.

ITALIAN SALAD

Serves 4

1 cos lettuce, torn into bite-size pieces
½ cup (70 g) pitted black olives,
chopped
⅔ cup (85 g) red capsicum, diced
⅔ cup (85 g) green capsicum, diced
¼ cup (35 g) pine nuts
½ cup (85 g) canned or boiled chickpeas

1. Mix all the ingredients together in a large salad bowl.
2. Toss with fat-free dressing and serve.

TIPS FOR COOKING PASTA

The biggest challenge in cooking pasta is preventing it from sticking together. Follow this advice for perfect pasta.

- Use a large pan – big enough to hold 12 to 24 cups (3–6 litres) of water for each 225 g of dry pasta.
- Bring the water to a rolling boil before adding the pasta (salting the water is optional but not recommended if you are watching your sodium intake). Adding oil will not prevent sticking.
- Turn up the heat so that the water continues to boil gently after the pasta is added. Stir from time to time.
- Cook until al dente (see packet for suggested time). Reserve ½ cup (125 ml) of the cooking water. Drain pasta in a colander; do not rinse.
- Toss with sauce immediately, or place in a bowl with reserved cooking water and keep covered until ready to serve.

ABOUT PASTA PRIMAVERA

With so many vegetables, pasta primavera can be wonderfully healthy.

- Asparagus, a popular primavera vegetable, is a good source of energy-releasing B vitamins, including folate, which lowers the risk of heart disease and stroke. With calcium and magnesium to maintain strong bones, asparagus is an all-around super food.
- To add more fibre, make this dish with wholemeal or buckwheat pasta.
- Mixing in broccoli, spinach, tomato and other vegetables would add flavour and colour, but few additional kilojoules.
- Enjoy this dish with frozen vegetables when fresh are out of season. Frozen vegetables are just as rich in vitamins and minerals.

Instead of primavera

Although primavera means springtime, this dish is delicious year-round. What makes it so versatile is that you can mix and match ingredients almost any way you like.

Instead of	Try	Why
Fresh asparagus and zucchini	Frozen mixed vegetables	Always in season
Parmesan	Mature pecorino	Sharper flavour
Milk	240 g ricotta cheese Tomato sauce	Creamier Kids may prefer it
Fettuccine	Buckwheat pasta	More fibre
Fresh basil	Dried rosemary or oregano	Heartier, deeper flavour

Parcel cooking

It's not a widely used method, but parcel cooking (or 'en papillotte') is surprisingly easy and delicious. Combine healthy foods and flavourings in a sealed parcel, pop it into the oven or on the barbecue, and then just sit back and wait to enjoy it!

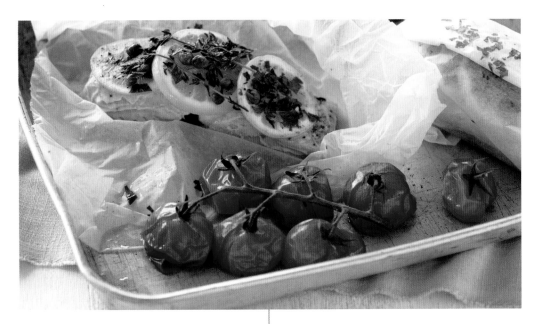

Fish parcels with Spanish rice

1 salmon parcel with tomatoes

Spanish rice (1 cricket ball)

1839 kJ, 439 kcal, 36 g protein, 16 g fat (3 g sat fat),
78 mg cholesterol, 36 g carbohydrate (9 g sugars),
7 g fibre, 294 mg sodium

BAKED SALMON PARCELS

Serves 4
4 x 150 g salmon fillets
12–16 sprigs fresh thyme
2 lemons, cut into thin slices
1 tablespoon capers
4 tablespoons chopped fresh parsley
1 tablespoon olive oil
2 cloves garlic, finely grated
500 g cherry tomatoes on the vine
freshly ground black pepper

1. Preheat the oven to 200°C.

2. Cut a 30 x 30 cm piece of foil for each salmon fillet; place on a clean surface; put a square of baking paper of top. Place the fish in the middle. Top with the thyme sprigs, lemon slices, capers and parsley and drizzle with some of the olive oil. Season with freshly ground black pepper.

3. Carefully wrap each parcel, bringing the edges of the foil to the centre and folding down firmly to secure the top and the sides.

4. Place each fish parcel on a lined baking tray, with the cherry tomatoes alongside. Drizzle the tomatoes with the remaining olive oil and season with pepper. Bake for 20 minutes for medium-cooked fish, or 25 minutes if you prefer it well done. Serve with Spanish rice.

SPANISH RICE

Serves 4

1 medium onion, finely chopped
1 medium green capsicum, finely chopped
1 celery stick, finely chopped
2 garlic cloves, finely chopped
115 g button mushrooms, sliced
125 g long-grain white rice
1 cup (250 ml) tomato juice
1 cup (250 ml) salt-reduced chicken stock
¼ teaspoon black pepper
1 bay leaf
4 roma tomatoes, halved, seeded
  and diced

1. Lightly coat a deep non-stick frying pan with cooking spray. Cook the onion, capsicum, celery and garlic for about 3 minutes or until the onion is almost soft. Stir in the mushrooms and rice, and cook for 2 minutes or until the rice turns golden.

2. Stir in the tomato juice, stock, black pepper and bay leaf. Bring to the boil over medium-high heat. Cover, reduce the heat and simmer, stirring occasionally, for 15 minutes. Stir in the tomatoes.

3. Cover again and cook for a further 10 minutes or until the rice is tender and all liquid is absorbed. Fluff with a fork to separate the rice grains. Discard the bay leaf before serving hot.

Instead of salmon

Ling or trevalla (200 g per serve): Parcel cooking works particularly well for delicate fish that tends to fall apart with other cooking methods. Season with a squeeze of lemon juice, along with salt and pepper.

Snapper fillet (170 g per serve): Try using a drizzle of Asian flavourings such as hoisin sauce or sesame oil.

Prawns (170 g per serve) and scallops (200 g per serve): These shellfish stay moist and succulent with parcel cooking. Flavour with finely chopped garlic and a light drizzle of olive oil.

Chicken breast (170 g per serve): Combine strips of chicken breast with sliced red capsicum and onion, and flavour with a teaspoon of salsa, for a new twist on the popular Mexican wraps called fajitas.

Lean steak (115 g per serve): Stays juicy and flavoursome when sliced into strips and tossed with thinly sliced onion. Season with a little teriyaki sauce.

Tofu (115 g per serve): Cut into 2.5 cm cubes and combine with snowpeas and mushrooms. Marinate first for extra flavour.

TIPS ON COOKING IN PARCELS

Cooking in a parcel retains moisture and flavour and minimises washing-up after cooking.

- Use foil, baking paper or greaseproof paper to hold the food.
- Add little or no liquid, since the parcel retains all the moisture from the food itself.
- Fold over parcel edges well to prevent cooking juices from escaping.
- Cook in the oven or over a charcoal fire. Cooking time will vary with the type of fish or meat and vegetables you are cooking. Root vegetables like carrots take longer than softer vegetables like peas or mushrooms.
- New potatoes are delicious cooked in a parcel. Scrub, then toss with 2 teaspoons olive oil, pepper and rosemary. Wrap in foil or paper parcels and bake or cook on the barbecue until the potatoes are soft. (Cooking time depends on the size of the potatoes.)

Asian noodles

Chinese and Southeast Asian cuisines are as rich in noodle dishes as the cooking of Italy. Brimming with interesting flavours and fresh ingredients, Asian noodle dishes make great one-pot meals at any time of year.

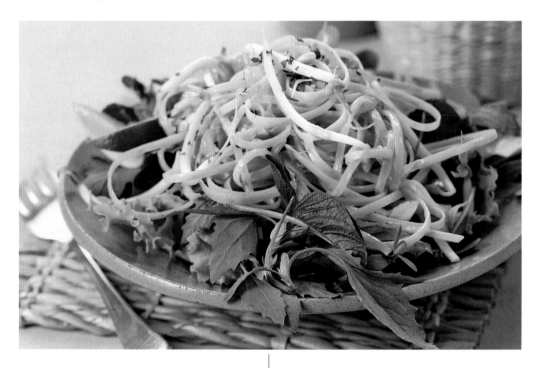

THAI NOODLE SALAD

Serves 4

225 g rice noodles
1 teaspoon peanut oil
2 cloves garlic, finely chopped
1 medium onion, thinly sliced
4 tablespoons salt-reduced vegetable stock
2–3 spring onions (scallions), sliced
1½ cups (160 g) bean sprouts, rinsed
⅓ cup (85 g) crunchy peanut butter
4 tablespoons reduced-fat coconut milk
8 cups mixed salad greens
2 tablespoons (15 g) fresh coriander, chopped
2 limes, juiced
2 tablespoons chopped peanuts

1. Cook the noodles according to packet directions. Reserve ½ cup (125 ml) cooking water. Drain the noodles, then place in a bowl with the reserved cooking water.

2. Heat the oil in a large non-stick frying pan. Cook the garlic for about 30 seconds. Add the onions and stock and cook for 5 minutes or until the onions are tender. Add to the noodles.

3. Add the spring onions and bean sprouts to the noodles and toss gently to mix.

4. Stir together the peanut butter and coconut milk. Add to noodle mixture. Toss to coat. Before serving, divide into four equal serves (cricket ball) and refrigerate extra.

5. Place an equal serve of salad greens on each plate. Top each bed of greens with the noodle mixture and garnish with chopped coriander, lime juice and chopped peanuts.

1874 kJ, 448 kcal, 12 g protein, 18 g fat (5 g sat fat), 0 mg cholesterol, 60 g carbohydrate (8 g sugars), 8 g fibre, 450 mg sodium

Instead of bean sprouts

If you prefer not to use mung bean sprouts, try one or more of these fresh Asian vegetables (cut into shreds, except for watercress, and fry or microwave briefly, just until the colour brightens). Alternatively, you can use canned water chestnuts or bamboo shoots.

Try	Features
Bok choy	Thick, light green stalks, dark green leaves, mild cabbage flavour
Gai choy (Chinese mustard greens)	Small leaves, zesty flavour (older, larger leaves are more pungent)
Wong bok (Chinese cabbage)	Light green leaves, lacy veins, delicate cabbage flavour
Watercress	Small leaves, crisp stalks, sharp and refreshing taste
Snake beans	Extremely long; resemble and taste like green beans

ABOUT NUTS AND NUT BUTTERS

If you've been avoiding nuts, give them another look. A growing number of experts recommend nuts as part of a healthy diet. The main form of fat in nuts – monounsaturated – has been linked to lower blood cholesterol levels. Like meats, nuts supply protein along with fibre, something not found in meats. Here's the catch: weight for weight, nuts have more than three times the kilojoules of meat, so use them wisely. Here's what you get from some favourites:

Type	kJ per 2 tablespoons (2 thumbs)
Almonds	135
Cashews	395
Peanuts	405
Crunchy peanut butter	785
Cashew butter	790
Smooth peanut butter	800
Almond butter	855

TIPS FOR ASIAN SEASONINGS

Countries that share a continent don't necessarily share a cooking style, as you see in Asia. Each country uses its own unique combination of sauces and seasonings. Our recipe features the classic flavours of Thailand: coconut, peanut, coriander and lime. To travel through the other cuisines of Asia, experiment with different flavours.

China: soy sauce, five-spice powder, hoisin sauce, oyster sauce, garlic.

Japan: soy sauce, rice wine, sugar, fish stock, ginger.

Korea: soy sauce, sesame oil, garlic, chillies, fermented soya paste.

Vietnam: fish sauce, lemon grass, coriander, garlic, shrimp paste.

Indonesia: ginger, tamarind, sweet soy sauce, coconut, lemon grass.

The Philippines: coconut milk, garlic, ginger, vinegar, fermented shrimp paste.

continued from page 99

predict how good a golfer you can be in 12 weeks? You need to learn some of the skills and practise them before assessing that. Only then will you be able to determine a reasonable path to success.

The same is true for *ChangeOne*. These first four weeks you have been learning new skills and practising them every day. We assume you have been losing weight and also reaping other personal rewards. Now that you know your weight-loss strengths and weaknesses, isn't it a smarter time to set a realistic goal?

The second reason for the delay is that goal-setting is serious business. Rightly or wrongly, your performance against your goals defines success for you, motivates you and, too often, lets you down. Goal-setting is so important, in fact, you'll discover that we devote a whole week to it a month from now. But until then it's time for some basics.

Take that initial weight-loss goal you set yourself and think about it for a few minutes. Ask yourself three questions:

1. Is my goal a reasonable one, something I can realistically achieve based on the progress I'm making so far?
2. How long is it likely to take to reach my goal?
3. What weight would I be satisfied with if I can't quite hit my ideal goal?

After you've given these weighty questions some thought, set out your goals for the coming months. We recommend your having a goal in mind for the end of the 12-week program, about two months from now. If that's not *your* ultimate goal, set another target on a longer time frame.

Think TRIM

As you think about workable goals for the coming two months and beyond, keep in mind the acronym TRIM. It stands for:

Time-bound. An effective goal should have a deadline – a time by which you expect to reach it. Choose a date two months from now, when you will have completed the 12 weeks of the *ChangeOne* program. Select a specific date and mark it on the calendar.

Realistic. We've said it before, but it's worth repeating: if you set a goal you can't reach, there's no point in setting it. Choose a target that you're pretty sure you can hit. Odds are you won't go from a size 18 to a size 10 in the next few months. But you could get to a size 16, or maybe even 14.

Inspiring. Your goal should be something that really matters to you – attainable, but ambitious enough to excite you. Maybe you don't really care all that much about kilos on the scales, for instance; what you're concerned about is getting into shape so that you can keep up with the kids on bushwalks and bike rides.

Measurable. A worthwhile goal has to be measurable. If it isn't, obviously, you'll never know when you've reached it. The first step is to make it as specific as possible. The next is to describe exactly how you plan to measure your progress. Here are a few examples.

Instead of	Make your goal to:
Lose as much weight as I can before summer begins	Drop 4.5 kg over the next two months
Be better about my diet	Follow *ChangeOne* at least six days out of seven each week
Get back into shape	Jog for 45 minutes at least three times a week in preparation for a 10 kilometre charity run
Try to be more active	Walk at least 30 minutes five days a week over the next two months
Eat fewer desserts	Treat myself to just one dessert a week over the coming month
Feel less embarrassed by the way I look	Lose 4.5 kg and join an aerobics class within two months

In addition to kilos on the scales, give yourself at least two other goals. Dropping several dress sizes, for example. Or fitting into a pair of jeans you wore two summers ago.

It's not all about the scales

Why have another goal in addition to kilos on the scales? Because while weight is the measure that most people use, it's not necessarily the best one. Who really cares what the bathroom scales say? What most people really want is to look better. And the scales can lie.

For example, let's say you're doing a great job on your slimming diet, dropping kilojoules and burning fat. At the same time, you've become so keen on exercise that you've started going to the gym. You're tightening up flabby muscles and even adding some strength. You look great! You feel terrific!

But when you step up on the scales, you find your weight has barely moved. Why? Because you're replacing fat with muscle, which actually weighs more than fat, volume for volume. You're changing your body composition for the better. The reflection in the mirror shows it. Maybe you've dropped a waist size or two as well. You feel stronger and fitter. But if you have no other gauge than kilos on the scales, you'll be disappointed.

Once you've settled on realistic and measurable goals, fill out the *ChangeOne* contract on page 342. Why a contract? Because while it's one thing to decide on a set of goals, it's another to really commit to them. Make a deal with yourself in writing. The form even includes a place for you to sign. For extra motivation, get a witness to sign it, too.

Silly? You may be surprised. There's something powerful about putting your signature on any agreement, even one you make with yourself. Before you sign it, make sure the goals you've set for yourself pass the TRIM test. Check again to be sure they're goals you are willing and able to work towards over the next few months.

What's your healthy weight?

One target worth keeping in mind is your healthy weight. Since height and weight are related, experts don't rely on weight alone. Instead they use a formula called body mass index (BMI). On page 343 you'll find information on how to calculate your current BMI and the weight you'll need to lose to reach a healthy BMI.

Because individual body types differ, the official BMI chart offers a recommended range, not a single magic number. Having your healthy weight in mind can often serve as a great motivator.

But keep your perspective. If you're overweight, losing just a little will make you healthier. Studies show that people who lose 5 per cent of their body weight significantly improve their blood pressure and cholesterol levels, thereby reducing the strain on their heart and arteries. They also lower their risk of diabetes. The closer you get to your recommended BMI, the healthier you'll be.

Changes ahead: eating out

More and more of our meals are eaten away from home – in restaurants, pubs and fast-food outlets. The only problem with eating out these days is that the food often comes in large serves that are loaded with fat and kilojoules. This week, while you focus on dinner, make a list of a couple of restaurants you'd like to try. Next week we're going to invite you to go out to practise a few simple strategies to cut those serves down to size.

More dinner choices

Can't find something you like from among the dinners suggested in this chapter?
Starting on page 318, you'll find more quick and delicious *ChangeOne* dinner ideas.

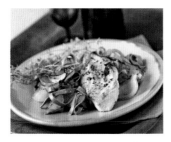

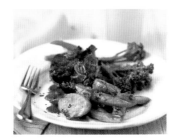

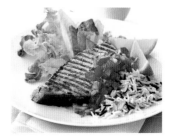

Chicken and caramelised onion stir-fry
page 319

Wine-braised beef
page 320

Barbecued fish with salsa
page 322

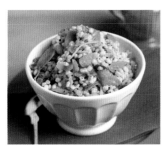

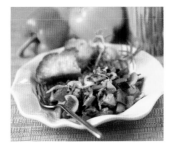

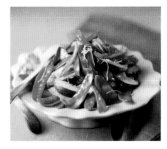

Barley pilaf with herbs
page 324

Summer ratatouille
page 324

Snowpeas and apples with ginger
page 325

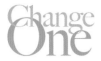

WEEK 5

Eating out

Even though you're watching what you eat, that's no reason to deny yourself the pleasure of eating out. Certainly, the serving sizes may be large, and in many restaurants the notion of a sauce is one loaded with butter and cream. But if you approach eating out with common sense and confidence, you can order what you want, and exactly how much you want, while sticking with your plan.

This week, eat out at least twice. Order exactly what you want, and don't take no for an answer!

Who knows? You might find it great fun getting the waiter and chef to serve you a more personalised meal. If you don't, just forget the experience and move on. There's no need to feel inhibited – you are the customer, paying to get what you want. So enjoy it, take your time and savour the flavours – as you'd like them.

A *ChangeOne* dinner date

Eating out has become one of the great national pastimes. In Australia and New Zealand, one in four meals is currently eaten outside the home, and this appears to be a rising trend. And never before have we had so many tempting choices, from Thai, Chinese, Japanese and Vietnamese to Indian, Italian, Greek, Lebanese and contemporary Australian and New Zealand cuisine – to name just a few!

But there is a downside to eating out. Restaurant food typically contains 22 per cent more fat than food consumed at home, say experts. And serve sizes have spiralled out of control, particularly at fast-food places. Serve 'creep' has happened so gradually that most people don't realise exactly how big their meals have become.

An American organisation called the Center for Science in the Public Interest (CSPI) began conducting clever sting operations several years ago. The group studied meals from restaurants just like those many of us eat in regularly.

Eating out serves

These meal plans use both standard measurements and the *ChangeOne* serve-size guide. In this chapter, we've focused on dinner. It's the meal people typically eat out, and it often delivers the biggest serves. When you're going out for breakfast or lunch, you can review the serve sizes in the preceding chapters. For a complete dinner meal (1900 kilojoules), choose one of each type of food, in the serve suggested:

Type of food	Example	Amount	*ChangeOne* serve
Starch or grain	Rice, pasta, noodles	⅔–1 cup (140 g)	Tennis ball
	Bread roll	Medium	Tennis ball
Protein	Prawns, scallops, crab	115 g	Cricket ball
	Chicken, turkey	85–115 g	Surface of palm
	Beef, veal	85 g	
	White fish	170 g	Chequebook
	Oily fish: salmon	85 g	
Vegetables	Green beans, with oil or butter	½ cup (65 g)	2 golf balls
	Peas, with butter	½ cup (80 g)	2 golf balls
	Steamed or raw	Unlimited	

One study found that, in some cases, an individual restaurant main course exceeded the kilojoules you should eat in a whole day.

In one operation, CSPI sampled almost two dozen Chinese restaurants. In another, its investigators ordered from the menus of a variety of Italian restaurants.

What they found made headlines in the USA. Serve sizes and fat content at many American restaurants have become so bloated that many meals are health hazards. In some cases, CSPI found, a single main dish exceeded what many of us should eat in a whole day. At some Chinese restaurants, for instance, an order of kung pao chicken (a spicy Szechuan dish) had 5880 kilojoules. Looking at Italian food, researchers discovered that spaghetti with meatballs at some restaurants came in at almost 4200 kilojoules. Pasta in a cream and cheese sauce soared to almost 7560 kilojoules in a single serving. Even half of one of these dishes puts you over your *ChangeOne* dinner target. And if you were to eat a couple of pieces of bread spread with butter, or dipped into olive oil, you could add 1470 or more kilojoules to the total.

If you eat out a lot – and many of us have about four meals a week in restaurants, pubs or fast-food outlets – numbers like those can be discouraging. But even though the chef rules the kitchen, remember that you rule the table. You're the customer, after all. You choose what to eat and how much of it you want. You decide how quickly or how slowly to enjoy a meal. You say when you've had enough. In some restaurants, you can even give the chef specific instructions as to how you want your meal prepared.

Many of the strategies you'll use to take charge in restaurants are those that you've already been practising: planning ahead. Monitoring hunger and fullness signals. Keeping an eye on serve sizes. This week, keep them in mind when you take yourself out to eat. They'll help you sit down to a *ChangeOne* meal you'll enjoy without regrets.

Do your menu homework

If you're considering a restaurant you've never tried before, stop by and look over the menu before you go in to make sure you'll be able to order the meal you want. Most establishments display their menus outside. Some even post them online. You won't be able to learn much about serve sizes, of course, but at least you'll know whether the menu includes some possible options. You could even pick the safest choices before you go in. That way you won't have to look at the menu and be tempted by fillet steak smothered in hollandaise sauce or tarts made with butter puff pastry.

If you eat out frequently, keep your own personal list of diet-friendly places in your area – restaurants where you know you'll be able to get a great-tasting, low-kilojoule meal.

Clearly, there are some kinds of restaurants you should avoid altogether – unless you have an iron will. Buffet-style restaurants, carveries, 'all you can eat' places, even sprawling salad bars pose a hazard. Salad bars sound healthy enough, but many of them are stocked with high-kilojoule dishes such as pasta salads with creamy dressings. Better to order a simple green salad with the dressing served separately. What about fish and chip shops? Most of what's on the menu there is so high in kilojoules and fat that you'll bust your kilojoule budget before you satisfy your hunger. Fast-food restaurants? Unless you're willing to eat half a burger or chicken sandwich and wash it down with a diet drink, you'll have a tough time finding one that doesn't overdo the kilojoules.

And remember, you're aiming to have at least two servings of vegetables. With your takeaway hamburger you'll be lucky to get a piece of lettuce and thin slice of tomato.

But don't worry. There are still plenty of places where you can sit down to a good meal, as you'll discover as you look through this week's suggestions.

Check-in

What meal do you typically eat out? Breakfast? Lunch? Dinner? All of the above? If you eat out a lot, take a fresh look at the serve sizes in the first four weeks of *ChangeOne* so that when that plate of pasta or a burger lands in front of you, you'll know just how much to eat and how much to leave or take home for later. Many dieters find that keeping a visual equivalent size in mind – a chequebook or a tennis ball, for example – helps prevent serve creep. If you only treat yourself to a restaurant meal once or twice a month, definitely use the tips in this chapter to guide you when you open the menu. But enjoy yourself, too. Have that steak or chop. If dinners out are an occasional treat, you don't have to worry. Still, pay attention to how full you feel. When you're satisfied, put your cutlery down and savour the feeling of being in control of your eating.

Italian

Antipasto, pasta and main dish with dessert is a standard meal in many Italian restaurants. Can you fit it into *ChangeOne*? Yes, as long as you pay attention to courses, serves and include lots of vegetables. Check out our sample meals below.

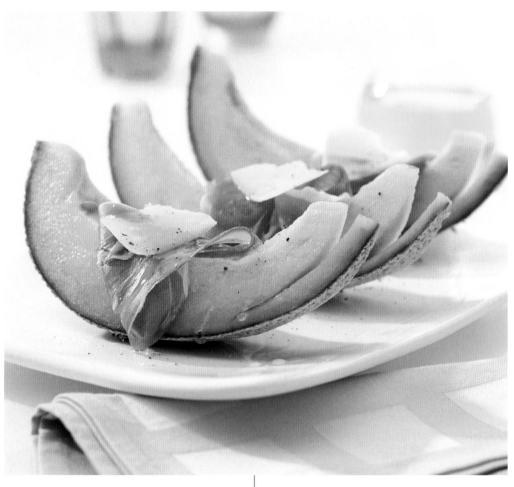

Menu 1

Melon with prosciutto ham
   (*pictured above*)

Pasta arrabbiata (spicy tomato sauce)
   with 1 tbsp grated parmesan

Large mixed salad

2 fresh figs

Approximate serve info (based on *ChangeOne* sizes):
2587 kJ, 618 kcal, 26 g protein, 21 g fat (6 g sat fat),
6 mg cholesterol, 83 g carbohydrate (41 g sugars),
13 g fibre, 1379 mg sodium

Menu 2

Tomato bruschetta

Small serve of spaghetti with seafood

Fruit-based (non-fat) gelato

Approximate serving info (based on *ChangeOne* sizes):
1960 kJ, 468 kcal, 27 g protein, 13 g fat (3 g sat fat),
112 mg cholesterol, 60 g carbohydrate (25 g sugars),
7 g fibre, 787 mg sodium

Choosing your meal

Soups

Italian soups are hearty, almost filling enough to be a meal in a bowl if paired with a slice of crusty Italian bread and a green salad. Minestrone – a tomato-based soup with vegetables, beans and pasta – is the best known. Pasta e fagioli features a fibre-rich combination of beans (fagioli) and pasta in a savoury broth. Top either with a sprinkle of parmesan for richer flavour.

Starters

Often listed as 'antipasto' on the menu, starters run the gamut from marinated seafood salad to deep-fried mozzarella. Choose fresh seafood, steamed or boiled, or a virtually kilojoule-free fresh vegetable salad. If you're wondering how some of your current favourites stack up, here are some typical serves, ranked from best to worst in terms of kilojoules and nutrition:

Olives (5 stuffed olives)	105 kJ/3 g fat
1 bread stick	105 kJ/0.5 g fat
Melon and prosciutto ham	630 kJ/5 g fat
Garlic bread (small piece)	840 kJ/10 g fat
Fried squid (starter size)	1260 kJ/12 g fat

Main dishes

Serves in many Italian restaurants are big enough to feed at least two. Limit your pasta serve to about a tennis ball. Salad niçoise is a good choice, but ask for the dressing to be served on the side. If you opt for pasta, choose a tomato-based sauce. Other good main courses include chicken cacciatore, seafood or grilled calves' liver. Resist the temptation of cream- or cheese-based dishes such as spaghetti carbonara. Here's a sample of Italian main courses and desserts with their nutritional values:

Spaghetti carbonara	2520 kJ/42 g fat
Spaghetti with pesto	1910 kJ/13 g fat
Spaghetti with tomato sauce	1260 kJ/6 g fat
Large mixed salad	210 kJ/3 g fat (1 tablespoon oil)
Tiramisu	2100 kJ/30 g fat
Zabaglione	840 kJ/11 g fat
Granita	420 kJ/0 g fat
1 fresh fig	70 kJ/0 g fat

HEALTH IMPOSTERS

- Pasta primavera: many restaurants make this pasta and vegetable dish with lots of cream.
- Eggplant parmigiana: crumbed and fried eggplant soaks up the oil.
- Stuffed mushrooms: the stuffing is usually a mixture of cheese, fatty sausage and plenty of cream.
- Antipasto: mostly meat and fatty salami slices.

ORDERING FOR A FAMILY OF FOUR

- One large salad, dressing served separately
- One starter
- Two pasta dishes
- Two non-pasta main dishes
- Two vegetable side dishes

DON'T FORGET

- Parmesan: just 1 tablespoon adds an extra 295 kilojoules and 5 g fat, but with its strong flavour, a little goes a long way.
- Desserts: many, like tiramisu and zabaglione, are heavily laden with fat and sugar.

Chinese

Although the traditional Chinese diet is considered to be one of the healthiest in the world, many of the dishes that appear on restaurant and takeaway menus are deep-fried, which makes them very high in kilojoules and fat. Because it can be hard to resist temptations like spring rolls, take the agony out of ordering by choosing one of the typical Chinese meals below.

Menu 1

Hot-and-sour soup

Prawns stir-fried with ginger and spring onions (scallions)

Small serve plain boiled rice

Fresh pineapple

Approximate serve info (based on *ChangeOne* sizes): 1579 kJ, 377 kcal, 18 g protein, 5 g fat (1 g sat fat), 103 mg cholesterol, 64 g carbohydrate (8 g sugars), 3 g fibre, 1238 mg sodium

Menu 2

Chinese chicken noodle soup
  (*pictured below*)

Stir-fried beef or chicken with oyster sauce

Fresh lychees

Approximate serve info (based on *ChangeOne* sizes): 2735 kJ, 653 kcal, 54 g protein, 22 g fat (5 g sat fat), 117 mg cholesterol, 63 g carbohydrate (17 g sugars), 8 g fibre, 1091 mg sodium

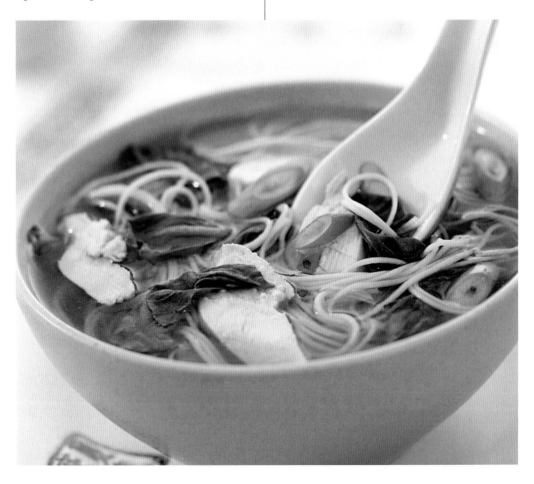

Choosing your meal

Starters

There's no need to say no to starters but it pays to choose carefully. Avoid deep-fried dishes such as spring rolls, wontons, deep-fried dumplings and prawn crackers. Soups such as wonton or eggflower are a terrific choice – they fill you up without an overabundance of kilojoules. Steamed dumplings (dim sum) are another excellent selection.

Chicken noodle soup	175 kJ/1 g fat
Sesame prawn toasts	295 kJ/6 g fat each
Spring roll	525 kJ/9 g fat
Prawn crackers (bowl)	1615 kJ/27 g fat

Main and side dishes

Most Chinese restaurants offer a good selection of healthy low-fat main courses. Stir-fried vegetables are probably the safest option – with chicken, beef, tofu, pork or seafood. An average serving of sweet-and-sour chicken can contain the equivalent of 8 teaspoons of sugar – so is best avoided – as is anything that is covered with batter or contains nuts. Opt for a small serve of plain boiled rice rather than special egg fried rice and boiled rather than fried noodles.

Sweet-and-sour pork (battered)	3000 kJ/42 g fat
Sweet-and-sour chicken	2455 kJ/30 g fat
Chicken chow mein	2165 kJ/25 g fat
Stir-fried beef with capsicums and black bean sauce	1575 kJ/20 g fat
Stir-fried vegetables	775 kJ/14 g fat
Egg fried rice	2310 kJ/15 g fat
Plain boiled rice	1040 kJ/2 g fat
Szechuan prawns with vegetables	1300 kJ/16 g fat
Chicken chop suey	1635 kJ/21 g fat
Chicken with cashew nuts	2225 kJ/35 g fat

TIPS FOR ORDERING

- Order a one-pot soup. The serve is generous, with lots of soup broth to fill you up.
- Order a side dish of steamed vegetables to mix in with a saucy main course. The extra vegetables add fibre and other nutrients and also make your serve look more generous.
- Order dumplings steamed rather than pan-fried. They taste just as good and have fewer kilojoules.

HEALTH IMPOSTERS

- Lemon chicken: chopped chicken with the skin on. The skin is high in fat and too fiddly to bother removing.
- Anything with cashews: nuts are great, but not with the extra fats and kilojoules they pick up when they are caramelised (sugared and often fried), as happens in many Chinese restaurants.
- Fruit fritters: these are not only deep-fried but often coated in caramel as well.

Bistro and pub food

Most good modern restaurants and pubs should have a selection of dishes suitable for the *ChangeOne* diet – simply cooked fish or poultry with vegetables is always a good choice. If you're not sure from reading the menu exactly what a dish is or how it is cooked, ask the waiter or waitress, and don't forget you can always request that a dish be served without the sauce or dressing.

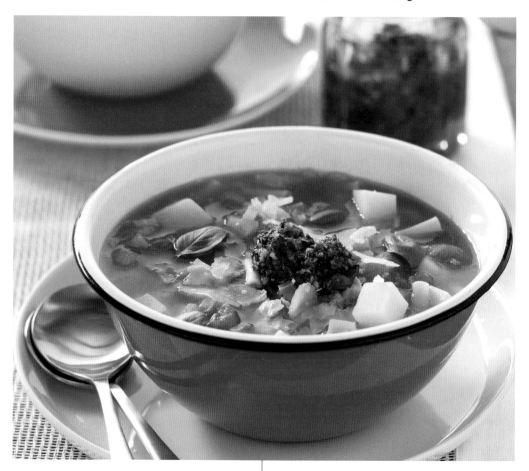

Menu 1

Vegetable soup, with pesto (optional)
  (*pictured above*)

Grilled tuna or chicken with
  mango salsa

Steamed broccoli

Fresh fruit salad

Approximate serve info (based on *ChangeOne* sizes):
2187 kJ, 522 kcal, 52 g protein, 18 g fat (6 g sat fat),
72 mg cholesterol, 38 g carbohydrate (22 g sugars),
10 g fibre, 168 mg sodium

Menu 2

Steamed mussels

Salmon fishcakes

Large mixed salad

Fresh berries

Approximate serve info (based on *ChangeOne* sizes):
2100 kJ, 502 kcal, 36 g protein, 15 g fat (5 g sat fat),
20 mg cholesterol, 60 g carbohydrate (11 g sugars),
2 g fibre, 1200 mg sodium

Choosing your meal

Starters

Seafood starters are a popular offering in many restaurants. As long as the seafood isn't fried or swimming in butter or olive oil, it's hard to go wrong with prawns or steamed mussels. Avoid high-fat starters like avocado and pâté. Choose melon, soup, salad, shellfish or smoked salmon, and skip the accompanying bread and butter. A leafy salad is always an option – try topping it with prawns and dressing with a tomato vinaigrette.

Vegetable soup	315 kJ/1.5 g fat
Smoked salmon	355 kJ/3 g fat
Melon	105 kJ/1 g fat
Marinated prawns	420 kJ/2 g fat
Asparagus with prosciutto	125 kJ/3 g fat

Main dishes

Chargrilling is a diet-friendly cooking technique which disposes of some fat as the food cooks and imparts delicious smoky overtones. But stay alert: the standard fillet or rump steak may be two or more full *ChangeOne* serves, and that's not counting the potatoes with it. Keep in mind that just one tablespoon (20 g) of melted butter has more than half the kilojoules of the main dishes below. Avoid creamy sauces, pastry and anything fried. Vegetarian options may not be lower in kilojoules – so watch out for dishes that contain cheese or nuts.

Salmon steak	960 kJ/15 g fat
Tuna steak	670 kJ/6 g fat
Grilled chicken breast	840 kJ/10 g fat
Medium jacket potato	670 kJ/6 g fat
Mashed potato	525 kJ/2 g fat (120 g serving)
Summer pudding	630 kJ/1.5 g fat
Lemon sorbet	335 kJ/0 g fat (1 scoop)
Fresh strawberries	210 kJ/0 g fat (1 bowl)
Fresh fruit salad	335 kJ/0 g fat
Ice-cream	505 kJ/6 g fat (1 scoop)

Love it or skip it?

Love it	Why?
Blackened	Rubbed with black pepper, paprika and other spices and chargrilled
Steamed	Cooked without fat in a steamer
Reduction	Sauce made by boiling down stock, wine or balsamic vinegar
Brochette	Meat, fish, poultry or vegetables on a skewer
Skip it	**Why?**
Béarnaise	Sauce made with butter and egg yolks
Beurre blanc	Light-coloured butter sauce
Chateaubriand	Large serve of beef fillet, usually for two
Dijonnaise	Dijon mustard and cream sauce

HEALTH IMPOSTERS

- Avocado: especially if served with a high-fat dressing.
- Fruit crumbles: mostly low on fruit and high on kilojoule-rich topping.

Indian

Traditionally, Indian food is quite healthy and balanced, with plenty of complex carbohydrate and vegetables, but many Western restaurants cater for Western palates. At around 2940 kilojoules and 40 g fat per serving, dishes like chicken korma, lamb rogan josh or anything with nuts or a creamy sauce should be given a wide berth by dieters. But if you choose wisely, healthy options are available.

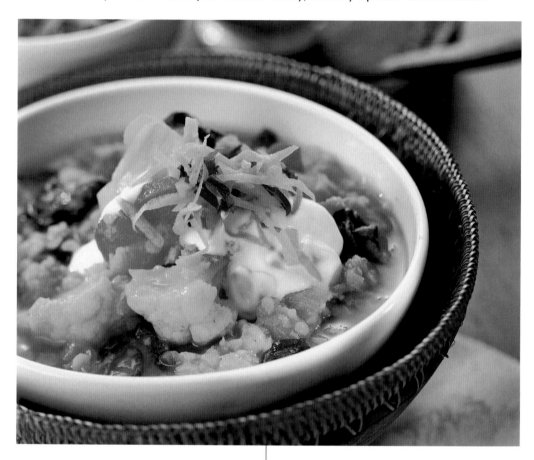

Menu 1

Chicken tikka

Vegetable curry

Raita

Plain boiled rice or 1 chapati

Fresh mango

Approximate serve info (based on *ChangeOne* sizes):
2099 kJ, 501 kcal, 21 g protein, 20 g fat (5 g sat fat),
52 mg cholesterol, 60 g carbohydrate (14 g sugars),
4 g fibre, 277 mg sodium

Menu 2

Vegetable samosa with salad
  (half a samosa)

Tandoori king prawns

Spicy lentil dhal, with chutney and
  raita (optional) (*pictured above*)

Fresh fruit salad

Approximate serve info (based on *ChangeOne* sizes):
1708 kJ, 408 kcal, 30 g protein, 6 g fat (3 g sat fat),
60 mg cholesterol, 62 g carbohydrate (23 g sugars),
18 g fibre, 483 mg sodium

Choosing your meal

Starters

Tandoori chicken or prawns are the best choice. If you can't resist a bahji or samosa, ask for a half serve or split a starter with your dinner guest. Avoid pappadams unless you're assured that they have been baked, not fried. They can add up to a whopping 840 kilojoules each before you even start your meal.

Tandoori chicken	1090 kJ/8 g fat (starter size)
Samosa	1990 kJ/45 g fat
Onion bhaji	1490 kJ/24 g fat

Main course

Chicken dopiaza, jalfrezi, tikka or sag are all good choices. Vegetable, fish or shellfish-based curries and dishes like matar (or mutter), paneer (peas with cheese) and sag aloo (spinach and potato curry) are relatively low in kilojoules and saturated fat as well. Balti-style curries are fairly low in fat and provide useful amounts of iron, absorbed from their cooking pots. Peshwari naan, paratha and pilau rice are made and/or cooked using lots of ghee (clarified butter), so choose chapatis and plain boiled rice instead. Cucumber raita, made with yogurt, is the best choice of accompaniment.

Lamb biryani	3780 kJ/20 g fat
Chicken korma	3360 kJ/40 g fat
Chicken dhansak	3150 kJ/41 g fat
Prawn biryani	2520 kJ/15 g fat
Prawn balti	1890 kJ/21 g fat
Tandoori chicken	1470 kJ/10 g fat
Chapati	825 kJ/8 g fat
Plain boiled rice	1040 kJ/2 g fat
Pilau rice	1640 kJ/10 g fat

Dessert

After a hot, spicy meal, there's nothing quite like a fresh fruit salad to cool you down. Many Indian restaurants also offer platters of fresh orange or melon slices following a meal.

Family restaurants

Restaurants and fast-food outlets that cater for families with children are a godsend for busy parents, but it can be difficult to know what to choose when almost everything seems to fall outside the *ChangeOne* guidelines. But with our menu choices, you can relax and enjoy yourself.

Menu 1

Garlic mushrooms

Grilled ham with pineapple

Jacket potato

Peas

Fresh fruit salad

Approximate serve info (based on *ChangeOne* sizes):
1859 kJ, 444 kcal, 24 g protein, 10 g fat (2 g sat fat),
17 mg cholesterol, 66 g carbohydrate (32 g sugars),
20 g fibre, 450 mg sodium

Menu 2

Tomato soup

Large mixed salad with
   low-fat dressing

Grilled chicken with herb sauce
   (*pictured below*)

Potato wedges

1 scoop ice-cream with
   fresh strawberries

Approximate serve info (based on *ChangeOne* sizes):
2364 kJ, 565 kcal, 55 g protein, 21 g fat (7 g sat fat),
158 mg cholesterol, 40 g carbohydrate (22 g sugars),
8 g fibre, 892 mg sodium

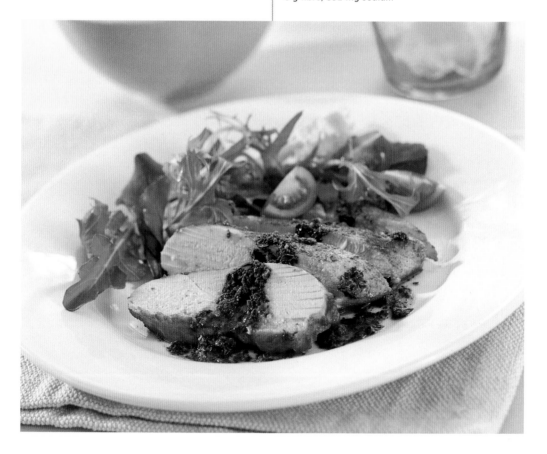

Choosing your meal

If you choose a burger, go for a small one and skip the cheese and bacon – you'll save greatly on kilojoules and fat. Don't think that by ordering a salad you're taking the healthy option – a Hungry Jack's Tendergrill Chicken Salad (with dressing) has 7.5 grams of fat more than a Hungry Jack's Cheeseburger, and a McDonald's Classic Salad with Crispy Chicken has 2 grams more fat and about the same kilojoules as a McDonald's Filet-O-Fish. Your healthiest option is to order your salad without dressing.

In family restaurants grilled chicken, fish or lean meat, such as pork, is always a safe choice. Avoid anything that is fried or coated with breadcrumbs or batter. Potato wedges are a good alternative to chips – a jacket potato is an even better option, as long as you don't smother it with butter or sour cream. Ask for it to be served plain, with a serve of grated cheese on the side, so that you can decide how much to add. Look at the chart below to help you work out your best choices.

HJ Cheeseburger	1359 kJ/14.3 g fat
McDonald's Cheeseburger	1180 kJ/12.4 g fat
HJ Whopper®	2889 kJ/40.7 g fat
Big Mac™	2060 kJ/26.9 g fat
HJ Bacon Deluxe™	2363 kJ/35.2 g fat
McDonald's Quarter Pounder	2280 kJ/30.2 g fat
HJ Tendergrill® Chicken Salad (with ranch dressing)	1342 kJ/21.8 g fat
McDonald's Classic Salad with Crispy Chicken	1250 kJ/15.1 g fat
McDonald's Filet-O-Fish™	1270 kJ/13.1 g fat
McDonald's McChicken®	1710 kJ/18.7 g fat
HJ medium fries	1566 kJ/19.5 g fat
McDonald's medium fries	1540 kJ/19.8 g fat
HJ Onion Rings, medium	1259 kJ/13.8 g fat
McDonald's large chocolate milk shake	2110 kJ/12.4 g fat
HJ Chicken Nuggets (6)	974 kJ/11.4 g fat
Chicken McNuggets® (6)	1160 kJ/17.9 g fat

Take control of the table

1. Ask and you shall receive

The waiters should know how a dish is made, what the ingredients are and how big the serve size is. So ask. Then have it the way you want it. If you'd like the grilled chicken breast without the skin, say so. If the vegetable side dishes are usually prepared with lots of butter, request yours lightly sautéed in olive oil or better still, steamed. Do you fancy a pizza? They should be more than willing to make yours with half the normal cheese, or none, and with an extra topping of vegetables.

2. Order one course at a time

One of the pleasures of eating out is taking your time – or at least it should be. Unfortunately, at too many restaurants waiters snatch up one course and rush in with the next before you've had time to put your fork down. There's a reason. Most restaurants want to turn tables round as quickly as they can to squeeze in as many seatings in an evening as possible. That's their business. Yours is to sit back, relax and take the time you need to eat only as much as you want – and no more. If you're worried about being rushed, order just one course at a time, not the whole meal. Once you've finished your starter, look back at the menu to consider what you'll have next. A useful rule of thumb: allot at least 20 minutes per course – the time your body needs to send satiety signals. Do you feel full? You're under no obligation to keep ordering.

3. Draw the line

Ask whether the kitchen can prepare half serves. Many restaurants are more than willing to do so. While you are waiting to order, take a quick look at the size of the serves that other diners are eating. If serves seem very large, you could even ask for a child's serve. Don't wait until you've started to nibble. Don't depend on your will-power to eat only half of what's in front of you. This is supposed to be dinner you're enjoying, not a test of your determination.

4. Rule the table

When you're eating out, you're in charge – not only of what you eat but of what's on the table. Lots of restaurants start you off with a basket of bread or rolls. If you're very hungry when this arrives, you'll automatically start eating it, probably slathered with butter and loaded with kilojoules, without even giving it a second thought.

Why waste the kilojoules? Politely tell the waiter, 'No bread, thanks'. If you're famished when you sit down, then order something more sensible to take the edge off your hunger – a side salad, a vegetable side dish or a glass of spicy tomato juice, for instance. At the same time, ask for a glass of water. Or, even better, a jug of iced water or a bottle of mineral water. Then you won't have to wait for anybody to fill your glass, and you can drink plenty of water with your meal. Always remember who's boss. If something arrives at the table that you don't want, politely decline it. No one will mind.

Manage the menu

Order wisely, and you can put together a meal that's long on flavour and short on kilojoules. Here are five things to consider when you open the menu.

1. Be colourful

Meat and creamy sauces are usually beige, aren't they? Where do most dishes get their brightest colours? From vegetables and fruit, of course. Choose the most colourful dishes on the menu, and chances are you'll order the healthiest, lowest-kilojoule selections. Spicy red salsas, purple-red beetroot, leafy green salads, golden yellow sweetcorn, purple eggplant and bright red and yellow capsicums all turn your plate into a rainbow of colours. As long as vegetables arrive without lots of added fat, they're free on *ChangeOne*. Help yourself. And there's another reason for filling your

Help!

'I know going out for fast food isn't the smartest thing to do. But sometimes there's no other choice, especially if the kids have anything to say about it. Is there any way to order off a fast-food menu and still keep kilojoules down?'

Yes, as long as you can resist the messages to add this and supersize that. Be a contrarian. Choose the smallest sizes. Avoid the secret sauce. Double up on lettuce and tomatoes. Order diet soda or water instead of sugary drinks. Here are 10 meal options to choose from.

- Chicken nuggets (four pieces), sauce (one packet), vegetable salad with fat-free dressing
- Grilled chicken flat bread sandwich (without sauce), vegetable salad with fat-free dressing
- Small hamburger, vegetable salad with fat-free dressing
- Plain baked potato, small Caesar salad with low-fat French dressing
- Veggie burger, vegetable salad with fat-free dressing
- Grilled vegetable sandwich (without mayonnaise), bean or lentil soup
- Zesty chicken salad bowl (no dressing)
- Taco salad with salsa
- Minestrone soup with French bread
- Toasted sesame bagel with smoked salmon and salad (no dressing)

plate with colour. Many of the substances that provide fruits and vegetables with their colours are anti-oxidants – potent disease-fighters that have been shown to lower heart disease and the risk of cancer.

2. Order starters and side dishes

Another favourite dieting strategy: forgo the main dish section of the menu and order only from the starters and side dishes. With large restaurant serves, a starter or side dish often makes the perfect meal by itself.

3. Dip into the sauce

Ordering salad dressing to be served separately and drizzling it on sparingly is one of the oldest tricks in any slimmer's handbook, of course. Remember that you can order other sauces on the side, too, from gravy to guacamole. Give yourself no more than a tablespoon. And put your fork to good use. Instead of pouring on the sauce or salad dressing, dip the tips of your fork into it and then spear a bite-size serve. You'll make a little bit of a good thing go a long way.

4. Create your own selection

If you're eating out with friends who share your concern about overdoing it, agree to order and share dishes. If there are four of you, order two or three main dishes. You'll get a chance to try a wider variety of items on the menu and keep serves down to size. Be careful, though: some people offered a lot to choose from end up eating a lot more. Decide in advance to sample only two or three forkfuls of each dish. With lots of dishes on the table, it's especially important to be aware of hunger and satiety signals. Sit back from time to time, take a deep breath and think about whether you've had enough – if you have, put your fork down, raise a glass of water and spend the rest of the time enjoying conversation.

5. Be a discerning food critic

Remember the credo of smart dining: if it doesn't taste great, don't eat it. Yes, of course, you paid for it. Of course it's a shame to waste food. But to finish something you don't really like is the true crime. It only means you won't get to eat something else that you'd really savour. When you're eating out this week, be a tough critic. Pay close attention to the first few bites. Decide whether it's good enough to finish or whether you'd just as soon set aside some kilojoules for something else. If you eat out frequently, consider keeping a diner's diary, with mini reviews and notes on what you had. Use a star system to award top restaurants your own *ChangeOne* rating. You'll find yourself paying closer attention to the food you eat – and enjoying it more.

Changes ahead: weekends and celebrations

Restaurant meals are meant to be savoured and enjoyed. So is the weekend. Whether it's a calm day at home or a wild outdoor excursion, so many of us use weekends for relaxation, family and good food. Once you master the art of restaurant ordering, *ChangeOne* style, your next task will be to take on your weekend eating habits.

For some of us this will be difficult. When we get together with friends and family, food seems to magically appear, in copious amounts. It's time to start thinking about the role food plays in your social and family life. Look back to last weekend and think through all you did and the role food played in things. Where were the temptations, the times when food was too available or the centre of attention?

As you will see, we've taken on the subliminal message that food equals love – that mum serving you an extra plate of dessert is her way of showing how much she cares for you. When you are ready to move on, we'll show you how to say no to all those food offerings, without feeling guilty or sacrificing taste and enjoyment. Plus, you'll learn techniques for handling celebrations and special occasions as well.

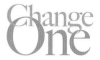

Weekends & celebrations

We almost called this chapter 'Family and friends'. Why? Because at weekends and celebrations, that's who you'll be spending your time with, and these people will have an incredible amount of influence over what you eat – and how much. In many cases they'll be instrumental in determining your long-term dieting success, either through their support or lack of it.

Weekends are also when the usual work-week routine is up for grabs. New temptations arise from every side: fancy dinners out, sausages or pies at a football match, Sunday lunches, tempting barbecues and birthday cakes.

This week, dive into your weekend with gusto. We're proposing just this one change: focus less on food and more on active fun.

We'll show you that you don't have to hide from friends, family or fun to stick to your new eating habits.

Get together with family and friends

By now you know that the real secret of losing weight isn't as complicated as a lot of diet books would have you believe. Like a lot of the volunteers who tested *ChangeOne*, you may have found that making just two or three changes was all you needed in order to start slimming down.

The same principles that have guided you up to now will serve you well when your routine switches gear at weekends and celebrations. Yes, you'll need to be a little creative. But that's not such a bad thing. Learning to be flexible is important. Life, after all, has a way of throwing us a curve now and then. The more confident you feel about adapting your diet to new situations, the better your chances of success. Weekends and celebrations are a great way to discover that you can control what you eat in almost any situation.

Why not take the weekend off?

If you've tried a deprivation-type diet in the past – the kind built around diet drinks or long lists of forbidden foods – you were probably tempted to take a holiday from it when weekends and celebrations rolled round. But by making a distinction between days when you follow a diet and days when you're on 'holiday' from it, you tell yourself that your diet is some kind of unnatural chore – it makes you eat one way to lose weight, but you really want to eat another very different way in your everyday life. That's the recipe for a diet that will fail. Too many dieters lose weight, then go off their diets and return to the way they used to eat. Almost immediately the weight begins to pile on again.

ChangeOne isn't about deprivation, as you know by now. It's about good food and a rational way of eating that you

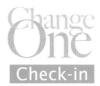

Check-in

Frustrated that you're not losing weight faster? There's no need to be, if you're dropping half to one kilo a week. That's a pace that will keep you on track not only to lose weight but to keep it off. Wish you were losing that much? Look back at the Fast Track suggestions in the breakfast, lunch, snack and dinner chapters. Choose two to put into effect this week. Fast Track turned out to be one of the most popular features of *ChangeOne* among our volunteers. Many followed them all.

can enjoy every day while you lose weight – and will continue to enjoy and benefit from long after you've lost those kilos. It is a diet you can live with every day.

That's the key. The more consistently you make smart eating choices, the more quickly they'll become second nature to you. That's why it's so important, at weekends and at celebrations, to find ways to use *ChangeOne* strategies to guide you even when your normal schedule is disrupted and you find yourself in situations where plates are piled high and drinks are flowing freely.

If you're celebrating something special – your birthday, an anniversary or a big wedding, for example – live it up. And plan ahead. Strike a deal with yourself in advance. In return for getting the chance to indulge a little, agree to skip snacks during the day; set aside 45 minutes for a kilojoule-burning activity; put together any combination that lets you, in effect, pay as you go. Keep track of what you eat during the day. Fill in a detailed food diary if you have time.

And remember, one indulgence doesn't mean you've failed. It doesn't even have to bring bad news on the scales. To gain 500 g, you have to consume about 14,700 kilojoules more than you burn. That's a lot of kilojoules. Even the biggest special-occasion feast isn't likely to pack that many. The truth is, a big blowout isn't what typically spells trouble for slimmers. The real danger is eating a little too much every day or every weekend. If you do indulge yourself this weekend, just be sure to follow the *ChangeOne* meal plans more closely during the coming week and you'll be fine.

When food is love

One big reason weekends and celebrations are difficult for slimmers is that in all the world's cultures, food equals love. Food is a celebration. Food is a reward. Food is comfort. What do we do for someone's birthday? Bake a cake. How do we celebrate a wedding? With a feast. The simple act of offering someone food is a way of showing love and affection. There's nothing wrong with that. We just need to keep a clear view of why we're eating.

This week and at the weekend, notice the role that food plays for you when you are with your family and friends. If the people who love you encourage you to eat more

Practising the art of saying 'no thanks'

'Eat up', your doting mother-in-law says. 'You're going to waste away to nothing if that's all you have.'

'Didn't you like my casserole?' your Aunt Ellen asks. 'You've always loved my casserole. Come now, just one more little helping. Dessert? But it's a special occasion. You can't say no!'

Of course you can say no – but sometimes only at the risk of hurting someone's feelings. Or so it may seem. But you don't have to let well-meaning urgings to eat cause you to overeat. You can always say no thanks. And by being diplomatic you won't hurt any feelings in the process. Here's how.

Be honest. Casually mention to everyone in advance that you're on a diet and watching serve sizes. Make it clear that you don't want to offend anyone, but that it's very important for you to keep an eye on how much you eat.

Compliment early – and often. If you're oohing and aahing after the first bite, it won't seem as if you didn't appreciate the dish when you turn down seconds later.

Pace yourself. If you know Aunt Ellen's feelings will be hurt when you don't sample her apple pie, plan your meal accordingly. Help yourself to smaller serves of the main course so that you have a little extra room – and some extra kilojoules to spare – when dessert is served.

Say yes to a little. Sometimes it's easier to say yes to a little than to say no and find yourself staring at an empty plate while everybody enjoys something sweet. But be sure that you control the serve size, not your Aunt Ellen.

Use delaying tactics. Sometimes you can avoid offending people by saying, 'Maybe later.' Or, 'I'm so full right now I wouldn't be able to enjoy it. Let me wait a little while.' Once the plates are cleared away and the festivities move on to the next stage, no one will remember that you didn't have dessert.

Take it home. Another strategy to avoid eating more than you want is simple flattery. When the offer for seconds comes along, rave about how great everything was – and ask if you can take a serve home rather than have seconds now. Remember: taking seconds home doesn't mean you have to eat them. If you don't intend to, make sure you dispose of them right away. We won't tell.

'I'm so full right now I wouldn't be able to enjoy it.'

than you want or need, look for alternatives. If your mother says, 'Eat, eat', to show she cares, say: 'No thanks, mum, I'm full right now – but let me help you clear the dishes so we can have a chance to talk.' If your friends' main device for getting together is a meal out, suggest alternatives that don't have to centre round food: playing cards or a board game, or a game of golf, tennis or squash, or a walk in a nearby park, for instance.

continued on page 136

Seafood on Saturday

Saturday brunches are often casual affairs enjoyed with friends. Simple, no-fuss dishes, such as fishcakes and smoked salmon with bagels, are perfect.

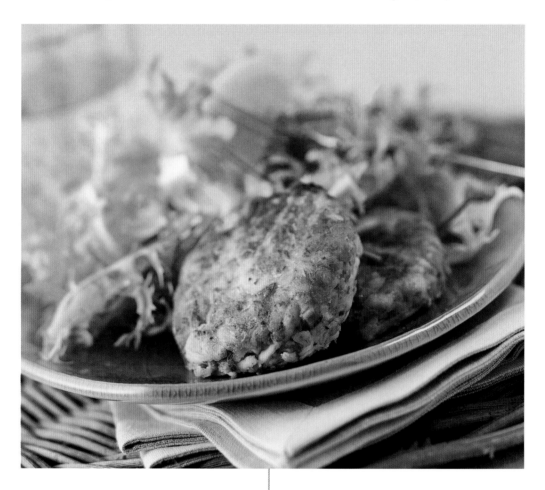

Fishcake brunch

2 crab cakes

tossed green salad with vegetables and non-fat dressing (unlimited)

1 small bread roll (tennis ball)

1 cup (125 g) seasonal berries (e.g. raspberries, strawberries and blueberries)

1603 kJ, 383 kcal, 30 g protein, 10 g fat (1 g sat fat), 137 mg cholesterol, 41 g carbohydrate (17 g sugars), 11 g fibre, 884 mg sodium

CRAB CAKES

Serves 4

20 g fresh breadcrumbs
1 celery stick with leaves, finely chopped
1/3 cup (45 g) finely chopped red capsicum
2 tablespoons finely chopped French shallot
1 tablespoon chopped parsley
2 tablespoons grain mustard
2 tablespoons reduced-fat mayonnaise
1 egg
1 teaspoon mixed dried herbs
450 g white crab meat
25 g plain flour
2 teaspoons vegetable oil

1. Mix together the breadcrumbs, celery, capsicum, shallot, parsley, mustard, mayonnaise, egg and herbs in a large bowl. Gently fold in the crab meat.

2. Preheat the oven to 180°C. With floured hands, divide the crab mixture into 8 and shape each portion into a small cake. Dredge the cakes with flour.

3. Lightly coat a large non-stick frying pan with cooking spray and set over medium-high heat until hot but not smoking. Add 4 crab cakes and cook for about 2 minutes on each side or until browned. Immediately after turning the cakes over, drizzle 1 teaspoon oil around them and gently shake the pan to spread the oil. Transfer the cakes to a plate lined with kitchen paper. Repeat with the remaining crab cakes and oil.

4. Lightly coat a baking tray with cooking spray. Place the crab cakes on the tray and bake for 8 to 10 minutes or until very hot in the centre. Serve hot.

5. One serve equals 2 crab cakes.

Smoked salmon and bagel brunch

1 bagel, any flavour, split in half and topped with

1 tablespoon reduced-fat cream cheese
2 slices smoked salmon
2 slices tomato
2 slices red onion (optional)
Capers or caviar (optional)

½ cup (125 g) fresh fruit salad

1 Buck's Fizz (equal parts orange juice and champagne or sparkling water)

1602 kJ, 383 kcal, 21 g protein, 4 g fat (1 g sat fat), 28 mg cholesterol, 54 g carbohydrate (28 g sugars), 6 g fibre, 1192 mg sodium

HEALTH TIP

When shopping for reduced-fat cream cheese, check the labels to compare the kilojoule and fat contents of different brands. They can vary considerably.

BRUNCH MENU TIPS

Try some or all of these ideas for your brunch menus.
■ A basket of mini muffins or crusty rolls

Salad variations

■ Baby spinach with reduced-fat dressing
■ Sliced cucumbers tossed with rice vinegar, sesame oil and a sprinkle of caster sugar
■ Cubed tomatoes drizzled with balsamic vinegar and extra virgin olive oil
■ Baby lettuce and watercress

Cheese choices

■ Low-fat cottage cheese mixed with chopped cucumber, capsicums and radishes
■ Ricotta flavoured with pure vanilla essence, cinnamon and caster sugar
■ Assorted sliced reduced-fat cheeses

Fruit treats

■ Fresh fruit salad
■ Tri-colour melon ball salad (rockmelon, watermelon and honeydew melon)
■ Sliced peaches drizzled with Amaretto

Eggs on Sunday

A leisurely Sunday breakfast or brunch with family or friends is among life's great pleasures. And since you're combining two meals in one, you have a lot more kilojoules to play with. These two menus feature egg dishes as the centrepiece.

The Sunday omelette

1 vegetable cheese omelette

1 serve chunky oven chips
(see opposite)

1 wedge of melon

1549 kJ, 370 kcal, 25 g protein, 19 g fat (6 g sat fat),
387 mg cholesterol, 25 g carbohydrate (13 g sugars),
6 g fibre, 366 mg sodium

VEGETABLE CHEESE OMELETTE

Serves 1
2 eggs
2 teaspoons chopped fresh herbs
 (e.g. oregano, dill, basil, parsley),
 plus extra leaves to garnish
freshly ground black pepper
½ cup (30 g) fresh baby spinach leaves
2 tablespoons grated reduced-fat cheddar
1 large tomato, chopped (optional)

1. In a bowl, whisk together the eggs with the herbs, 1 teaspoon water and freshly ground black pepper to taste. In another bowl, toss the spinach with the cheese and tomato, if desired, and set aside.

2. Lightly coat a non-stick omelette pan or small frying pan with cooking spray and set over medium heat for 1 minute. Pour the egg mixture into the pan and cook until the eggs begin to set on the base. Lift up the edge of the omelette and push the cooked part towards the centre to let the uncooked portion run onto the pan. Cook 3–5 minutes, or until the omelette is set underneath and almost set on top.

3. Spread the spinach filling over half of the omelette. Fold the omelette over in half and cook for 2 more minutes. Slide the omelette onto a plate and garnish with the reserved herbs.

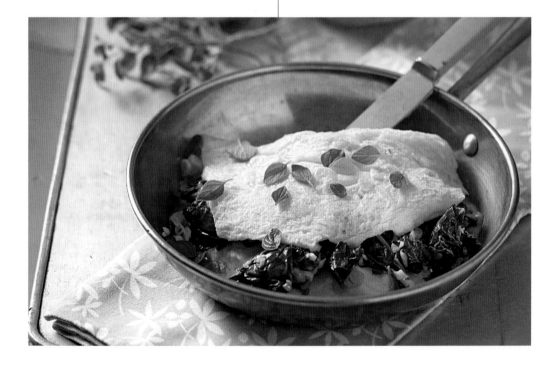

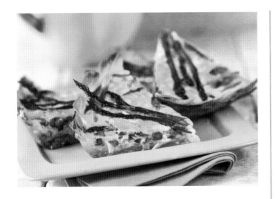

Quiche with fruit bread

1 slice asparagus and cheddar quiche

1 slice peach and yogurt loaf
(recipe on page 311)

150 ml orange juice

1160 kJ, 277 kcal, 17 g protein, 10 g fat (5 g sat fat),
86 mg cholesterol, 28 g carbohydrate (20 g sugars),
3 g fibre, 364 mg sodium

ASPARAGUS AND CHEDDAR QUICHE

Serves 6

1 tablespoon dried breadcrumbs
225 g potatoes, peeled and very
thinly sliced
2 teaspoons olive oil
450 g asparagus, trimmed
100 g grated reduced-fat mature cheddar
3 spring onions (scallions), sliced
1 can (about 350 g) reduced-fat
evaporated milk
2 eggs
2 eggwhites
2 teaspoons melted butter
1 teaspoon dry mustard
freshly ground black pepper

1. Preheat the oven to 200ºC. Coat a 23 cm flan tin with cooking spray and sprinkle with the breadcrumbs. Beginning in the centre of the tin, arrange the potato slices in slightly overlapping circles to cover the bottom. Lightly brush with the olive oil and press down gently. Bake for 10 minutes.

2. Set aside 8 to 12 asparagus spears. Cut the rest into 2.5 cm pieces.

3. Sprinkle the potato base with a third of the cheddar. Cover with the asparagus pieces, then sprinkle with the spring onions and another third of the cheese.

4. Whisk together the evaporated milk, eggs and eggwhites, butter, mustard and freshly ground black pepper to taste. Pour into the tin and sprinkle with the remaining cheese. Arrange the whole asparagus spears on top. Bake for 35 minutes or until a knife inserted in the centre comes out clean.

ABOUT EGGS

Although eggs contain relatively high levels of cholesterol, it's the amount of saturated fat in a food rather than the amount of cholesterol that has the most impact on cholesterol levels in the blood. A medium egg (the standard for recipes) contains about 315 kilojoules and 30 times more cholesterol than 25 g chocolate, but because the chocolate contains about twice as much saturated fat as the egg, it's more likely to raise blood cholesterol levels. And eggs have a lot to offer nutritionally – they're one of the few dietary sources of vitamin D and they also provide good amounts of vitamins A, E, B_2 and B_{12} (one medium egg provides almost 100 per cent of the recommended adult daily intake of B_{12}).

CHUNKY OVEN CHIPS

For each serve, cut a scrubbed small baking potato (with skin) into thick chips or wedges. Put into a polythene bag with 1 teaspoon olive oil and freshly ground black pepper to taste, and shake to coat the potatoes. Spread out in a hot roasting tin and bake at 240ºC for 45 to 50 minutes, turning once or twice, until crisp and well browned.

continued from page 131

When you do find yourself at the table with friends and family, remember that you don't have to overeat to show you care. Food is only part of what makes sitting down with friends and family a pleasure. We get together to talk and laugh, to catch up on the latest news, to reinforce the ties that bind by expressing our feelings for one another. If you're engaged in conversation, no one will notice that you've put your fork down and are sipping from your water glass. Food may nourish our bodies, but it's laughter and expressions of caring, after all, that nourish our souls.

Nurturing yourself

Family and friends aren't the only people who urge food on us as a reward or show of affection. Some of us do it to ourselves. We eat to reward ourselves, or to feel better when we're a bit low. Especially if you grew up being offered food to feel better, you may have internalised the same reflex. Feel bad? Eat. The trouble, of course, is that you'll almost certainly overeat. When you do, you'll feel bad. And what do you do then? Well, eat some more.

How to escape? You may already have found part of the answer in becoming aware of genuine hunger cues, and distinguishing them from environmental and emotional triggers. But if you still have trouble resisting the urge for food rewards, make a list of alternatives to edibles. What else will make you feel better? If your day is full of stresses, reward yourself with five minutes of quiet time to relax and de-pressurise. (You'll find more stress-busting strategies in Week 9, Stress Relief, which begins on page 182.) If you love music, take a few minutes out to play a favourite piece. If you really, really, really want something to eat, reward yourself with a stick of sugar-free gum, a suggestion we've made before because it *really* works. Make it a habit, in fact. Over time, whenever you get the urge to treat yourself to food, you'll think 'sugar-free gum'.

> Music, quiet, a phone call, a walk – all of these serve as small personal rewards.

Have a plan in place

Routines may change at weekends and when you're celebrating, but that doesn't mean everything is thrown up in the air. It's likely that you've already made at least a few plans for this weekend. Before it gets underway, think ahead. Write down a schedule for breakfast, lunch and dinner, and fill in as many blanks as possible. Think of it as a reverse food diary. Let's say your weekend plans include a trip to your mother's house to celebrate her 70th birthday with a big family do. Your schedule might look something like this.

Saturday

Breakfast: *ChangeOne* breakfast at home
Lunch: on the way
Dinner: Mum's house

Sunday

Breakfast: Mum's house
Lunch: family celebration
Dinner: on the way home

continued on page 139

Smart holiday tricks

When the Christmas season arrives, it's usually difficult to avoid being surrounded by food as you catch up with relatives and friends. Here's how to cope.

Be helpful anywhere but in the kitchen. This is tough, especially if you're at the in-laws' house. But it's all too easy to nibble when you're surrounded by food in various stages of preparation. Volunteer for other duties: setting the table, fixing drinks, clearing up, running errands – anything that doesn't involve food.

Be the activity director. Take the lead in suggesting non-eating activities that the family can do together.

Grab a water bottle. When there are lots of high-kilojoule drinks around, it helps to have an alternative available. Keep a glass or bottle of water handy.

> Volunteer for any job that doesn't involve food.

Keep 'free' snacks and drinks on hand. Satisfy your hunger before the meal with low-kilojoule crudités – carrots, celery, capsicums, radishes – and diet drinks. That way you won't have to rely on your will-power alone to steer clear of all those diet-busting rich foods.

Stay with the kids. If all the adults are circling the food table, spend time with the children. At most ages, kids are more likely than adults to be doing something active. Their energy and playfulness can help distract you from wanting food. Help them to make decorations or lead a game of hide-and-seek.

Go out. If the sight and smell of all that food becomes just too much for you, excuse yourself and get out of the house. Take a walk or go for a drive.

137

ChangeOne

Success Stories

Surpassing her goals

Kathy Bennett has been spending a lot of money on clothes lately. Since she started *ChangeOne*, Kathy has gone down three sizes, so she's had to buy a completely new wardrobe.

Not that she's complaining about it. 'My original goal was to fit comfortably into my pants, but I eventually lost 14 kilograms and over 12 centimetres from my hips', she says.

And the benefits for Kathy go well beyond kilos lost and brand-new outfits. 'My cholesterol count made a significant drop without any medication', she says. 'I also found that I have more energy and less stress, which I'm sure is related to the exercise program suggested by *ChangeOne*.'

Kathy, who has two children, aged 20 and 23, started with *ChangeOne* because she liked that it was a well-balanced program that allowed her to eat anything, with no prohibited foods.

'I ate everything I loved through my weight-loss process, including penne à la vodka and hot dogs – I just had less of it', she says. 'The portion-control tricks are great. The easiest one for me was cutting my main meal in half when I went out to dinner – except I ate all the vegetables. Because it was so easy, it just became a new way of life for me.'

Exercise was also a key to Kathy's success. 'I increased my aerobic exercise from once a week to six times per week and used every opportunity to burn kilojoules, including walking up and down

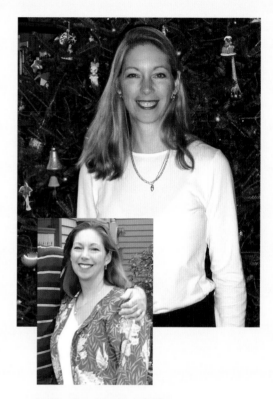

Kathy Bennett lost 14 kg, dropped three sizes and lowered her cholesterol.

20 flights of stairs on my way to and from the cafeteria every day', she says.

Kathy's family has been extremely helpful with her weight-loss efforts. 'My children and my husband were wonderfully supportive through the process, eagerly anticipating my weekly weigh-ins and never once trying to tempt me to eat something off my plan', she says. 'It's a real ego boost to have family and friends, even my aerobics instructor, comment on how thin I look.'

continued from page 137

Once you've written up a schedule, identify meals that are likely to pose the toughest challenge and think up ways to prepare in advance to make them easier. In the example above, Saturday breakfast is a breeze, but lunch on the way could be treacherous, given the sorts of places to eat that you are likely to come across. Family dinners are always a challenge – too much food, too many people urging you to eat. And a celebration lunch on Sunday! The table will be laden with all the family's favourite dishes.

Never fear. There are plenty of ways to plan ahead for a weekend like this. Here's what to consider.

1. Do it yourself

The best way to control what you eat is to make it yourself. If there's not much chance you'll find a healthy meal en route, consider packing your own in advance. You'll save money, frustration and time. If the weather's good and you can find a nice place to stop, you can turn a packed lunch into a picnic. When the weekend includes a shared meal, where everyone brings something, contribute a *ChangeOne* dish. Fix two if you have the time. That way you'll have a choice of dishes you know you can rely on to be low in kilojoules. Don't forget to bring along sugar-free drinks or sparkling mineral water.

2. Celebrate special occasions with special food

At most big family gatherings and celebrations, people lovingly prepare home-made delicacies like Aunt Margaret's chicken pie or your grandmother's baked custard tarts. Spend your kilojoules wisely by skipping potato chips, nuts and other savoury snacks before the meal and choosing only the most special foods for the special occasion. As much as possible, plan your entire meal in advance.

3. Practise pacing yourself

The big meal at Christmas is one time when just about everyone relaxes and enjoys a leisurely feast. It's a great chance to practise all your best tortoise skills. For a long meal, you may have to use every delaying tactic in the book. Drink a sip of water between each bite. Put your fork down frequently. Sit back in your chair and enjoy the conversation for a few minutes without eating anything.

4. Watch the alcohol

Wine, punch, beer and other alcoholic drinks have a way of flowing freely at special meals. Don't let too much alcohol dissolve your best intentions to stick to your diet. Limit yourself to one glass with your meal. The rest of the time, have sparkling mineral water with a slice of lemon or lime, or sugar-free soft drinks. Want an icy cold beer on a hot summer's day? Obviously, 'lite' or alcohol-free beer are options, and they're getting better and better.

5. Get out and about

The extra leisure time at weekends offers a great opportunity to plan activities that involve burning more kilojoules – gather your relatives for a bushwalk or a walk to an historic lighthouse or some other place of interest, a game of beach cricket or volleyball, a game of tennis, a fun run in the park, a bike ride, Frisbee throwing. Burn 2100 extra kilojoules this weekend and you can treat yourself to a big piece of blackberry and apple pie without worrying about upsetting your kilojoule balance. Activities that the whole family can join in are also a great way to enjoy time together that doesn't centre around food.

6. Take time for bedtime

Weekends are a wonderful opportunity to catch up on sleep you may have lost during the week. Remember: lack of sleep can erode your will-power and your determination. Obesity experts believe it can even cause you to put on weight. Get to bed a little early one night this weekend. If that doesn't work, allow yourself to sleep a little later than usual one morning.

7. Fine-tune your expectations

If the coming week holds a crowded schedule of holiday parties, be realistic about your goals. Instead of trying to continue losing weight, for instance, relax your goal and aim to maintain your current weight. Then, when the holidays are finished, you can start shedding weight again. Setting standards that are impossible to meet is setting yourself up for failure. Unless you have an upcoming modelling session for the cover of *Vogue*, odds are you don't have to lose a certain amount of weight by any particular date. Remember, this is a plan for your entire life. Don't put yourself under more pressure than you need. It's far better to take a little while longer reaching your goal than to put yourself under unnecessary stress.

Should you enlist family and friends?

A bit of encouragement, a helping hand, or perhaps someone joining you on your morning or evening or lunchtime walk can be a great morale booster. So can a shoulder to lean on when things aren't going your way. Help from family and friends can also take the pressure off and eliminate unnecessary stresses in your life.

How important are the people around you when it comes to slimming success? At first, behavioural scientists assumed the answer would be 'very'. The more support dieters had, the assumption went, the better their odds of losing weight and keeping it off. But the results of studies looking at social support and weight loss have been mixed. Some people do better when they have a strong social network. Others do just fine on their own.

Knowing whether you tend to be a team player or a solo flyer is the first step in finding the kind of support and encouragement you need to succeed. To find out, answer the questions in the quiz on page 147.

Your friends in need

Social support comes in many forms, from the neighbour who joins you on your morning walk to the partner who decides to do the *ChangeOne* program along with you. The first step in getting the help you need is deciding what kind of help you need. Tick one or more of the following categories.

❏ An activity partner
❏ Someone to talk to when I'm feeling down or discouraged
❏ Someone who can answer specific diet questions
❏ Help in the kitchen
❏ Help around the house
❏ A lunch or dinner companion
❏ Other: _____

continued on page 146

Cooking outdoors

What better way to entertain than with a barbecue. But prepare yourself: meals you make for friends and family at weekends tend to be larger than everyday meals, so eat less at the other two meals that day.

Barbecued chicken feast

Crudités platter (unlimited)

Spicy chicken (1 breast, or 1 drumstick plus 1 thigh)

Grilled summer vegetables (coffee mug)

Warm potato salad with dijon vinaigrette (2 golf balls)

2 small sesame breadsticks

1 piece seasonal fruit

2033 kJ, 486 kcal, 41 g protein, 12 g fat (3 g sat fat), 116 mg cholesterol, 52 g carbohydrate (28 g sugars), 14 g fibre, 675 mg sodium

GRILLED SUMMER VEGETABLES

Serves 4

2 small bulbs fennel, about 225 g each
1 eggplant, about 450 g, cut lengthwise into 1 cm thick slices
4 tomatoes, halved
3 large capsicums, preferably 1 each green, red and yellow, cut into strips
1 red onion, cut into 8 wedges
¼ teaspoon salt
¼ teaspoon freshly ground black pepper
1 tablespoon orange juice
8 fresh basil leaves, thinly sliced
1 clove garlic clove, finely chopped
1 teaspoon grated orange zest

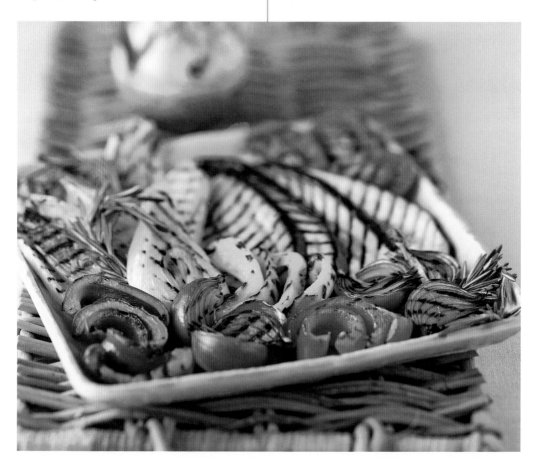

1. Prepare a charcoal fire (or preheat the grill or a ridged cast-iron chargrill pan).

2. Cut the leafy tops off the fennel bulbs and set aside. Trim the bulbs and cut vertically into 1 cm slices. Coat the fennel, eggplant, tomatoes, capsicums and onion with cooking spray, or brush them with a very light coating of olive oil, and sprinkle with the salt and pepper.

3. Barbecue (or grill) the vegetables for about 4 minutes on each side, or until tender and browned. Transfer to a serving platter and sprinkle with the orange juice.

4. Finely chop the reserved fennel tops and mix in a bowl with the basil, garlic and orange zest. Sprinkle over the vegetables.

5. Serve warm or at room temperature.

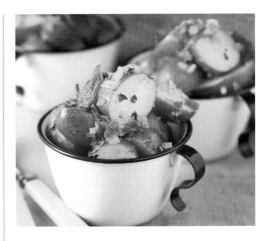

SPICY BARBECUED CHICKEN

Serves 4

1 chicken, 1–1.3 kg
3–4 tablespoons dry spice rub, made with equal parts paprika, onion and chive seasoning and garlic granules, plus pepper to taste
1 can beer

1. Prepare the barbecue, placing the coals around the outside edge. If using a gas barbecue, leave one burner off.

2. Rub the chicken inside and out with the spice mixture. Loosen the skin slightly and sprinkle a bit of the spice rub between the skin and the flesh.

3. Open the can of beer and pour out half. Place the beer can on the barbecue, in the centre if using charcoal or over the unlit burner on a gas grill. 'Sit' the chicken on top of the beer can (the can should fit inside the chicken cavity) with its legs spread to form a 'tripod' on the rack.

4. Close the barbecue lid and cook the chicken for 45 to 60 minutes or until thoroughly cooked. Carefully remove the chicken and can from the barbecue.

5. Cut the chicken into 6 pieces – 2 thighs, 2 drumsticks and 2 breasts. One serve equals one breast, or one drumstick plus one thigh. Remove the skin before eating.

WARM POTATO SALAD WITH DIJON VINAIGRETTE

Serves 4

300 g red-skinned or waxy new potatoes, scrubbed and quartered
3 thin slices smoked chicken or turkey
1 small onion, chopped
3 tablespoons cider vinegar
1 1/2 tablespoons caster sugar
1 tablespoon dijon mustard
1/2 teaspoon olive oil
1/2 teaspoon freshly ground black pepper
1/4 cup (45 g) sweet-and-sour gherkins, finely chopped
1/4 cup (45 g) finely chopped red capsicum
4 tablespoons chopped parsley

1. Cook the potatoes in a large saucepan of boiling water for about 10 minutes or until tender. Drain and keep warm.

2. Meanwhile, cut the chicken slices in half, then cook in a large non-stick frying pan (add cooking spray if necessary) until crisp. Transfer to a paper towel to remove excess moisture, then crumble. Cook the onion in the same pan (respray if necessary) for 7 minutes, or until golden.

3. Place the vinegar, sugar, mustard, oil and pepper in a screwtop jar, shake to combine, then whisk into the onion in the pan. Bring to a simmer and cook for about 2 minutes. Add the potatoes, gherkin, red capsicum and half the crumbled chicken. Cook, stirring, for about 2 minutes, or until the potatoes are coated and hot. Sprinkle with the parsley and the remaining crumbled chicken. Serve warm or at room temperature.

Holiday classics

Holidays and food go hand in hand, and most of us look forward to enjoying the same foods year after year. It's fine if you choose to leave *ChangeOne* behind for a feast day celebration. To continue following *ChangeOne* during the holidays, check out our sample menu and some new variations on old favourites.

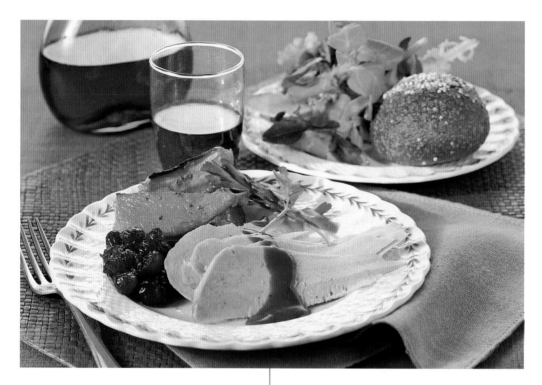

Christmas lunch

85 g apple-stuffed turkey breast
(deck of cards)

2 tablespoons turkey gravy, bought or home-made (golf ball)

2 tablespoons cranberry sauce
(table tennis ball)

Orange-glazed carrots and sweet potatoes (2 golf balls)

Green salad with fat-free dressing
(unlimited)

1 crusty bread roll (tennis ball)

1770 kJ, 423 kcal, 25 g protein, 7 g fat (1 g sat fat),
25 mg cholesterol, 75 g carbohydrate (39 g sugars),
4 g fibre, 959 mg sodium (Note: figures do not include
starter, dessert and drinks.)

ABOUT FEEDING A CROWD

■ Select at least two starters, one vegetable (like stuffed mushrooms or a crudités platter) and one based on low-fat or reduced-fat cream cheese.

■ Offer a green salad as a low-kilojoule filler. Make the dressing optional, and offer a fat-free alternative.

■ Main course choices should include one or two dishes, a starch side dish (pasta, rice, potatoes), rolls or bread and one or two cooked vegetables.

■ Prepare each recipe for about half the number of people expected. For example, if you have 16 guests, prepare each dish to serve 8.

APPLE-STUFFED TURKEY BREAST WITH ORANGE MARMALADE GLAZE

Serves 8

1 whole turkey breast joint on the bone (1.2–1.5 kg)
1 teaspoon freshly ground black pepper
2 celery sticks, cut into 2.5 cm pieces
2 large dessert apples, peeled and thinly sliced
1 large onion, thinly sliced
5 sprigs fresh thyme, plus 1 teaspoon chopped fresh thyme
2 teaspoons olive oil
2 cups (500 ml) apple juice
½ cup (150 g) low-sugar orange marmalade
½ cup (125 ml) white wine or apple juice

1. Preheat the oven to 180ºC. Rinse the turkey, pat dry with paper towels and rub the skin all over with pepper.

2. Combine the celery, half the apples and onion, and 3 thyme sprigs in a roasting tin, piling in a mound in the centre. Toss the chopped thyme with the remaining apples and onion in a bowl. Stuff half of the mixture under the turkey skin; place the remaining mixture in the neck cavity.

3. Set the turkey on top of the vegetable mixture in the tin. Lightly brush the turkey with olive oil and top with the remaining thyme sprigs. Pour the apple juice into the tin. Roast for 1 hour. Discard the thyme sprigs, and baste the turkey with half the marmalade. Continue roasting for about 15 minutes or until the turkey is golden brown and cooked through, basting twice with the remaining marmalade. An instant-read thermometer inserted in the thickest part of the breast, not touching bone, should reach 75ºC. Transfer the turkey to a platter and allow to rest for 10 minutes, then carve. Discard the skin.

4. Stir the wine or juice into the apples and vegetables in the tin and boil, scraping up the browned bits from the tin, until liquid is reduced by half. Serve with the turkey.

ORANGE-GLAZED CARROTS OR SWEET POTATOES

Serves 8

1 kg carrots or sweet potatoes, peeled
1½ cups unsweetened orange juice
2½ teaspoons ground coriander
¼ teaspoon salt
1 tablespoon olive oil
2 tablespoons (20 g) fresh mint, chopped

1. If using carrots, halve lengthwise and cut into 5 cm lengths. If using sweet potatoes, cut into eighths lengthwise and then cut into 5 cm lengths.

2. Combine the carrots or sweet potatoes, orange juice, ground coriander and salt in large frying pan. Bring to the boil over medium heat. Reduce to a simmer, cover and cook for 15 minutes.

3. Uncover the pan, increase the heat to high and cook for a further 7 minutes or until the vegetables are tender.

4. Stir in the oil, and cook for 1 minute, until the vegetables are glossy and the sauce is creamy. Stir in the mint and serve. (Note that one serve is 2 golf balls.)

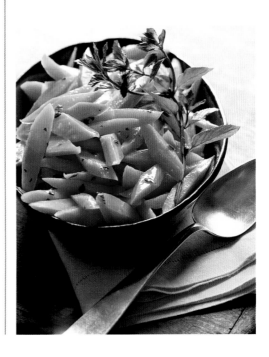

continued from page 141

Now, make a list of possible candidates to fill the positions you've ticked. Keep in mind: sometimes support comes from unexpected places. A work colleague may be more useful to you than a close family member. A neighbour you meet on one of your walks – someone who's also trying to slim down – may offer more help than a close friend.

If you're looking for emotional support, identify someone you're willing to confide in, even if that means admitting weakness or failure. If you're looking for practical help around the house, you probably already know who to ask. So ask. Be specific about what you need, and why you need it. If you're asking someone to do a real favour, think about – and ask – what you can do in return.

Beware of saboteurs

In a perfect world, family and friends would support you 100 per cent. But we live in an imperfect world. Sometimes the people closest to you may be threatened by your efforts to change.

Often it's especially the people closest to you, in fact, who have trouble with your decision to lose weight. A husband or wife, for example. A brother or sister. Why? If your husband or wife tends to be jealous, your decision to lose weight could be interpreted as a desire to be found attractive to other people. If your spouse could stand to lose a little weight, too – but isn't willing to try right now – he or she may resent your determination and success.

There are plenty of reasons that don't take a psychiatrist to figure out, of course. Following a diet requires changes in the kitchen and at the table. Some family members may not want to be bothered by those changes. They may not like the extra time you spend planning lunches or dinners. They may feel uncomfortable finishing everything on their plate when you eat only half of what's on yours.

Take a moment to think about the people closest to you. Among them, is there anyone who:

- Urges food on you even when you say that you're not hungry?
- Belittles your efforts to lose weight?
- Throws obstacles in the way of your being more active?
- Seems resentful or threatened by the fact that you've begun to lose weight?

Change One Quiz

Team player or solo flyer?

Some people need the support and advice of people around them. Others do best on their own. To determine whether you're best suited to be a soloist or a team player, answer the following true or false questions. Your score will help you choose the best strategies to overcome obstacles and to keep your motivation high.

1. I'm comfortable talking to other people about my weight.
- ○ True
- ❏ False

2. If things aren't going well for me, I typically turn to family or friends for advice.
- ○ True
- ❏ False

3. I'm embarrassed talking about my feelings with other people, even people close to me.
- ❏ True
- ○ False

4. Getting a little pat on the back now and then would help motivate me right now.
- ○ True
- ❏ False

5. When I make up my mind to do something, I don't really need other people to push me.
- ❏ True
- ○ False

6. I have at least one person in my life with whom I can talk about almost anything.
- ○ True
- ❏ False

7. I tend to keep my feelings to myself.
- ❏ True
- ○ False

8. The people around me are part of the reason I've had trouble losing weight in the past.
- ❏ True
- ○ False

9. I've always tended to tackle problems on my own.
- ○ True
- ❏ False

10. I'm not really sure that the people around me have my best interests in mind.
- ❏ True
- ○ False

11. Just being able to talk things over with someone when I've got a problem can make things seem better.
- ○ True
- ❏ False

12. I'm very uneasy about letting people see my weaknesses.
- ❏ True
- ○ False

13. I've joined groups in the past, and they've really helped me.
- ○ True
- ❏ False

14. Frankly, I don't really trust people to be honest with me or tell me what they're really thinking.
- ❏ True
- ○ False

Turn to next page to add up your score.

Quiz score

Add up the number of coloured shapes you ticked according to colour.

○ Orange _____

❏ Green _____

○ Orange circles show team players, people who benefit from the support of others. The more you've ticked, the more likely you are to benefit from a strong support network of friends and family. If you wish you had a little more help from those around you now and then, read on for tips on how to get the support you need.

❏ Green boxes indicate solo flyers – people who typically go it alone. The more you've ticked, the more likely you are to depend on yourself.

Most of us are a little of both, of course – we turn to friends or family sometimes and depend on ourselves at other times. So don't be surprised if your score falls somewhere in the middle. Read on for advice on how to strengthen your social network, along with tips on how to make a better job of helping yourself.

■ Undermines your efforts with negative messages, saying things like 'I don't know what makes you think you'll be able to lose weight this time' or 'Once the holidays start, you're going to gain it all back again anyway'?

■ Gets angry or frustrated when you leave food on your plate?

■ Constantly reminds you that you're on a diet and clucks over every bite you eat? That's not help, it's a constant irritation that could wear you down over time.

If so, you may be struggling against someone who's trying to sabotage the change that you want to make. Often the hardest part in dealing with a saboteur is acknowledging that your personal relationships aren't perfect, and that someone close to you may be standing between you and the improvements that you want to make. It's easier to blame yourself or your lack of will-power. But it's crucially important to recognise when someone is making life harder for you rather than easier. Otherwise, they can undermine your chances of success.

Talk it over

This week, if you spot a problem like that and you think it comes mainly from a lack of communication, ask your problem person for a heart-to-heart talk. Explain why losing weight is so important to you – and why the sincere support and enthusiasm of people around you matters so much. Point out things that make it hard for you or hurt your feelings. And be specific about the kind of help you need. For instance:

■ 'I'd rather you didn't offer me more. When I say no, I feel as if I'm hurting your feelings. But it's very important to me right now to cut back on the amount I eat.'

How to be your own best friend

Can't find a support team? Doing just fine on your own? Whether you're a soloist or a team player, a few strategies can help you get through the inevitable rough patches. The key is to be your own best friend. Here are four ways to do that.

Banish negative thoughts. Most of us have heard that little voice that whispers: 'You're never going to be able to do it' or 'You just don't have what it takes.' Learn to recognise such negative thoughts and replace them with the kinds of positive messages a good friend would offer. 'Yes, you can do it.' 'One slip-up is no big deal.' 'Keep up the good work.'

Keep a journal. If that negative voice in your head just won't let up, try carrying a small notebook with you this week and jot down every negative thought that occurs to you. You may be surprised to find that the simple act of writing these thoughts down makes you see how irrational they are. If you can't dismiss them, take a moment to come up with a positive counter-message. 'I'm trying to improve myself.' 'I've stayed

'No one's perfect. I'm doing my best.'

with a diet for five weeks, which isn't bad.' 'No one's perfect. I'm doing my best.' By keeping a diary, you'll also become aware of the situations and circumstances that trigger negative thoughts. Avoid them if you can. If you can't, have your positive counter-messages ready.

Reward yourself for a good job. When you reach one of your goals – even if it's something as simple as sticking to *ChangeOne* through a long holiday weekend – give yourself a reward. For a little extra motivation, decide in advance what the reward will be: a new pair of walking shoes, a new item of clothing, a spa or massage treatment, or tickets to a big match or concert.

Learn to laugh at your foibles. Having a sense of humour can go a long way when you're trying to make a big change in your life. Take yourself too seriously and you'll slip into the kind of all-or-nothing thinking that makes people give up before they've even given themselves a chance.

■ 'I'd really like you to join me for a walk after dinner instead of watching television. Maybe we can make a list of the programs we really want to see and work out a schedule around them.'

■ 'It would help me a lot if we put snack food in the cupboard rather than on the benchtop where I see it all the time. I have a tendency to eat when there's food out.'

■ 'It really hurts my feelings when you say that I never stick with things. I'm really trying this time. Your encouragement means a lot to me.'

■ 'I appreciate that you want to help me lose weight, but continually reminding me I'm on a diet is driving me to distraction. For the most part, I want to handle this on my own. Let me ask for help when I need it.'

Ask your spouse or partner to talk about their own feelings. Explore what you can do to make the situation easier. If a loved one feels threatened, make it clear that your love hasn't changed.

In some cases, you may know that all the talk in the world isn't going to solve the problem. Then the best strategy is learning to recognise acts of sabotage and to find ways to defuse them. This week, try to avoid tense situations that involve food. Spend less time in the kitchen, for instance, and more in other parts of the house. If leaving food on your plate is a flash point, serve yourself only as much as you want to eat.

No advice will fit every situation. Use your best judgment. And remember: if you can't get the support from one source, you can often find it from another. And you can always learn to lean on yourself for motivation and encouragement, too.

> Be sure to have fun at weekends. It makes healthier eating so much easier.

Enjoy yourself

It should be easy to enjoy yourself at weekends, during the holidays and at times of celebration. But if you're constantly worried about being tempted by too much food, it's easy to forget that the whole point of weekends and celebrations is to relax and have a good time. The meal suggestions on these pages offer plenty of great flavour and serves guaranteed to satisfy even a weekend appetite.

So this weekend, make sure you relax and have fun. Being physically active at weekends and on other days off also adds enjoyment and gives you an opportunity to relax.

Why make a point of having a good time when you're on a diet? Because the more you're able to find pleasure in food, the easier you'll find it to stay on the program, turning healthy eating into a lifelong habit.

Changes ahead: fixing your kitchen

Some of us love to cook, the rest of us don't. But cook we must, almost every day. Next week, we will be focusing on having a kitchen that is as friendly and simple as can be, so that making *ChangeOne*-style meals is child's play.

So even as you work through your strategies for weekends and celebrations, ponder your kitchen set-up. Are you overstocked with snacks and unhealthy prepared foods? Or is your pantry so bare that making a healthy, fresh meal guarantees a trip to the shops? Do you own a can of cooking spray? If yes, is it easier to get to than the butter in the refrigerator?

We think you'll be surprised at how much easier cooking healthily can be, once you make a handful of small tweaks to the way you buy and store your food and supplies.

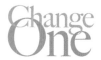

Fixing your kitchen

'On days when warmth is the most important need of the human heart', the author E.B. White once wrote, 'the kitchen is the place you can find it...' These words still hold true. Even in today's world of takeaway pizzas and microwave meals, the kitchen is still the warm heart of most households.

This week you'll transform the kitchen by tossing out the devilish foods on hand, replacing them with *ChangeOne* choices, and rearranging for easier, healthier cooking.

Why the changes? Because we don't ever want you to think of your kitchen as a place to be avoided. In *ChangeOne*, we want the kitchen to remain a place of warmth, a place that encourages happiness and healthy eating at the same time.

Stocking up

Making sure you have plenty of food in your pantry may sound like strange slimming advice. Who wants more temptations around when you're trying to eat less?

In fact, as many dieters discover, a bare cupboard can spell trouble. No matter how scant your provisions are, chances are there's a bag of potato chips from last week's party or a box of chocolates left over from a dinner party lurking somewhere. And if that's all there is to eat, guess what you're going to grab if you get hungry enough. Exactly.

By keeping plenty of healthy foods around, you'll have plenty of choices, not just for snacks but for every meal of the day. And with some clever kitchen organisation, you can make sure the best choices are in front of you when you open a cupboard or the refrigerator door. What's more, a well-stocked, well-organised kitchen can save you time and spare you frustration. With the right selection of essentials on hand, you can put together a simple and delicious meal without having to rush out to the corner shop for provisions. Many home cooks are inspired to make interesting dishes simply by opening the refrigerator, checking what's there and conjuring up tasty combinations. (You'll find three from-the-pantry recipes on pages 158, 161 and 164.)

How can your kitchen help you? To find out, answer the questions in 'Inspecting your kitchen'.

The first step in designing a diet-friendly kitchen isn't shopping; it's clearing your shelves. So get the rubbish bags ready, along with a box for items you can give away to a charity shop. It's time to get rid of food you don't want and don't need around to tempt you.

Start with the pantry. For each item, ask yourself, 'Would I eat this?' If yes, then ask, 'Should I eat this?' Keep in mind your family's tastes, of course. But don't be too generous. If you shouldn't eat it, chances are your loved ones shouldn't, either. Focus in particular on items that have sat around for more than six months.

Move to the refrigerator and freezer next. Clear out those old jars of condiments, those squishy old capsicums, those eight-day-old leftovers.

If it feels good to clear the shelves, it should. And it'll feel even better when you fill up the space with foods that are healthier, fresher and more interesting.

> Ask yourself, 'Would I eat this?' Then ask, 'Should I eat this?'

Go shopping

Your next step is a trip to the supermarket to buy essentials. Exactly what those essentials are will depend on your taste, how often you prepare meals at home and the kinds of foods your family likes. You'll find a master shopping list of pantry essentials on page 159 to use as your guide. You won't want them all, of course. The more choices you have on hand, though, the easier it will be for you to put together a *ChangeOne* meal or snack on the spur of the moment.

Before you go to the supermarket this week, keep in mind the six essential strategies for smart shopping.

1. Have a snack before you leave. You'll get some exercise pushing your trolley down the aisles and hauling bags, so go ahead and take the hunger edge off before you get there. An empty stomach can make you empty-headed. Nothing weakens will-power faster than being hungry. You've probably seen shoppers so hungry that they dip into the bag of potato chips or packet of biscuits even before they've reached the check-out. Avoid trouble by shopping after you've eaten a meal. If you absolutely have to shop for dinner on an empty stomach, help yourself to a *ChangeOne* snack before you set off for the supermarket.

2. Start with a list – and stay with it. Your local supermarket is full of temptations that can be hard to resist. Supermarkets are in the business of selling food, especially items with a big profit margin. The biggest money-makers are often the items that are prominently displayed at eye level or at the ends of aisles around the store. The chances are you'll see row after row of snack foods, potato chips, biscuits, soft drinks and highly sweetened cereals. Steer your trolley down almost any aisle and you'll be surrounded by brightly coloured packages specifically designed to entice you to grab them

Check-in

Is someone making it harder rather than easier for you to eat as you should? If you realised last week that you have a saboteur in your midst, consider taking an extra week to resolve the situation as best you can. Keep a diary and write in it every time someone says or does something that seems designed to sabotage your efforts. At the end of each day, look over your entries and devise ways to free yourself. Strategies include avoiding situations that involve food, countering negative messages with positive ones, or simply learning to ignore criticisms or unwanted enticements. The best approach sometimes is to talk about it. At other times, separating yourself from the source of trouble is a better solution. Use your judgment. Just remember: you're in charge of what you eat – no one else. Be considerate of other people's feelings, but stick to your resolution.

Change One Quiz

Inspecting your kitchen
How diet-friendly is your kitchen? There's only one way to find out.
Put on your kitchen inspector's cap and fill out the following checklist.

1. What are the first three things you see when you open the refrigerator door?

    1. _____

    2. _____

    3. _____

2. What are the first three things you see when you open the freezer?

    1. _____

    2. _____

    3. _____

3. List the three handiest snacks in your kitchen:

    1. _____

    2. _____

    3. _____

4. How many different kinds of fresh vegetables does your refrigerator or vegetable rack contain?

❑ None

❑ One or two

❑ Three or more

5. Is there a bowl of fresh fruit on the work surface?

❑ Yes

❑ No

❑ Usually, but not today

6. Do you have the makings of a *ChangeOne* dinner in your pantry and refrigerator?

❑ Yes

❑ No

❑ Usually, but not today

7. Where do you keep your shopping list?

❑ Posted on the refrigerator door or in another prominent place

❑ Tucked away somewhere in the kitchen

❑ What list?

8. Rate your collection of storage containers

❑ Plentiful, in a variety of different sizes

❑ Enough for a few leftovers

❑ What storage containers?

9. How many 'too-tempting-to-resist' foods are stored in your kitchen right now?

❑ None

❑ One or two

❑ Three or more

10. Which of the following are absent from your kitchen?

❑ Measuring spoons

❑ Kitchen scales

❑ A non-stick frying pan or wok

❑ A set of sharp knives

❑ A vegetable steamer

❑ Microwave oven

❑ Rice cooker

❑ Set of small bowls and plates

Turn to next page to add up your score.

Quiz score

Assessing your answers:

1, 2, 3. If the first items you see fit into the *ChangeOne* menu, your kitchen is in great shape. If not, your kitchen is working against you. Either get rid of the stuff you'd rather not be tempted by, or tuck it away where you have to work to get it.

4. Vegetables are free, so keep a tempting variety to make it easy to throw together a low-kilojoule meal without having to go to the shop.

5. Put a bowl of fruit out where everyone in the family can see it. That way, it will be the first place everyone goes when a snack attack strikes.

6. If you don't have the ingredients for a *ChangeOne* meal in your pantry, you should. If you do, you'll be ready for anything, from a stormy night to a surprise visitor.

7. Invest in a wipe-clean shopping list you can mount on the refrigerator. It's a great way to keep track, so you won't be caught short when you want to cook a quick and simple meal.

8. Keep plenty of storage containers handy. They're great for keeping leftovers. But you can also use them to divide up giant-sized packets into reasonably sized serves as soon as you get home.

9. Why drive yourself mad keeping foods you can't resist? Throw them out. Or put them so far out of reach that you'll have to make a really big effort to get them. One of our *ChangeOne* volunteers tucked his treat foods behind a couple of rows of wine glasses.

10. Invest in a few time-saving, slimmer-friendly kitchen tools.

and pop them into your trolley. All natural! Two for one! Giant family-size economy pack! Choose me!

To avoid the hard sell, put together a shopping list in the quiet and comfort of your own kitchen. Build your list around recipes and meal plans. Use the guide to kitchen essentials on page 159, along with our shopping strategies on page 340.

Once you get to the supermarket, stick to your list. If fresh peaches or perfectly ripe tomatoes are in season, help yourself. Don't be afraid to tweak your meal plan if you find something irresistible in the produce section or a good bargain at the fish counter. But don't reach for that jumbo-size bag of cheesy wotsits just because it's on special offer this week. If it's not on your list – or your diet – it doesn't belong in your trolley. If you don't find what you're looking for, talk to the manager. Most supermarkets are happy to stock what customers want.

3. Steer your trolley around the perimeter.

In most supermarkets, the healthiest choices are arranged around the perimeter of the store. That's where you'll find dairy products, the produce section, and the meat and fish counters. Processed foods, including those rows upon rows of brightly coloured snack food packets, are usually in the centre of the store. The more shopping you do around the perimeter, the less processed food you're likely to eat – and the more food that fits your *ChangeOne* diet.

4. Think small.

Special outlets have grown up around the notion of saving money by buying in bulk. There's nothing wrong with saving a few dollars. But if you have a hard time stopping yourself once a big bag of potato chips is open, take heed. If you're buying food to eat right away, buy a small packet – preferably a single-serve size. If you buy jumbo sizes to save money, divide them into single-serve-size, resealable plastic bags or containers as soon as you get home.

5. Read the small print.

With few exceptions, all processed and packaged foods are required to carry detailed food labels that list ingredients and nutrition information. Learning to read a label will help you shop wisely. When your goal is to lose weight, the most important number on the label is kilojoules per serve (but do look at fat and fibre too). Be sure to check how the label defines a serve size. The amount can vary widely even within the same category.

continued on page 160

Managing your food

1. Use opaque storage containers for 'treat' foods so you won't be lured by the tempting sight of the contents.
2. Put notes on food containers to remind yourself of what a sensible serve should be.
3. Decide in advance how much you plan to eat – before you open the container.
4. Attach a list of your favourite *ChangeOne* snacks to the refrigerator door as a reminder.
5. Put a date on leftovers – and a reminder on your calendar of when you plan to eat them.
6. Once a week tour your kitchen, ensuring the healthiest foods occupy the most prominent positions.
7. Keep a list of essential items that are running low so that you won't be caught unprepared.

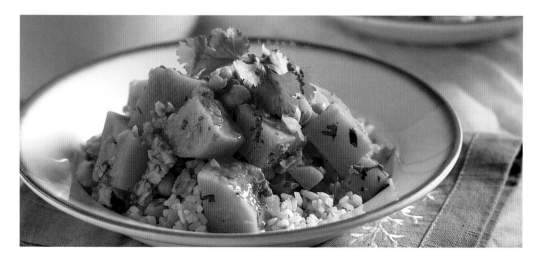

Pantry stew

Here's an easy vegetarian dish made from the pantry with a few fresh herbs and some long-life vegetables.

Easy midweek dinner

Chickpea, sweet potato and carrot stew (2 cricket balls)

1 slice garlic bread (palm-size)

1826 kJ, 436 kcal, 16 g protein, 12 g fat (2 g sat fat),
2 mg cholesterol, 66 g carbohydrate (16 g sugars),
13 g fibre, 525 mg sodium

CHICKPEA, SWEET POTATO AND CARROT STEW

Serves 4
- **1 tablespoon olive oil**
- **3 teaspoons cumin seeds**
- **3 teaspoons ground dried turmeric**
- **2 teaspoons coriander seeds**
- **1 bunch (125 g) fresh coriander, roots discarded, stems and leaves separated and finely chopped, plus 4 sprigs to garnish**
- **2 sweet potatoes (kumara) (about 800 g), peeled, cut into small chunks**
- **2 large carrots, cut into small chunks**
- **2 cloves garlic, crushed**
- **finely grated zest of 1 lemon**
- **¼ cup (60 ml) lemon juice**
- **2 cans (about 400 g each) chickpeas, rinsed and drained**

1. Heat the oil in a large deep heavy-based saucepan over medium–high heat. Add the cumin, turmeric and coriander seeds and stems. Cook for 2 minutes, or until aromatic.

2. Stir in the sweet potatoes, carrots and garlic. Sauté for 10 minutes, or until the vegetables begin to softened. Add the lemon zest, lemon juice and 2½ cups (625 ml) water. Stir, then bring to a boil. Reduce heat and simmer for 25 minutes, or until the vegetables are tender.

3. Add the chickpeas. Cook for 20 minutes, or until the chickpeas are very soft and the mixture has thickened. Serve garnished with coriander sprigs.

GARLIC BREAD

Serves 4
- **2 cloves garlic, finely chopped**
- **2 teaspoons olive oil**
- **4 slices ciabatta or French bread** (palm-size)
- **4 teaspoons grated Parmesan cheese**

1. Preheat the grill. Mix together the garlic and olive oil. Spread one-quarter of the garlic mixture on each slice of bread. Top each slice with 1 teaspoon grated Parmesan.

2. Grill for about 1 minute, or until the topping is golden brown.

Kitchen essentials

Use this guide to make sure your kitchen has all the items you'll need for healthy snacking and easy-to-cook meals. Here, we list some everyday staples – the basic provisions you should have on hand to be sure you can always put together a quick meal from a well-stocked pantry and refrigerator. For a guide to perishables – the fruits, vegetables, dairy products and meats that you use in *ChangeOne* meals – look at the shopping strategies on page 340.

In the pantry
- Oils: olive, peanut, sesame and sunflower
- Herbs, dried
- Any spices, dried
- Stock cubes or powder*: chicken or vegetable
- Flours: wholemeal, plain and self-raising
- Sugars: white and brown
- Tomatoes, canned*
- Tomato sauce*
- Tuna, canned*
- Baking powder
- Bicarbonate of soda
- Soups, canned*: mushroom, minestrone or vegetable
- Vinegars: balsamic and red wine
- Cocoa powder, unsweetened
- Cornflour
- Vanilla essence
- Cooking spray
- Peanut butter*
- Mushrooms, dried

Condiments
- Salt and pepper
- Tomato sauce or ketchup*
- Mayonnaise, reduced-fat*
- Mustards*: dijon and English
- Soy sauce
- Tabasco sauce
- Pickles and relishes*
- Capers*
- Olives*

Cereals, grains and beans
- Cereal: ready-to-eat, wholegrain
- Porridge oats
- Couscous
- Legumes canned or dried: kidney beans, chickpeas, black beans, cannellini beans, etc.
- Pasta
- Rice: brown and white
- Polenta

Snacks
- Low-fat wholemeal crackers
- Water biscuits
- Nuts, mixed
- Popcorn kernels
- Wholegrain snacks like rye or multigrain crispbread

Fruits and vegetables
- Fruit canned in juice*
- Fruit, assorted fresh
- Sultanas
- Garlic, fresh
- Onions
- Potatoes: new, baking or roasting
- Celery
- Capsicums, green or red

In the refrigerator
- Eggs
- Butter
- Cheeses for grating, such as parmesan

- Milk: skim or reduced-fat
- Yogurt, natural: low-fat or non-fat

In the freezer
- Bagels
- Breads: wholegrain and pita
- Berries and other fruit, frozen
- Fruit sorbet, frozen fruit bars or fruit juice ice blocks
- Beef or chicken bones for home-made stock
- Chicken breasts, individually portioned
- Lean chicken mince
- Lean beef mince
- Veggie burgers
- Pizza bases, frozen
- Prepared dinners: low-kilojoule, frozen
- Vegetables, frozen

Miscellaneous
- Carbonated water
- Vegetable juices
- Sugar-free drinks
- Herbs, fresh
- Tomato salsa
- Green chillies
- Tortillas, small: corn and flour

These items may need to be refrigerated after you've opened them.

The single most important change of habit for many ChangeOne volunteers was learning to shop smart.

continued from page 157

Some cereal boxes list 30 grams as a serve, for example, others 40 grams. Some foods may look as if they're low in kilojoules – until you discover that their suggested serve size would fit into a thimble.

6. Keep treats as a treat.

Don't buy high-kilojoule items you have trouble resisting once they're under your roof. Do you really want them tempting you all the time? To ensure that treats remain treats, make them part of a special occasion. When the family wants ice-cream, say, go out to get it. Don't make it too easy by keeping tubs in the freezer. Kids clamouring for biscuits? Take them to the bakery section of the supermarket and buy a couple of good ones. Decide in advance how much you'll have. One small bite of everybody else's ice-cream will let you sample a range of flavours and still keep you within the recommended serve size for dessert. A nibble or two on the kids' biscuits will satisfy your sweet tooth.

Breaking the chain

The single most important change of habit for many of our *ChangeOne* volunteers was learning to shop smart. If you prepare a lot of your meals at home, the decisions you make at the supermarket go a long way towards determining what you eat and don't eat.

To understand how important smart shopping is, visualise a chain. Scientists who study behaviour talk about chains of behaviour – individual decisions that connect like links on a chain. Let's say you give in to temptation one night and eat that whole 500 ml container of toffee pecan ice-cream in the freezer. At first, that may seem like a single impulsive act. But in reality, it's the end of a long chain of choices.

Think back to the beginning. That toffee pecan ice-cream didn't find its way into the freezer on its own, after all. The links in the chain might look something like this.

- You go shopping when you're hungry.
- Rushing out of the door, you forget to take your shopping list.
- At the store, you see a sign that says SPECIAL OFFER ICE-CREAM! Uh-oh.

continued on page 162

Quick beans and rice

A dish of beans and rice goes with just about anything – here we've served it alongside grilled chicken. You can make the dish mild or spicy.

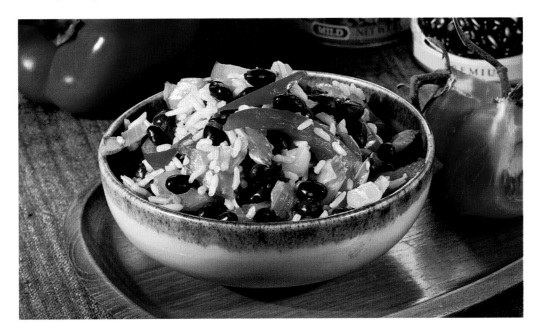

Chicken, beans and rice

Quick beans and rice (2 golf balls of rice and 1 tennis ball of beans)

1 grilled chicken fillet

Mixed green salad (unlimited) **with 1 tablespoon fat-free dressing**
(1 salad-dressing cap)

1890 kJ, 451 kcal, 41 g protein, 15 g fat (3 g sat fat), 99 mg cholesterol, 51 g carbohydrate (9 g sugars), 8 g fibre, 531 mg sodium

QUICK BEANS AND RICE

Serves 4
2 teaspoons olive oil
1 red capsicum, diced
½ medium onion, diced
1 stick celery, diced
1 clove garlic, finely chopped
1 can (about 400 g) black or red kidney beans, drained
1 tablespoon chopped green chilli or 1 teaspoon Tabasco sauce (optional)
2 cups (400 g) hot cooked brown rice

1. In a large non-stick frying pan, heat the olive oil and cook the capsicum, onion, celery and garlic for about 5 minutes, or until soft. Add the beans and chilli or Tabasco sauce, and heat until warmed.

2. Combine with the brown rice. Serve hot.

GRILLED CHICKEN FILLET

Serves 4
4 skinless chicken fillets, about 150 g each
2 teaspoons olive oil
lemon juice
freshly ground black pepper

1. Place the chicken fillets in a shallow dish in one layer. Sprinkle with the olive oil, and lemon juice and freshly ground black pepper to taste (or use your favourite marinade). Set aside for 10 minutes.

2. Cook under the grill or on a ridged cast-iron chargrill pan for 7 to 10 minutes or until cooked through, turning once.

continued from page 160

- You pop a container in your trolley.
- You pop that same container into the freezer, telling yourself you'll only have a little, and only on special occasions.

Change One Success Stories
Lots of little packets

'I know I could probably find something a little grander, or maybe a little healthier for me', says Paul Rodriquez, 'but for me, convenience matters at lot. If something takes too long to put together, I'm not going to do it.'

So after trying a variety of *ChangeOne* breakfasts during the first few weeks, Paul settled on the ultimate in convenience: individual-sized breakfast cereal packets that he can buy 30 to a box at his local bulk outlet. 'I can have one at home or take it to work if I'm running late. I don't have to worry about pouring a certain amount into a bowl.'

The same solution helped steer him away from the high-fat, high-kilojoule snacks he used to eat. Paul now buys oat-based cereal bars – 420 kilojoules each – in bulk at the same shop. He takes one or two with him to have as a snack every day.

'Maybe later I'll want to branch out and be a little more creative.

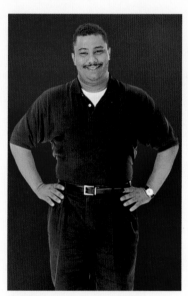

Paul Rodriquez lost 7 kg over the first five weeks on *ChangeOne*. He puts part of his success down to the convenience of the diet.

But right now it helps not to have to decide what I'm going to eat for a snack. If I get hungry, I just reach for a cereal bar. It's been great.'

After years of putting on weight, Paul was thrilled to see it beginning to slip away – 7 kilograms over the first five weeks.

- You're feeling low one night. You know you should get up and out for a walk to feel better, but …
- You're hungry. You open the refrigerator door, but because you haven't gone shopping recently there's not much there that you want.
- You open the freezer door and what's this? A container of toffee pecan ice-cream! It leaps into your hands.
- You know you should serve up just one small scoop and put the container back, but you're feeling lazy, so you open the lid and grab a spoon.
- You know you should sit down at the table and eat the ice-cream slowly, savouring every bite. But the TV is on and you wander into the sitting room. Instead of paying attention to the ice-cream, you eat while you're watching TV. The next thing you know, the whole 500 ml is gone.

How can you make sure that doesn't happen? Of course you can break the chain at any one of its links. You can get the ice-cream home, realise your mistake and give it away. Or you can pause with your spoon in hand and decide not to dig in. Yes, you can *but* if you're like most people, the best time to stop the chain is at the supermarket. You won't have to resist eating something you didn't buy. That's something to remember the next time you're tempted by something you know could overwhelm your will-power and set your diet back.

Put food in its place

Once you're back from your shopping trip, it's time to take a serious look at your kitchen. The strategy is simple. Put the healthiest choices in the most prominent places on your kitchen shelves

Help!

'I have three teenage kids, and the kitchen is filled with foods they love – potato chips, ice-cream, soft drinks and all the rest. How can I slimmer-proof my kitchen against that kind of temptation?'

You can't, not entirely, but you can certainly make your kitchen more comfortable for yourself. If your kids are tall enough, ask them to keep their snack foods on the upper shelves. Assign them a shelf out of reach for soft drinks and other sweetened beverages in the fridge. Insist on reserving the most accessible shelf in the refrigerator for foods that are on your menu. Ask the kids not to leave bowls and packets of junk food lying around. When they've finished eating, tell them to put the food away.

Don't stop there. Try to encourage the rest of the family to follow your example and eat food with fewer empty kilojoules. Yes, it can be an uphill struggle. But many kids these days are surprisingly health conscious. And since weight problems typically begin early in life, you'll be doing them a favour.

Sit down with your kids and explain why losing weight really matters to you. If your children are still young, you can nudge their tastes in the right direction. Only keep healthy choices around, and in no time, they'll be eating healthier foods without a battle. One *ChangeOne* participant regularly offered his four- and six-year-olds wholemeal bread rolls, broccoli, asparagus, grilled fish and, well, macaroni cheese. Okay, so it was lots of macaroni cheese. But getting the kids to eat broccoli and asparagus was a big victory.

Penne with tuna

Just add vegetables to these pantry staples for an easy, hearty dinner.

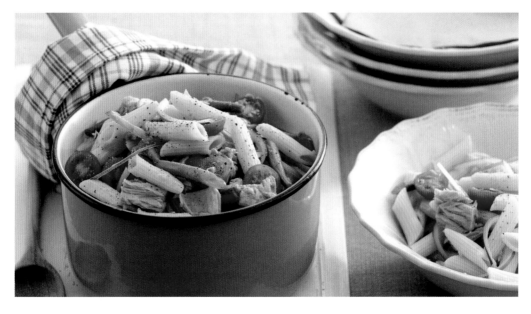

Quick tuna pasta

Penne with tuna (2 tennis balls)

Rocket salad (4 cricket balls)

1839 kJ, 439 kcal, 23 g protein, 7 g fat (1 g sat fat),
15 mg cholesterol, 69 g carbohydrate (4 g sugars),
6 g fibre, 189 mg sodium

PENNE WITH TUNA

Serves 4
375 g penne or other short pasta
150 g green beans, trimmed and halved
**1 small red onion, halved and finely
   sliced**
200 g cherry tomatoes, halved
**1 can (about 185 g) tuna in water, drained
   and flaked with a fork**
1 tablespoon extra virgin olive oil
freshly ground black pepper

1. Fill an electric kettle with water (about
1.5 l) and bring to the boil, then pour the
water into a large saucepan. Return to
boiling over high heat, add the pasta and
cook, stirring often, for 8 minutes. Add
the beans to the pan, cover and return

to the boil. Uncover and cook for a further
2 minutes, or until the pasta is al dente and
the beans are cooked.

2. Drain the pasta and beans, then return
to the saucepan. Drizzle with the oil and add
the onion, tomatoes and tuna. Season with
freshly ground black pepper, gently toss
together and serve.

ROCKET SALAD

Serves 4
400 g or more rocket tossed with
4 teaspoons olive oil
2 teaspoons balsamic vinegar, or to taste

Instead of	Try
Tuna	Canned salmon
	Cooked peeled prawns (450 g)
	Tofu
Green beans	Broccoli florets, sliced zucchini or peas
Penne	Egg noodles

and in your refrigerator. Put 'treat' foods – the items you only want to reach for now and then – out of sight, even out of reach.

Let's say you like to treat yourself to an oat and raisin biscuit from time to time. Now imagine that those biscuits are stored in a clear glass jar on the kitchen counter. Every time you come into the kitchen for a snack, they're the first thing you see. Which means every time you enter the room you've got to rely on your will-power to resist turning a special treat into an everyday occurrence.

Why put yourself through that? Imagine, instead, that you keep a bowl of fruit on the counter and a few plastic containers with carrot and celery sticks at the front and centre of the refrigerator. The biscuits are safely stored away on the very top shelf of the cupboard in a container with a lid that snaps shut – high enough that you need to get the step ladder when you want them. Suddenly it's easy to grab something low in kilojoules and rich in nutrients – an apple or a handful of carrot sticks.

By the end of this week, your kitchen will be a place where you can relax, not a place where you have to constantly feel you have to resist temptations.

Changes ahead: how am I doing?

In a typical conversation about weight loss, you talk about losing kilograms. It's the easiest, clearest measurement of how you are progressing. But is it the best measurement? Certainly not.

Once you have your kitchen under control – and it might be wise to take extra time on that task, given how important it is, and how many habits might need tweaking – we'll turn to the subject of measuring progress.

Sounds too simple to be important? Not at all. Examining yourself and assessing progress can be a tricky business. We tend to be very hard on ourselves. We forget the important criteria – energy, attitude, overall appearance – and focus on unrealistic statistical measurements. So to prepare for this examination, think again about why you really want to lose weight. Think about how you judge your success or failure. And be prepared to look at yourself in a whole new way.

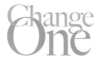

WEEK 8

How am I doing?

'How long does getting thin take?' Winnie the Pooh asks anxiously in A.A. Milne's classic children's book. You may be asking the same question just about now. You probably have other questions, too. Why do you seem to lose weight some weeks and not others? Are you making reasonable progress towards your goal? What can you do to kickstart your diet when weight loss stalls?

This week, you'll assess how you're doing and find ways to get over or around trouble spots.

To get you started, take the 'Seven weeks of progress' quiz on the opposite page. You will use its questions in this chapter to focus on the best ways to overcome your unique weight-loss challenges.

Seven weeks of progress

Circle the appropriate number in the right-hand column to track your score.

1. How do you feel about your weight-loss progress so far?

Very satisfied	3
Satisfied	2
Disappointed	1

2. How would you rate your energy level since you began *ChangeOne*?

Improved	3
About the same	2
Slumped	1

3. How would you rate your self-confidence while on *ChangeOne*?

Better	3
About the same	2
Worse	1

4. How many days last week did you closely follow the *ChangeOne* menu for breakfast, lunch, dinner and snacks?

All or most	3
About half	2
Fewer than half	1

5. How often are you able to stick to sensible serves when you eat out?

All or most of the time	3
About half the time	2
Less than half the time	1

6. Planning is crucial to dieting success; how well are you doing when it comes to planning where and what you'll eat?

Very well	3
Good	2
Only so-so	1

7. Feeling hungry can whittle away at anyone's will-power. How would you describe your experience on *ChangeOne* so far?

Hunger isn't a problem for me	3
Now and then I get so hungry that I eat more than I should	2
Hunger is a problem for me a lot of the time	1

8. How often do you experience strong cravings for specific foods (chocolate, ice-cream, salty snacks or sweets, for instance)?

Never	3
Now and then	2
Frequently	1

9. What phrase best describes your family and close friends?

Behind me 100 per cent	3
Somewhat supportive	2
Not very helpful	1

10. How would you rate your overall motivation right now?

Excellent	3
Good	2
Shaky	1

11. Stress can often get in the way when people are trying to change. How are you dealing with stress?

Very well	3
Well enough	2
Not very well	1

continued on page 168

continued from page 167

12. **Sometimes it seems there's food everywhere. How would you rate your ability to deal with temptations?**

I'm getting better at eating only if I'm hungry	3
I give in to temptation now and then, but not as much as before	2
I still have a very tough time saying no	1

13. **Where did you eat in your house during the past week?**

Kitchen and dining room only	3
In front of TV or in the bedroom	2
Both in front of TV and in the bedroom	1

14. **How many days during the past week did you fit in at least 30 minutes' worth of physical activity (walking, jogging, bicycling, gym workouts, etc)?**

All or most	3
Three or four days	2
Fewer than three	1

Quiz score

Scoring:
Add up the sum of the numbers you've circled and use the guide below to start evaluating your progress:

A score of 32–42: A big gold star for you. Put a tick beside any questions that you scored as 1 and read the corresponding tip below for advice on how to move ahead.

21–31: A little extra help could improve your chances of success. Mark the questions you scored as 1 and read the numbered tips that follow for advice.

14–20: Okay, you're having a tough time. Many people do when they first try to lose weight. Put a tick beside responses you scored as 1 and read the numbered tips in the section that follows for advice on dealing with these trouble spots.

Succeeding your way

No single diet works for everyone. Even diet experts have been surprised to find how many ways there are to succeed, or fail, at slimming. Some people like to be told exactly what to eat, then follow a strict plan. Others can take a few basic principles and handle the rest. Some people need a lot of support from family and friends. Others go it alone.

We've seen the same thing among the volunteers who tested the *ChangeOne* program. Some began to lose weight right away with breakfast; others didn't hit their stride until they changed their approach to dinner. There were people who began to lose weight as soon as they changed the way they snacked. Others had their greatest success by paying attention to hunger cues. For some, *ChangeOne* was a breeze. For others it wasn't always easy.

The quiz you completed should help to clarify the challenges you've encountered on *ChangeOne.* To help you to overcome these challenges, we'll review the questions in detail, offering tips and advice as we go, to make sure you are getting all you can out of your efforts.

1 Disappointed in your results?
Reassess your goals. Renew your commitment.
If you've lost 3.5 kilograms or more since starting *ChangeOne,* there's no reason to be disappointed. Most experts say a healthy weight-loss plan should average 450 grams–1.5 kilograms a week. Eight weeks into *ChangeOne*, in other words, you can expect to have lost 3.5–12 kilograms. Losing weight more quickly than that means losing muscle tissue along with fat – and that, in turn, could slow your metabolism and make it harder to maintain your weight loss.

If you haven't started seeing the progress you'd like, there may be several reasons. If you've significantly increased the amount of exercise you're doing, you may be losing fat but adding muscle. That's fine. In fact, it's the sure-fire way to look firmer and shapelier. But because you're trading fat for muscle, you may not see much difference on the scales. One sign that you're making progress is your waist size. If it's going down, you're changing for the better.

The most important thing now is not to get discouraged. Make a pact with yourself to take a little extra time and expend a little extra effort this coming month to reach your goal – and make sure it's realistic. (We'll be assessing goal-setting in more detail later in this chapter.)

2 Energy at a low ebb?
Have a snack – and get moving.
While people usually feel much better when slimming, some people do experience periods of fatigue when they begin to

Eating more frequently can stabilise your energy levels, and being active can actually *increase* them.

lose weight. As you take in fewer kilojoules than you burn, you force your body to turn to the energy it has stored as fat. Falling short on kilojoules can make you feel tired and even grumpy. There's another kind of fatigue, too: some people begin to get tired of dieting. You don't have to allow either kind of fatigue to derail your weight-loss program.

If you're feeling deep fatigue every day, talk to your doctor. But if you simply have occasional slumps and less energy than you used to have, try eating smaller meals more frequently during the day. Save the piece of fruit from breakfast to eat midmorning. Keep aside the sliced vegetables you brought for lunch and have them as soon as you feel hungry in the afternoon. Eating more frequently can steady your blood sugar levels so you won't feel a slump when your energy supplies run low.

Another way to combat fatigue is to fit extra physical activity into your daily schedule. It seems paradoxical to be more active when you feel you have less energy, but research shows that physical activity can actually make people feel more energetic rather than less. Activity provides a psychological boost that can banish the blues. Getting up and moving also increases your self-confidence. And regular exercise increases stamina, so you'll build reserves of energy for more activity.

3 Need a boost of self-confidence?
Celebrate small victories.

It's easy to lose confidence if you're not reaching the goals that you have set and you're not quite sure why. There's always the temptation to blame yourself. You know how it goes. You tell yourself that you just don't have the staying power, or the will-power, to lose weight. Banish those negative thoughts. You haven't failed just because the weight is proving more stubborn than you'd expected. For the moment, focus on your successes.

Here's a trick that has worked for some of our volunteers. Let's say you've managed to lose 2.5 kilograms so far, which may not sound like a lot. But the next time you're at the supermarket, grab a 2.5 kilogram bag of potatoes. Carry it around under your arm as you shop. Getting heavy? That's the amount of excess weight you used to carry around all the time. On the scales 2.5 kilograms may not seem like a lot; but when you carry that much in your arms, and think of it as the fat you've lost, you'll realise that you have already accomplished a great deal. Remember, too, that kilograms aren't the only measure of your success. Make a list of other benefits you've gained by following *ChangeOne*. Maybe your clothes feel a little more comfortable. Maybe you're moving around more easily. Maybe you're simply eating healthier meals. Whatever your successes are, celebrate them. And remember: if you can make one change, you can make two. If you can make two changes, you can make three.

4 Struggling with a particular meal?
Go back for seconds.

If you're pleased with your weight-loss progress so far but you aren't following the *ChangeOne* menu for all of your meals, don't worry. Some people find they need to make only one or two small changes – giving up chips or switching to sugar-free drinks, for example – to start losing weight. If you're not satisfied with your progress, go back to the meal that's giving you trouble and take another week to master it. Set aside enough time so that you can follow that chapter's meal plans to the letter, at least for one week. Try a few suggestions you didn't try the first time round. Too rushed to have breakfast? Get everything ready the night before. Eating too many snacks during the day? Distract yourself for a few minutes with something other than food – a short walk, an errand or a household chore.

5 Is eating out your downfall?
Zero in on serve control.

If your parents praised you for cleaning your plate, you may still have trouble leaving food behind – especially when you've paid good money for it at a restaurant. With today's serve sizes, eating out can be a major challenge. Don't let the size of the serve put down in front of you determine how much you eat. Keep in mind the *ChangeOne* serve sizes we've been visualising – a tennis ball or a pack of cards, for example – to remind yourself what a reasonable amount of food should look like. Ask the waiter to take away what you don't want to eat (and perhaps pack it so you can take it home, if local laws

If you are not satisfied, take another week to master the meal that's giving you the most trouble.

allow). Pay attention to hunger and fullness cues. And eat slowly. For more tips on navigating restaurants, turn to Week 5 (page 110).

6 Trouble planning ahead?
Make a list. Check it twice.

Knowing where your next meal is coming from is critical to successful dieting. If you're having trouble planning ahead, try this: set aside 15 minutes the night before or first thing in the morning to make a list of what you'll need to do that day to stick with *ChangeOne*. Your list might include a quick shopping trip to buy what you'll need for dinner, a reminder of when and where you plan to get some exercise during the day, or a note to book a table for lunch at a restaurant where you know you'll be able to order a sensible meal. Or look for a frozen meal that meets the *ChangeOne* guidelines. Keep several in the freezer. If you're having trouble finding time to pack a lunch, choose a meal that's quicker and easier to prepare: for instance, a macaroni salad you can make in advance and even divide up into single-serve containers.

7 Famished?
Eat more often.

It's fine to be hungry just before your next meal. But if you're getting so famished that you're tempted to give up the whole idea of losing weight, it's time for a reassessment. For starters, this week fill out a Hunger Profile for a few days (you'll find it on page 344). Keeping tabs on your appetite will highlight when you typically feel the hungriest during the day, and what you do about it. Next, begin helping yourself to a snack during those moments when you're feeling especially ravenous. Choose low-kilojoule snacks, rich in fibre, as these will fill you up without putting you over your kilojoule target. If you're still hungry after lunch or dinner, help yourself to an additional serve of vegetables. Keep an eye on your weight. If you continue to lose weight, even if it's a little more slowly than before, that's fine. You're more likely to stick to a diet that doesn't force you to go hungry. If your weight remains steady, that's fine, too. Consider attacking the other side of the kilojoule equation by increasing your activity level. Add 15 minutes of walking a day to what you already do. Keep

You're more likely to stick to a diet that does not force you to go hungry.

this in mind, as well: many of our volunteers reported feeling hungry at first, but very quickly, their appetites adjusted to *ChangeOne* serve sizes, and they began to feel perfectly satisfied. So don't give up.

8 Caving in to cravings?
Forge a new association.

Food cravings aren't hunger pangs. When you're genuinely hungry, you want food and any food will do. Food cravings are usually for something special – chocolate, ice-cream or a salty snack, for example. Sometimes food cravings are part of emotional eating. You want chocolate because it makes you feel better when you're a bit low. Food cravings can also be reactions to environmental triggers. You want ice-cream after dinner or popcorn when you get to the cinema simply because all the cues remind you of a particular food.

The solution is to teach an old dog a new trick by creating a different, healthier association. Instead of having dessert after dinner this week, get up from the table and go for a 15-minute stroll. Instead of popcorn at the cinema, bring along a *ChangeOne* snack. It won't take long before you associate cinema-going with a cereal bar or a piece of fruit instead of popcorn. For more on food triggers, emotional eating and environmental cues, look back at Week 6, which begins on page 128.

> Food cravings aren't hunger pangs. They are caused by emotional and environmental triggers.

9 Need a helping hand or a friendly word?
Ask for it.

When the going gets tough, the tough often call on friends and family. If you're not getting the support you need, take this week to explore ways to enlist help and encouragement. The best way to get what you need is to ask for it. Be specific about the kind of help you need. Ask if there's anything you can do in return. Wishing you had an eating partner? How about starting a *ChangeOne* dinner club?

And keep in mind that even though the support of people around you can smooth the way, making a lasting change is ultimately up to you. Even without the active support of family and friends, you can make it on your own. Look back to 'Talk it over' on page 149 if you need more encouragement.

10 Motivation in need of a service?
Think back to the beginning.

Once the first flush of excitement is over, it can be tough to stay motivated on any diet. Now's the time to remind yourself why you wanted to lose weight in the first place. Write down your three top reasons for starting *ChangeOne*. Below that, make a list of the benefits you've noticed so far. These may include the way you feel, the weight you've managed to lose, the way your clothes fit, or the fact that you're getting more exercise than before. Assign each one a rating of one to three stars, depending on how important it is to you. Put up your list somewhere where you'll see it every day (on the refrigerator door, for instance). By reminding yourself of the reasons you started *ChangeOne*, and the benefits you've already gained, you may strengthen your motivation.

> For a super boost, remind yourself why you wanted to lose weight in the first place.

11 Feeling frazzled?
Find a way to let off steam this week.

Being on a diet can be stressful. Add to that the other strains and stresses in your life and the combination can seem overwhelming. If stress is threatening to derail your efforts to eat a healthier diet, it's time to take action. Next week, we'll zero in on ways to deal with stress.

For this week, think of one change you can make in your life that will relieve some of the pressure. Ask someone to take on one of your responsibilities at home or in the office. Rearrange your schedule to find time to relax. During this week, experiment with different ways to let off steam. Listen to your favourite music. Sit quietly and concentrate on your breathing. Take up yoga. Go for a walk or a workout. Exercise eases stress and burns extra kilojoules as well.

12 Surrounded by temptations?
Take control of your surroundings.

If your will-power is being tested every time you turn round, it's time to take charge of your environment. At home, put those tempting occasional treats out of sight and make sure the kilojoule-efficient choices, like fruit and vegetables, are the centrepiece of your kitchen. At work, don't keep food around your desk or work area. If you find yourself in a situation where you can't remove the temptations, remove yourself – go for a walk, do an errand or choose a *ChangeOne* snack. Remember, the less you have to rely on only sheer will-power to avoid temptation, the more likely you are to reach your goals.

13 Eating all over the house?
Practise the 'one room, one chair' rule.

If you eat in practically every room of the house, you're creating associations with food everywhere you go. You'll have no escape from the urge to binge. Set aside one room and one chair for eating at home. This week, make a pact with yourself to go there for every meal and every snack you eat at home.

14 Sitting on the sidelines?
Get in on the action

You don't have to start running marathons. All you have to do is find opportunities to walk. This week, work out how to add at least 15 minutes of walking during the main part of the day – before breakfast, in the lunch hour, running errands, or an evening stroll.

Give your will-power some help. Don't make cheating easy.

Goal-setting, part II

Back in Week 4 of the *ChangeOne* program, you signed a goal-setting contract with yourself. It's time to pull it out and give it a read. Were you fair on yourself? It's all too easy to have unrealistic expectations when you decide to lose weight – especially when it's the first time you've tried it in earnest. Even people who have dieted in the past tend to set goals that are tough to reach. And when they don't reach them, they give up.

By now you're an expert on what it takes to lose weight. You also know what you're willing and able to do. This is the perfect time to take a clear, no-nonsense look at what you want to accomplish from now on. In addition, by revisiting your goals and committing yourself to them afresh, you'll take a big step towards staying motivated. To start off, fill in the questionnaire, 'How do you spell success?', opposite.

Don't mistake success for failure

Almost anyone who sets out to do it can lose weight on a diet. The crazy thing about many slimmers is that when they succeed, they often don't realise it. Many people who succeed end up thinking they've failed. The reason: they get their minds wrapped round an unattainable goal and never see what they've achieved.

You probably guessed where we're going with the questions in 'How do you spell success?' Most people have several goals in mind when they decide to lose weight. A super-ambitious goal is great if it fires you up at the start. But if it's just too ambitious, and you begin to think you'll never reach it, you can begin to feel frustrated, then disillusioned. You may actually succeed in losing a lot of weight and getting all the benefits that go with it – looking and feeling better, for instance – but if you didn't reach that goal, you may consider the diet a failure. Then you might give up, go back to your old patterns of eating and gain back all the weight you'd lost.

To test the reality of the typical slimmer's expectations, researchers at the weight-loss clinic of the University of Pennsylvania in the USA carried out a clever experiment. They asked a group of women at the start of a diet program to describe four different goals. The categories will sound familiar. We borrowed them for the quiz you just completed.

Change One Quiz

How do you spell success?

Part I

1. **How much did you weigh when you began the *ChangeOne* plan?** _____

2. **What is your dream weight?** _____

3. **Let's say you can't reach your dream weight. What's the most you can end up weighing and still be happy with the results?** _____

4. **If you can't reach your 'happy' weight, what weight would you describe as acceptable?** _____

5. **Let's say that you lose weight, but still don't reach an 'acceptable' weight. What ending weight would leave you feeling disappointed?** _____

Part II

1. **Look again at your 'dream' weight. What is the number based on?**

❑ The lowest my weight has been as an adult

❑ My ideal weight given my height

❑ What I weighed when I was at school or college

❑ The lowest weight I've been able to reach on a slimming diet

❑ A healthy weight for me according to my doctor

❑ Other
_____

2. **Numbers on the scales aren't the only way to measure the success of a diet. Besides weight, what other measures are important to you? On a scale of 1 to 5 – not important to very important – rate the following items:**

Smaller dress or trouser size	1 2 3 4 5
How my clothes feel	1 2 3 4 5
How I feel (slimmer, more energetic, more attractive)	1 2 3 4 5
Specific health measures (blood pressure, for example)	1 2 3 4 5
Overall sense of health	1 2 3 4 5

3. **If dress or trouser size is an important measure of success for you, what goal do you have in mind?**

Dress size: _____
Waist size: _____

4. **What else do you hope to achieve by slimming? On a scale of 1 to 5 – not important to very important – rate the following:**

Feeling more self-confident	1 2 3 4 5
Feeling sexier or more attractive	1 2 3 4 5
Being happier about myself and what I look like	1 2 3 4 5
Feeling more in control	1 2 3 4 5
Not being embarrassed by my weight	1 2 3 4 5
Feeling fitter	1 2 3 4 5

Answers

Congratulations! You got every question correct. There are no wrong answers to the questions we just asked; they are too personal for that. But your answers do say a lot about your expectations. For insights on your comments and some thoughts about whether you are being fair to yourself, read on.

The researchers asked the women to specify:

■ Their dream weight – the amount they would like to weigh if they could choose the ideal number.

■ Their happy weight – a number on the scale that, even if it wasn't perfect, would make them happy.

■ Their acceptable weight – the number that they'd be willing to accept if they couldn't reach either their happy weight or their dream weight.

Weight-loss goals: myth vs reality

Myth 1: Your ideal weight is what you weighed when you were first married (or at university, or before you had children...)

If you're hoping to get back to what you weighed a year or two ago, fine. There's a chance you really might get close to that weight again. But if you're talking about what you weighed 15 or 20 years ago, you might want to reconsider. Many people put on weight as they get older. And no matter how hard they try, they have a hard time being as active as they were in their early twenties. Don't live in the past. Set a weight-loss goal that's appropriate for you now.

Myth 2: Your ideal weight is as indicated by 'Your healthy weight calculator' (page 343).

It is true that height and weight are often related. Taller people weigh more than shorter ones, all things being equal. But all things are never equal. Many other factors play a role in determining what you weigh. For example, your body type: big-boned and solid, small-boned and light, or in between. Your metabolism: whether you naturally burn brightly and move a lot, or take things more slowly. The number of fat cells you have. How much your parents and other relatives weigh. The numbers listed for someone your height in this chart are just an approximation of what your healthy weight should be. Don't let a number determine if you've succeeded or failed.

Myth 3: Your ideal weight is the lowest weight you've been able to get down to in the past.

Okay, so you've lost that much weight. But the fact that you're slimming again says you gained at least some or even all of it back again. If you set a weight-loss goal that's too low for you to maintain, you'll get caught in the trap of yo-yo dieting – losing weight, gaining it back, and then trying to lose it again. The best weight goal is one you can live with.

Myth 4: The less you weigh, the healthier you'll be.

Not true. In fact, many studies show that if you're overweight, even seriously overweight, losing just 5 to 10 per cent of your current weight is all you have to do to get the bulk of the health benefits associated with weight loss: lower risks of heart disease, stroke, diabetes and even some forms of cancer.

Myth 5: If you don't reach your dream weight, you'll never be happy.

You don't believe that, do you? A number is just a number. And if it's a number that leaves you frustrated and stuck in an endless cycle of losing and gaining weight, it's time to replace it with a more reasonable one.

Don't live in the past. Set a goal for the present.

■ Their 'disappointed' weight – a number that, even though it was less than what they currently weighed, would leave them feeling disappointed.

The women in the experiment had high hopes. They began the program weighing an average of 99 kilograms. Most of them hoped to get down to 68 kilograms – a 31 kilogram loss. If they couldn't have their dream weight, most said, they'd still be happy if they got down to 70 kilograms. If all else failed, they'd accept a final weight of 74 kilograms. They'd be disappointed if they ended the diet at a weight of 82 kilograms, an average loss of 17 kilograms.

How did they do? The women in the six-month program lost an average of 16 per cent of their starting weight. Most experts would call that a success. The average weight loss at that point in a successful diet program is around 10 to 15 per cent.

Though the researchers were thrilled, the women were not. Their 'disappointed' weight would have required losing 17 per cent of their starting weight. Even the number they described as merely acceptable represented a 25 per cent drop. Their dream weight would have required a 32 per cent weight loss.

Think about it. These women did fantastically well. They lost a significant amount of weight. But without a realistic goal to measure their progress by, most of them were likely to consider the diet a failure. That's crazy.

Divide big goals into milestones

'Oh no', you're probably thinking just about now, 'this is where they tell me I can't lose as much weight as I'd like.'

Not for a second. All we want to do is urge you to make sure your first goals are achievable. Especially if you have a lot of weight you'd like to lose, it's helpful to think in terms of milestones rather than the ultimate weight you want to be. Once you reach your first milestone, you can celebrate your success, take a deep breath and head on to the next one. This approach helps you to gain confidence. It also makes it easy to measure your progress step by step, rather than in a single leap. And that's what *ChangeOne* is about.

What's a reasonable first milestone? Many experts say you should first set your sights on losing about 10 per cent of your starting weight. To calculate that number, take your weight when you started *ChangeOne* and knock the last

ChangeOne Success Stories

Looking good, feeling healthy

Concerned about future weight-related health problems, Scott Montgomery had wanted to lose weight for a long time, but he just didn't know how to get started. After reading about *ChangeOne*, he was instantly intrigued and wanted to give it a try.

'It's a very sensible approach to dieting', he says. 'So many diets require you to change your eating habits overnight, which is very tough to do. It's a slow change, which is important.'

Scott began noticing results right away. So far, he's lost 32 kilograms on *ChangeOne*. 'Before, I wore 42-waist pants. Now I wear a 36 and can almost fit into a 34.'

He has also made some health improvements. 'I have a lot more energy!' he says. 'My blood pressure and cholesterol levels are down. I don't breathe hard when I work out.'

Scott has enjoyed experimenting with the many different meal and recipe options from *ChangeOne*. He found that eating a healthy breakfast was one of the most important changes he made. 'I never ate breakfast, but I never miss it now', he says. 'It's important to jump-start your metabolism in the morning.'

Exercise has also made a big difference. 'Working out helped me drop the weight a lot faster', he says. 'But make sure that it's something you enjoy doing and that it burns kilojoules.' He also kept track of what he ate, which helped him to

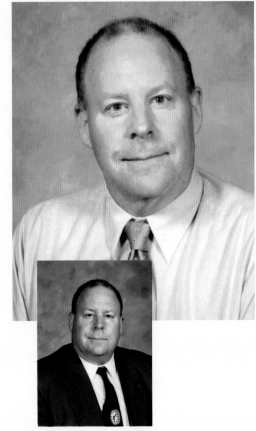

Portraits taken just one year apart show how losing 32 kg had a dramatic effect on Scott Montgomery's appearance.

avoid going off the plan during the day.

Scott is enjoying his healthy life and appreciates the compliments from people who notice his positive changes. 'People who haven't seen me for a while just stop and stare', he says. 'I have more pride in my appearance.'

number off. If you weighed 100 kilograms, for instance, 10 per cent is about 10 kilograms.

Once you reach your first milestone, allow yourself a few weeks to savour the new, slimmer you and to consolidate the changes you've made. Take the time to enjoy all of the other benefits you're likely to experience, from the way you look in the mirror to the way your clothes fit. Then, when you're ready, set the next milestone for weight loss. For many people weight loss slows as they shed kilos. That's perfectly natural. To avoid becoming discouraged, set subsequent milestones at about 5 per cent of your starting weight – 5 kilograms if you started out at 100 kilograms, for instance.

A contract with yourself

At the end of Week 4, we asked you to sign a *ChangeOne* Contract. Now that you've got a bit more experience under your belt – which you've moved up a notch or two, we hope – take a look back at your contract. How are you doing? Do the goals you set back then still seem reasonable? Are they the goals that matter most to you?

Write up a revised contract if your earlier goals aren't working for you. This is a contract with yourself, after all. You're doing what you're doing – eating better, being more active and losing weight – for your own sake, nobody else's. You decide the goals that mean the most and work the best for you. By putting them in writing, you'll be able to keep them in mind – and gauge your progress along the way.

Changes ahead: stress relief

Our lives are filled with stress, and that's not always a bad thing. Stress comes in many forms and intensity levels, and much of it is normal and healthy. The trouble comes when we are unable to balance our daily stresses with time to recuperate and relax. Next week, we will be looking at how stress can affect the way you eat and sabotage your weight-loss efforts. To prepare for the coming week, think about the ways you deal with stress. Do you turn to food when the going gets tough? Does your day allow for time to relax and enjoy life? Are excessive responsibilities and the interests of family getting in the way of caring for yourself?

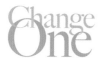

WEEK 9

Stress relief

All we're asking you to do this week is relax. That's right, relax. Take a moment or two to shake off the stresses and strains of daily life.

Sounds easy? If only it were so. Life can feel so hectic these days that even taking a minute or two off from the pressures of work and family seems impossible. While achieving a stress-free life is unlikely, you can definitely loosen the hold tension and anxiety have on you.

That's important, especially when you're trying to lose weight. A difficult period at work or tension at home has knocked many dieters off their program. Stress can rob you of the energy you need to stay focused and motivated. If the pressure gets fierce enough, you may be tempted to say 'I just can't do this' and give up your best intentions to stick to a healthier diet.

This week you'll identify sources of stress in your life and try out techniques to manage or even eliminate them.

Take the pressure off

Like a lot of people, you may find yourself reaching for something to eat when the demands get to be too much. That's hardly surprising. Just the act of eating can make you feel better when your nerves are frayed or you're feeling down. Recent studies have shown that eating – especially eating something high in carbohydrates – can lower your level of stress hormones and make you feel less frazzled.

In fact, you may feel better after eating because that's exactly what your body signals you to do: eat something. Scientists are learning that stress itself can actually trigger hunger. Here's how it works. Say you're on your way to a vital meeting. You're already running a little late when traffic comes to a sudden halt ahead of you. Instinctively, your body readies itself to do something to deal with the problem. Your brain signals your adrenal glands to churn out a variety of hormones, including the stress hormone cortisol. One of cortisol's jobs is to trigger the release of glucose and fatty acids, in case your muscles need energy.

Back in our hunter-gatherer days, this system made sense. Stress didn't take the form of traffic jams; instead, it was usually a real physical threat, such as a charging animal. A 'fight or flight' stress response evolved to prepare us, within seconds, to do battle or run away. These days, the challenges we face aren't as straightforward. Yes, you might be tempted to stop the car, get out and run the rest of the way to your meeting. If you did, you'd burn off the energy your body has made available. But chances are you sit there and smoulder until the traffic finally begins to move again.

Check-in

At about this point in *ChangeOne*, you're probably having an easier time with some of the changes you've undertaken than with others. That's no surprise. Our volunteers reported the same experience. Your natural reaction may be to target the part that's giving you the toughest time. That's great. But if you get so frustrated that you begin to wonder if it's worth the trouble, ease off. Focus on changes that feel a little bit more do-able right now. If fitting in activity every day just isn't on the cards, don't worry. Concentrate instead on reining in serves. If paying attention to hunger and fullness cues has made a big difference, focus your energy there and don't worry that you're missing breakfast now and then. Go with your strengths. Zero in on the changes that offer the biggest pay-off and concentrate on turning them into easy habits. Go easy on yourself.

Afterwards, the result of your surge in cortisol is an increase in appetite – your body's way of guaranteeing that you'll replace the energy it released in the form of glucose and fatty acids.

A flood of these hormones wouldn't pose much of a problem if it happened only now and then. But a steady tide of tense situations can keep cortisol levels high all day, making you feel hungry almost all the time. As if that's not bad enough, cortisol also triggers enzymes that activate fat cells, priming them to store energy as fat. The most susceptible fat cells are those around your middle, which are particularly sensitive to the effects of cortisol.

You see the problem. Stress makes you hungry. Eating makes you feel better. Stress promotes fat. And you put on weight instead of taking it off. Watching your efforts to lose weight come to nothing can create even more pressure and tension.

Now is the time to make sure you don't get caught in the upward spiral of stress and eating.

If stress is getting the better of you, remember that everyone's life has its hassles, small and large. One major difference between people who succeed and those who don't, psychologists say, is how we deal with everyday tribulations.

To see how well you handle stress, complete the test opposite. Your answers will help you to analyse how you cope with the challenges of daily life.

Help!

'I feel jittery and short-tempered a good part of the day. I thought it might be too much caffeine – but I have only a couple of cups of coffee in the morning, that's all. What's going on?'

Watch the caffeine you're getting from sources other than coffee. The caffeine in coffee is a stimulant, and in some people it can aggravate stress. But there's also caffeine in tea, colas, chocolate and some pain relievers – you may be getting a lot more than you realise. The best way to know if too much caffeine is a problem for you is to cut back on the amount you consume, but don't cut it out entirely. Caffeine withdrawal can cause headaches and may make you feel even more jittery and short-fused. A better bet is to begin mixing regular coffee with decaffeinated coffee. Over two or three weeks, gradually add more decaf and less of the high-octane brew. Then, if you decide to give up coffee altogether, you'll have an easier time.

Step one: solve problems that *can* be solved

The most direct way to deal with stress is to eliminate the situations that wear you down. Easier said than done? Yes, but the more irritations and annoyances you can unload, the easier it is to tackle the big issues. You may find there are plenty of petty aggravations you can fix quickly once you start paying attention to them. Every time you find

Stress test
Read each statement below and tick those that apply to you now.

❏ A lot of things in my life seem to be out of control right now.

△ I have several good friends I can call if I need to talk something through.

❏ When I'm feeling frazzled, I often have the urge to eat.

△ I'm feeling pretty good about my life right now.

❏ I often feel overwhelmed with the thought of everything that has to be done during the day.

△ I feel better once I've made a list of what I have to do.

❏ Trying to lose weight has definitely added to the pressures I feel.

❏ It's really been frustrating for me to try to find time to be more active.

△ Taking control of my diet has made me feel better about myself.

❏ Sometimes, I resent all the responsibilities I have.

△ I'm pretty good at taking problems in my stride.

❏ Lately, I notice myself losing my temper when even little things go wrong.

△ Even when things get a little crazy, I still feel as if I'm in control of what's going on in my life.

❏ If someone puts me on hold while we're talking, and then doesn't come back on the line fairly soon, it really makes me mad – angry enough to hang up sometimes.

❏ I don't have much patience with people who make mistakes.

△ Even though my life is pretty crowded, I'm good at keeping my priorities straight.

△ I don't worry much about things I can't control.

❏ When I'm under a lot of pressure, I sometimes find myself running in three different directions at once.

❏ I frequently wake up in the night feeling anxious about my life.

△ No matter how hectic the day has been, it's easy for me to relax and unwind once I get home.

❏ I wish I had more control over what happens in my life.

△ Exercise is a good way for me to let off steam.

❏ Social situations often make me nervous.

△ Frankly, I don't tend to worry about the little things – I reckon they'll take care of themselves.

Quiz score

What your score means:
How many of each colour did you tick? If you tallied more orange triangles than green squares, your responses indicate that you've got the pressures of everyday life well in hand. But if green outnumbers orange it could spell trouble – stress is hurting your life. If the numbers are about equal – and even if the orange slightly outnumber the green – be aware that a bad day could send you into the stress zone. Whatever your score, there are plenty of effective ways to keep cool, calm and collected. Just read on.

yourself getting agitated, stop and see if you can find a solution. If you can never seem to find the car keys or your specs, for instance, establish a place where you put your keys, glasses, mobile phone or whatever, every time you put them down. Post a reminder on the door, if you have to, until you get into the habit.

If preparing dinner makes your blood pressure rise because half the time you don't have on hand what you need, take the time at the weekend to stock up for the week. Make double batches of dishes that can be stored, to cut your cooking time.

If you can't stand the heat...

For people who compulsively turn to food when tensions reach boiling point, the simplest solution is to get away from the food. If there are problems at home, don't deal with them in the kitchen. Go to another room of the house to sort them out, and don't take food with you, either. Under pressure at work? Keep snacks out of easy reach. This week, remember a simple rule: don't eat to relax. Try one of these techniques first. Then wait 5 or 10 minutes to see if you're still hungry. If so, then go ahead and eat.

Not all problems are that easy to eliminate, of course. Let's say your boss gives you more work than you can manage. On top of that, you haven't been given the authority you need to do the job. That's a classic high-stress dilemma. What to do about it? The direct solution is to talk to the boss and explain the problem. Frame the talk not as a complaint ('You're asking too much of me') but as a search for solutions ('It would help me a lot if we could decide on priorities, and if I had your support for making a few key decisions').

Or say your problems are at home – tension in your marriage, for instance, or trouble with one of the children. Talking it through with the person closest to you might help you get to the source of the pressure and relieve it. Yes, it can be hard to ask for help – but it gets easier when you first ask yourself, 'What am I getting out of letting things go on the way they are?' You might explain to your spouse or kids why reducing tension in the household is so important to you now. If the problems are more complicated than the family can handle alone, consider enlisting the help of a counsellor.

Only you can know which problems you can confront directly and which you may have to learn to live with. Almost certainly there are going to be irritations (or situations that are worse than minor irritations) that you can't eliminate – at least at the moment. But you can learn to live with them without being overwhelmed by them, and without letting them derail your diet.

Step two: accept the things you can't change

There are people who can shrug off almost any setback. Others get frazzled when even the smallest things don't go right. In either case, the demands may be the same. The difference is in how you respond to them. Psychologists don't understand all the reasons people react so differently to stress. Having a sense of humour seems to help many people. Being able to distract yourself is a bonus. Just having something you really enjoy doing offers time out from the pressures of life. Playing a musical instrument, solving a crossword, reading a good book, volunteering at a charity shop – all can take your mind off problems and give you a much-needed holiday from fretting.

Naturally, you can't completely change your personality. But experts say you can change the way you react to hassles and frustrations. On the following pages we offer seven ways to cool down when your temper flares or the problems in your life feel overwhelming. This week, try out several of them. If one doesn't seem to work for you, move on to another. Your goal: to have at least two stress-busting techniques you can turn to when the pressure builds and your nerves begin to feel frazzled. Knowing how to relax and let off steam will help you stay focused and motivated.

1. Run away

One of the most effective ways to defuse stress is to run away from it – or at least walk briskly. In one study that asked 38 men and 35 women to keep diaries of activity, mood and stress, volunteers felt less anxious on days when they were physically active than on days when they didn't exercise. Even when stressful events occurred, people in the study said they felt less troubled on their physically active days.

Why? Exercise acts as an antidote to life's pressures in several ways. First, it is a simple distraction from problems. Second, it may change the chemistry of stress, blunting the effect of hormones like cortisol. Exercise has also been shown to ease the symptoms of moderate depression. That, in turn, may help people deal better with daily hassles. And then there's the fact that exercise burns kilojoules, an added bonus for slimmers. Physical activity makes it easier not only to lose weight but to keep kilojoules in balance once you go off your diet, and that's enough to make anyone feel good.

Virtually any kind of physical activity seems to relieve the effects of stress, although some researchers think that activities that involve repetitive movements – walking, running, bicycling or swimming, for instance – may offer the best defence. Many people consider swimming to be one of the most relaxing of all forms of exercise, a soothing way to literally go with the flow. Repeating a physical movement over and over again somehow seems to ease mind and body.

Think about some ways to make your work-out even more relaxing. If you're a walker, be aware of the way your arms swing from front to back and the rhythm of your gait. Repeat a soothing word or phrase each time you exhale.

An ancient cure for frayed nerves

Looking for a simple way to relax, refresh your energy, become more limber and tighten up muscles at the same time? Yoga may be the answer.

Exercise scientists have long known that yoga offers a great way to stretch, increase strength and improve balance. Now psychologists are discovering that it can also ease a troubled mind.

In one research study, Australian soldiers suffering post-traumatic stress disorder were divided into two groups. One group received five days of training in yoga and meditation. When compared to the group who did not receive the training, these soldiers had significant improvements in stress scores even six months later.

Another study conducted in Germany involved 24 women with high scores for stress, anxiety and depression. Half of the participants were asked to maintain their normal activities, while the others attended yoga practice for 90 minutes twice each week for three months. The women in the yoga group showed significant improvements in their perceived levels of stress, anxiety, depression, energy, fatigue, and general wellbeing after the three months. They also reported improved sleep, and less back pain and headaches.

Yoga is among the best stress-busters around.

How can you get started? On pages 282 to 283, 287 to 289, and 293 to 295 you'll find a simple stretching routine that includes several modified yoga poses. Aim to get started this week. If you enjoy the routine, you may want to sign up for a yoga class. Many fitness centres or yoga studios offer them. You'll also find helpful instruction for yoga in DVDs, videos and illustrated books.

If you work out on an exercise cycle or stair machine at a health club, you probably find yourself parked in front of a bank of television sets. Watching TV can prevent you from getting into the soothing rhythm of your work-out. Studies show that watching television makes people more jittery, not less. So ignore the screen. Concentrate on your breathing and the repetitive movement of your arms and legs. If the gym plays music that gets on your nerves, bring a personal stereo with headphones and your own favourite music, or use noise-blocking earplugs and enjoy a quiet interlude.

Don't watch TV when exercising. It distracts you and disrupts your rhythm.

2. Do one thing at a time

Chances are that you've heard of Type A behaviour – the hard-driven, competitive, take-no-prisoners personality type once thought to be linked not only to high levels of stress but to a greater risk of heart disease. The original term for Type A behaviour was hurry syndrome, because Type As tend to do everything faster than more relaxed personality types. Type As feel so rushed, in fact, that they often try to do three things at once. They're the ones you see eating lunch, talking on their mobile phones and driving – all at the same time.

If you find yourself falling into this behaviour, make an effort this week to focus on the task in hand. Instead of balancing your accounts while you're talking on the phone, give the phone call your full attention, then turn to the figures afterwards. If you're constantly being interrupted by phone calls while you're trying to work on something, let the answering machine take messages, instead of picking up the phone. Ring people back when the time is right for you. Do one thing at a time and you may feel your stress meter reading begin to fall.

3. Put out the fire

Anger can be stressful, especially the 'hot-headed' kind that lashes out and doesn't solve the problem that ignited it. However, never expressing your anger can be harmful to you as well. If you feel your temper about to flare, stop, take a deep breath and ask yourself three quick questions suggested by Dr Redford Williams, a researcher at Duke University in the USA, who pioneered work in anger control:

■ **Is this really important to me?** If the answer is no, leave what sparked your anger behind.

ChangeOne Success Stories

Taking control, one week at a time

Dianne Barnum was no stranger to dieting or diet books. 'I've read lots of them and tried lots of programs', says Dianne. More than 22 kilograms heavier than she wanted to be, she'd never found a plan that worked for her. When *ChangeOne* came along, she was among the first to sign up.

'Frankly, I wanted a lot from a diet. I wanted a program that was based on solid advice and the kind of foods I like. But I also wanted it to be doable. No counting kilojoules all the time. No adding up food points. I didn't want to have to spend all my time writing things down. I wanted to be able to go on living my life – going out to restaurants with my husband, socialising – and make sensible eating part of it. But I also really wanted to shed kilos.'

She did. She dropped 7.7 kilograms by the end of Week 9, and by the end of the first 12 weeks she was down 10 kilograms. But she didn't stop there: after five months on *ChangeOne* she had lost 18.2 kilograms. 'The most important thing I learned was how to take control. It's easy to blame other people or the things around you when you're overweight. But the simple truth is, you're the one who decides what you're going to put in your mouth, no one else. Once I knew that, all I needed was knowledge about smart choices and sensible serve sizes.'

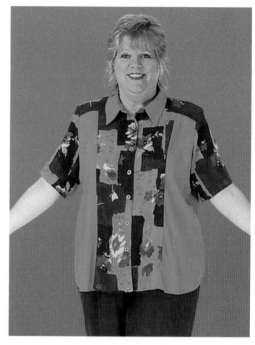

Dianne Barnum was no stranger to dieting or diet books, but *ChangeOne* was the first to offer her everything she was looking for, including favourite foods.

On course to lose the 22 kilograms she set as her goal, Dianne continues to look for one change a week to keep her on track. 'It may be something as simple as finding a new recipe I haven't tried. Or experimenting with a new food. I'll vary my exercise program just to keep it interesting. Whatever it is, every week I try to make one more change. And what a difference that's made in the way I look and feel. I look at myself in the mirror now and see a different person. And I love it.'

If the answer's yes, then ask yourself:

■ **Am I justified in being angry in this situation?** Argue the pros and cons, as if you had to make your case in court. If your answer is, 'No, I don't really have much to moan about', you're likely to feel your anger and stress dissolve. Of course the answer may be, 'Yes, darn right, that bloke nearly ran me off the road, and he's so busy talking on his mobile phone he didn't even notice it!'

Then ask yourself just one more question:

■ **Is there anything I can really do about it?** Honking the horn like mad isn't going to change anything. It's only likely to make you feel even angrier. Here's a case where the best response is to let it go, take a deep breath and keep out of the bloke's way.

If your answer to the last question is 'yes', then you're in luck. You have the chance to make a real change for the better. Let's say you're angry because one of the kids keeps leaving junk food out on the benchtop in the kitchen when you've specifically asked them to put it away. Lay down the law. Explain why you don't want junk food lying around. Get angry if you have to. Then let your anger go. If you have trouble doing that, ask yourself the first question again, but with a little twist: 'What do I get out of staying angry?' Chances are the answer is not much, except a load of unpleasant aggravation.

If all else fails, try this: imagine this is your last day alive and write down how you'd be dealing with the situation if you knew, assuming that you still have to go to work and do normal things. You're likely to find out you have better things to do than stay angry and tense.

4. Phone a friend

Of course, it sounds a little soppy. But talking to someone else – even just phoning someone to say a quick hello – does more than take your mind off your troubles. It can be powerful medicine. Swedish researchers have reported that people with a strong sense of social connection to other people were almost one-third less likely to die after having a heart attack than those who were socially isolated. Part of the reason, researchers believe, may be the stress-easing effect of close relationships. If you don't have a circle of friends to turn to, consider beginning to build one by volunteering for a local community

You'll find you can fix plenty of aggravations if you take the time to recognise them.

charity, joining a club or a church group, signing up for a departmental project at work or taking an exercise class.

5. Talk to yourself

Sometimes we're our own worst enemies. Instead of easing our pressures, we add to them by thinking in terms of absolutes, using words like 'never' or 'should' or 'always'. 'I should never have done that.' 'Things always go wrong for me.' 'I'll never be able to lose weight at this rate.' If that sounds like you, be alert to moments when you're being unreasonably hard on yourself and try to lighten up. Counter the negative messages with positive ones.

Don't be embarrassed to say them out loud if you're alone. 'Stop now. Easy there. Give it a rest.' Replace the harsh absolute with a more reasonable and forgiving thought: 'So it's going to take a while to lose the weight. So what? No one's pushing me but myself. I'm doing fine.' Take the broad view. Things don't always go wrong for you, after all.

The truth is, things occasionally go wrong for everyone. And when they do, everyone has the same challenge: to sort things out and get on with life.

6. Laugh it off

Laughter can be strong medicine, say researchers. The act of laughing eases muscle tension and relieves stress and has even been shown to lower the risk of stress-related illnesses such as heart disease.

In one study, researchers at the Center for Preventive Cardiology at the University of Maryland Medical Center in the USA tested some 300 volunteers' propensity to laugh at everyday events. The scientists found that those with a ready laugh were less likely to have heart problems than those who rarely smiled. Even among people with elevated blood pressure or cholesterol levels, the ability to laugh offered protection against heart attacks.

It's not always easy to laugh when things go wrong. But if you need a good chortle, try watching a DVD of a favourite comedy film, watching your favourite sitcom or keeping a humorous book handy - a collection of cartoons offers plenty of laughs. If you frequently fume in rush-hour traffic, try listening to an audio book – preferably a funny one.

'What do I get out of staying angry?' Chances are, not much.

7. Practise relaxation

Another proven way to ease stress is what cardiologist Dr Herbert Benson of Harvard University calls the relaxation response. According to Benson's studies, the method taps into an innate mechanism that can be used to counteract the human 'fight-or-flight' response that underlies stress. His research shows that it can lower blood pressure and ease muscle tension. Benson suggests setting aside 20 minutes and following these simple steps.

Find a quiet place where you won't be disturbed. Sit in a comfortable position, one that allows you to relax your body. Close your eyes.

Starting with your feet and progressing upwards through the body, relax your muscles. End with the muscles of your face. Take a moment to experience the feeling of being completely relaxed.

With your eyes still closed, breathe in and out through your nose, concentrating on each breath.

As you exhale, begin to repeat silently a short phrase or single word, such as 'peace' or 'calmness' or 'easy does it'. Choose a word that helps you focus your mind and banish distracting thoughts.

Continue repeating your soothing word or phrase and concentrating on breathing. The experts usually recommend doing this exercise for 10 to 15 minutes. Don't set an alarm, though, or you'll constantly be thinking about when it will go off. Have a watch or clock handy and open your eyes now and then to check the time. And don't be discouraged from doing the relaxation routine if you don't have a full 15 minutes. Even a few minutes will help.

Sit quietly for a few more minutes, first with your eyes closed and then with them open. Enjoy the way your body and mind feel.

Sounds easy? In fact, most of us have a hard time letting our minds go quiet and our bodies relax. You may need to practise relaxing a few times before you master the art. But with some practice, you'll find that you can slip quickly into relaxation and away from stress.

> Most of us have a hard time letting our minds go quiet and our bodies relax.

Making the change

Choose at least three of the strategies in this chapter to try this week. You probably already have an intuitive sense of which ones are best suited to your temperament. But don't be afraid to try at least one that sounds a little far out. You may be surprised at how effective it can be.

Whatever you choose, don't put added pressure on yourself by thinking you have to squeeze yet one more change into an already crowded schedule. Most of these stress-busting techniques take no time at all. Even those that do, like practising the relaxation response or exercising, are well worth the extra time. By taking a few minutes to relax, you may find you're more focused and productive when you get back to work. Certainly, you'll feel calmer. And that's a change that will help you stay in charge of your diet and your life.

Changes ahead: superfoods

Next week you'll find out which foods are super weight-loss winners. We'll introduce you to the 10 superfoods that will help you achieve your weight-loss goals. We also tell you how much of them you need to eat to lose weight, what their health benefits are and how to keep the menu interesting by preparing them in different ways.

ChangeOne offers the promise that you can still eat the foods you like, but after reading which foods are going to help you achieve your weight-loss goals, you'll want to make sure you add them to your list of favourites. Including one superfood in at least one meal a day is all you need to put you firmly on the path to reaching those goals.

So as you proceed through this week, think about how you can include weight-loss superfoods in your diet. The meal plans on pages 332 to 339 show you how to do that as part of a balanced eating plan.

Comfort foods for relieving stress

'Comfort food', we've come to call it – simple, satisfying, home-cooked meals that conjure relaxed family dinners in a cosy kitchen. Each of us has certain dishes we think of as comforting; usually they're recipes we associate with childhood. Sitting down to one of them can be a great way to relax and recover from a difficult day. Here's a sampler of four *ChangeOne* comfort-food meals guaranteed to transport you to easier times:

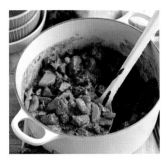

Beef stew
page 94

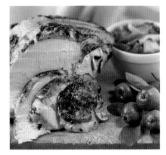

Apple-stuffed turkey breast
page 145

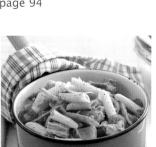

Penne with tuna
page 164

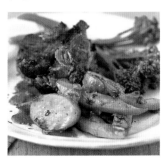

Wine-braised beef
page 320

WEEK 10

Superfoods

Yes, we know what we told you: On *ChangeOne,* you get to eat the foods you want – and we're not backing off from that promise! But we have a feeling that after reading the next few pages, you'll be eager to put these weight-loss superfoods on the menu.

Thanks to three decades of research, we now know that many delicious foods have an uncanny talent for helping people to lose weight.

The real weight-loss superfoods? Grilled salmon. Nuts. Barbecued chicken. (No kidding!) A bowl of cereal with fresh fruit. Crunchy salads and hearty soups. And that's just for starters. So this week, you can enjoy adding a *ChangeOne* superfood to at least one meal each day.

Over time, you'll learn how to make them your automatic choices when you are hungry, stressed out, pressed for time or find yourself in a situation that could encourage overeating.

ChangeOne Quiz

What's your superfood IQ?

We've studied the research, consulted the experts and come up with 10 foods that have the most significant weight-loss benefits. They're not always what you might think, so see if you can identify our superfood picks in this rather challenging quiz.

1. For weight loss and health, research shows that the best drink to have most frequently is:

a. Milk b. Fruit juice
c. Water d. Coffee

2. Which of the following breakfast foods was proven in a recent study to keep dieters feeling fuller longer?

a. Eggs b. Wholemeal toast
c. Porridge d. Cornflakes

3. Which snack helped dieters who ate it daily lose 18 per cent more weight than those who skipped it?

a. Pretzels b. Chocolate
c. Nuts d. Ice blocks

4. One study showed that starting lunch with this item reduced kilojoule consumption at the meal by an average of 420 kilojoules. Which item is it?

a. A bowl of soup b. A glass of water
c. A piece of fruit d. A garden salad

5. Another study showed that dieters who ate this food four or more times a week ended up losing more weight than those who didn't eat it. Which food is it?

a. Soup b. Prawns
c. Chocolate d. An apple

6. Yet another study showed that women who frequently consumed this common breakfast food weighed 4 kilograms less on average than those who generally didn't eat it. Which is it?

a. Grapefruit b. Orange juice
c. A banana d. Cereal

7. Which of the following common entrée choices has the fewest kilojoules per gram?

a. Prawns b. Lean pork
c. Chicken breast d. Salmon

8. Which of these protein superstars is so versatile that it plays a starring role in every popular weight-loss plan?

a. Tofu b. Pinto Beans
c. Chicken d. Lean beef

9. This low-kilojoule food is eaten for breakfast and dessert; added to sauces, dips and spreads; and even mixed into drinks. Plus, it contains nutrients that may speed up weight loss. Which is it?

a. Ricotta cheese b. Yogurt
c. Peanut butter d. Apricot jam

10. Of 20 foods that are commonly known to have the most fibre per gram, 15 are in the same category. What is this super-fibre food family?

a. Cereals b. Squashes
c. Beans d. Root vegetables

Quiz score

Welcome to the *ChangeOne* superfoods list! Each of the questions above corresponds to the superfood of the same number on the following pages. Be prepared for some surprises!

Food to the rescue

Our superfood highlights are a lot like superheroes – each has a unique power. In this case, those powers help you lose kilos and keep them off. Some superfoods trick your tummy into telling your brain that you're already full. Others are rich and satisfying to eat, yet their kilojoules don't seem to end up as fat on your hips. Some reset your appetite so you'll want to eat less at your next meal without even thinking about it. Others fine-tune your metabolism so your body burns energy effectively throughout the day.

To earn their places on our exclusive list, though, these foods had to do even more. Each offers special health benefits, such as protecting against heart attack and diabetes, boosting immunity, lifting your energy level or guarding your vision, for example. In summary, here's what we looked for.

■ **Easier weight loss** We scoured medical research to find out if any foods can truly help you lose more weight. There are plenty of products that claim to melt kilos, but could any healthy foods make the same claim? What we found surprised us. A snack food long seen as decadent – nuts – actually seems to help people shed weight. Nuts don't melt fat, of course, but they may help by making you feel so full that you simply eat less later on. Researchers are also looking into the possibility that their tough cell walls may block fat absorption.

■ **More satisfaction** Nothing torpedoes a new weight-loss plan quicker than cravings. You know how that goes. You eat a Spartan breakfast and a sensible lunch, and at 3 o'clock your body seems to propel you, as if in a dream, to the shop for a doughnut and a soft drink. That's the power of a craving – most often triggered by a slump in blood sugar. We've found the foods that keep blood sugar low and steady – thanks to fibre and protein – freeing you from the roller coaster of up-and-down blood sugar levels and a surge of food cravings.

■ **Better metabolic burn** Lots of research suggests that some foods, such as green tea and chilli pepper, turn up your body's fat-burning ability, but those effects are small or short-lived. We've found something better: low-glycemic foods. Low-glycemic foods not only keep blood sugar low, they also keep your metabolism higher while you're on a weight-loss program, according to amazing research from a major children's hospital in the US. You can actually burn 340 kilojoules more each day when you eat these foods as compared with eating a typical low-fat diet. The result is more weight loss, fewer cravings and more energy.

■ **Easier kilojoule reduction** We also wanted to help you eliminate unnecessary kilojoules from your daily eating plan without sacrificing pleasure or nutrition. We found the ultimate weapons – a first-course strategy proven to cut mealtime kilojoules and an age-old beverage that could save you hundreds of kilojoules a day. And we promise that there's no need to ever feel hungry.

For each of our fabulous 10, you'll discover their full range of benefits, some ideas for getting more into your diet and guidelines on how much to eat for optimal effect.

SUPER FOOD Water

Good old H_2O has all the right stuff: zero kilojoules, low cost and convenience (just turn on the tap or grab the bottled version, available virtually everywhere). Sipping this precious fluid instead of one soft drink per day can save you a whopping 5880 kilojoules in a week – and may help you lose 9.5 kilograms in a year, according to nutrition experts from the University of North Carolina in the US.

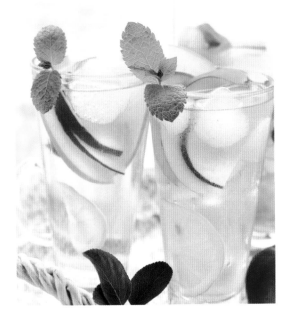

That's why water is the official *ChangeOne* beverage – we recommend that you make it your drink of choice at meals and between meals, too. (Read on for ways to add flavour without adding sugar and kilojoules.)

What about reports that Australians and New Zealanders are concerned about water and dehydration? Well, you don't see people falling over in the streets from thirst, but that's a silly way to look at it, isn't it? The truth is, only a third of us are getting enough for optimal health and weight.

And while foods, especially fruits and vegetables, do contribute to your daily fluid quota (as do tea and coffee), nothing keeps you hydrated as well as a refreshing glass of water. Unfortunately, though, we need to explode two myths right now: Water *won't* flush fat out of your fat cells, and it *won't* raise your metabolism enough to burn significant kilojoules, even if it's icy cold.

Water's real weight-loss power is that it keeps you hydrated, which can help you avoid overeating caused by 'stealth thirst' – unrecognised signals of early dehydration. It can help you feel full. It's the perfect substitute for snacks eaten out of habit, boredom or anxiety. And it can help you cut hundreds of kilojoules a day if you substitute it for sweetened soft drinks.

Health bonus: An American study found that drinking more than five glasses a day could significantly reduce the risk of a heart attack. Researchers think that staying hydrated may cut the risk of developing heart-threatening blood clots.

Keep it interesting: Sip soda water with a splash of orange or grape juice; add a slice of lemon, lime or even cucumber to ice-cold water; or make iced (or hot) herbal or green tea.

Get this much: How much do you need each day? About 30 millilitres of water for every 900 grams of body weight. This is just enough to replace fluid lost naturally through breathing, sweating and trips to the toilet. If you weigh around 70 kilograms, that's almost 2.5 litres. How many glasses is that? It depends on your glass! A teacup or small juice glass often holds just 175 millilitres; a large drinking glass could hold 700 millilitres. We suggest you find out how much liquid your everyday drinking glasses hold (surprisingly, few people know), then figure out how many glasses you need to drink. Probably, it'll be between 6 and 10.

Important note for exercisers: Drink an extra cup or two of water before you get started and again afterwards – and sip half a cup every 15 to 20 minutes during your work-out.

Hold the salt

Carbonated water goes by many names, including club soda, soda water, mineral water and effervescent water. While the names are often used interchangeably, the drinks aren't all the same. In particular, some types of carbonated water have salt added to them. Check the bottle's label and skip those. Too much salt in your diet can cause several health problems, including high blood pressure.

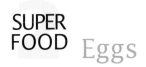
Eggs

Satiety – that satisfied, filled-up feeling that makes snacking and overeating the furthest thing from your mind – may be as close as the dozen eggs nestled in a carton in your fridge. In one US study, women who ate two eggs, toast and jam for breakfast reported feeling fuller longer than those who started the day with just a small tub of yogurt and a bagel slathered with cream cheese.

The egg eaters went on to eat 29 per cent fewer kilojoules at lunch and nearly 1150 fewer kilojoules for the entire day. (The bagel group had 8547 kilojoules each, while the egg group ate 7396 apiece.) And how's this for staying power: they even ate less the following day, according to researchers from the Rochester Center for Obesity Research in Michigan, USA. 'Eggs have a 50 per cent greater satiety index than breakfast cereal or bread', the researchers concluded.

Why? Ah, there's the mystery. It could be the balance of protein and fat or some other combination of nutrients in eggs. Experts aren't certain. They do know that eggs ranked in the same 'super-satisfying' category as cheese, meat and fish in a study of the 'fullness factor' of foods conducted at the University of Sydney in Australia.

Health bonus: Egg yolks are rich in lutein, an anti-oxidant that protects the eyes against age-related macular degeneration, a leading cause of blindness.

Keep it interesting: Store hard-boiled eggs in the fridge (they'll keep for up to five days), then slice some into your lunch or dinner salad to create a fast main course or chop and mix with low-fat mayonnaise and a little relish for egg salad (add a sprinkle of curry powder for an exotic taste). Make a two-egg omelette with a dusting of grated cheese and some roasted vegetables for lunch or dinner.

Get this much: If you're not at risk for heart disease, it's okay to have a few eggs a week.

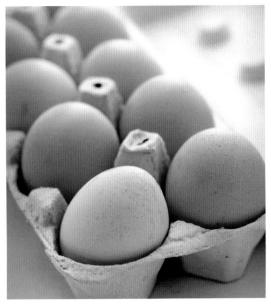

SUPER FOOD Nuts

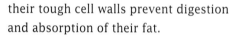

At last, there's no reason to feel guilty about thoroughly enjoying a handful of nuts. Once a forbidden food, these little nuggets are packed with good fats, protein, fibre and a variety of important vitamins and minerals. We've known this for a while, but the 'new' news is that a growing stack of studies shows that nuts can help you lose weight, too.

In one eye-opening US study, people who snacked daily on oily, salty peanuts for eight weeks didn't gain weight. Why? Scientists suspect that those who munched nuts were so satisfied by the fat, protein and fibre that they ate less at meals and other snack times without even knowing it. There were even signs that the nuts boosted metabolism ever so slightly. And in another amazing study, dieters who added almonds to their daily menus lost 18 per cent more weight than those who didn't, according to researchers in California, USA. The magic? Almonds, like other nuts, make you feel full. And, researchers say, it's possible that

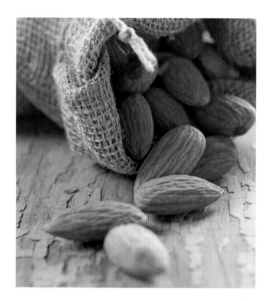

their tough cell walls prevent digestion and absorption of their fat.

Health bonus: Good fats in nuts can prevent blood clots, promote a healthy heartbeat and lower blood pressure.

Keep it interesting: Pack nuts in single-serving portions in small plastic bags as soon as you buy them. Buy several varieties and combine them. That way, you'll get a wider variety of beneficial nutrients and fats.

Get this much: As we mentioned earlier in this book, eating nuts requires a little planning – otherwise, this weight-loss strategy becomes a kilojoule binge. If you snack on nuts or plan to add some to a salad, we suggest counting out your allotment, then putting the container away before you start munching. A handful of nuts provides about 840 kilojoules; a 420-kilojoule serving equals about 8 walnut halves, 15 almonds, 10 to 12 cashews, 5 or 6 macadamia nuts, 10 pecans, 12 hazelnuts or 1 tablespoon of peanut butter.

Change One Success Stories

Inspiring others, one step at a time

Susan Miller started *ChangeOne* with hopes of losing some weight. 'I needed to change how I ate, and I really liked the concept of changing only one thing at a time', she says.

A busy mother of four kids under the age of 11, Susan liked the fact that she could be on *ChangeOne* without preparing special foods or altering her entire diet overnight. 'There's a clear understanding of how much I can eat, and I learned to do this with the foods I normally eat', says the 36 year old. 'I was able to do it at my own pace and be successful in baby steps.'

Now 70 centimetres smaller overall and 19.5 kilograms lighter, Susan is thrilled with her progress. And she's using her success and enthusiasm for the program to help and inspire others, encouraging them to get started and stick with it. 'I've seen women from all walks of life be successful at this – if we can, you can, too!' she tells them.

Susan has passed healthy *ChangeOne* tips on to her kids, too. 'I've learned what the correct portion sizes are, which I can now teach to my children.'

Susan is also a lot more active than she used to be. 'I am willing to try new things since I don't feel "conspicuous" anymore', she says.

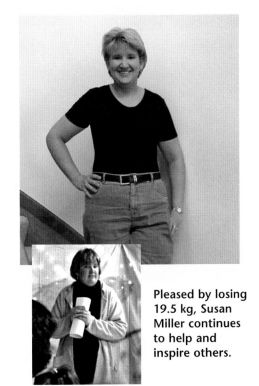

Pleased by losing 19.5 kg, Susan Miller continues to help and inspire others.

Another bonus is the frequent compliments she gets from friends and family. 'They're thrilled for me!' she says. 'It's fun to see someone I haven't seen for months and hear comments on how good I'm looking.'

Susan continues to lose weight, and she plans to stick with her new healthy habits. 'I really love *ChangeOne*', she says. 'It's not a diet – it's a way to relearn how to eat.'

SUPER FOOD

Salad

Mixed greens could be a surprisingly simple secret to successful weight loss. In one US study, researchers found that dieters who started their lunch with a large serve of mixed salad vegetables with fat-free dressing ended up eating 420 fewer kilojoules overall at that meal. How can this be?

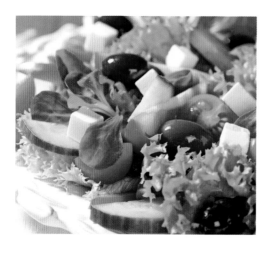

Well, salads made with ingredients such as lettuce, carrots, tomatoes and capsicums are big in size (and flavour) but low in kilojoules, due in part to their high fibre and water content. Dieters in the study filled up on 3 cups of salad – nearly a day's worth of nutritious vegetables – without eating more than 150 precious kilojoules. Just as important, the salad influenced how much they ate for the rest of their meal. Crunchy vegetables are satisfying to munch, and their chunky shapes and sizes stretch your tummy so that receptors on the stomach lining send 'all full' messages back to your brain. For added benefits, sprinkle your salad with vinegar. Nutritionists found that this condiment can cut blood sugar by up to 30 per cent after a meal – an effect that could reduce cravings later in the day. And a few drops of quality olive oil will help your body absorb additional nutrients from the salad without adding too many extra kilojoules. Avoid sugary commercial 'fat-free' dressings.

Health bonus: Eating more vegetables will increase your daily intake of fibre and anti-oxidants, cutting your risk of heart disease, diabetes and even some cancers.

Keep it interesting: Try baby spinach, radicchio, mixed field greens, spicy rocket or other interesting lettuces from the produce section. Each has a unique character.

Get this much: We suggest starting lunch or dinner every day with a high-volume, low-kilojoule salad, especially if you tend to overeat. Start with a generous bed of lettuce, top with chopped tomatoes, grated or sliced carrots, cucumber rounds, and cut-up green or red capsicums, and add any of these: shredded zucchini, sliced raw mushrooms, onions, fresh herbs (basil is heavenly), celery, fennel or shredded cabbage. Top with a splash of vinegar and a little olive oil, or about one capful of low-fat dressing.

SUPER FOOD Soup

When you're craving comfort food but want to avoid fat and kilojoule minefields such as macaroni and cheese or lasagna, simply start with soup. Hot, hearty and a pleasure to eat, soup's a proven weight-loss star that fills you up so you eat fewer kilojoules during the rest of the meal. In one study of 500 dieters, those who ate soup at least four times a week lost more weight than those who ate it less often. The study's researchers found that eating a 840-kilojoule bowl of soup before lunch was more satisfying than having the same number of kilojoules from biscuits and cheese – and helped dieters eat less during their meals. Why? Think quantity: the biscuits and cheese appetiser was less than 55 grams; the soup was a satisfying 550 grams.

Soup is a great alternative to salad as a first course during cold weather, it makes a satisfying snack and it's the perfect kilojoule-control secret weapon when dining out. Just look for stock-based soups made without cream and with little butter or fat. At home, start from scratch or use fat-free, salt-reduced stock. Add fresh or frozen vegetables to first-course soups. For a main course, pump up the nutrition and kilojoules with lean meat, beans and even whole grain noodles, barley or lentils. For a low-kilojoule 'cream' soup, puree the liquid and half of the cooked vegetables in a blender, then add to the rest of the vegetables. Top with plain yogurt instead of sour cream.

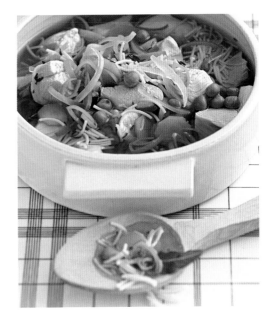

Health bonus: Extra fluid, plus healthy vegetables that help protect your heart and cut the risk of cancer.

Keep it interesting: Add extra frozen vegetables to canned chicken vegetable soup; toss fresh or dried herbs into soup to intensify the flavour (try dill in chicken soup, rosemary in white bean soup and coriander in black bean soup); keep salt-reduced stocks and canned beans on hand as the base for quick, healthy soups.

Get this much: We suggest having soup on days when you don't feel like starting lunch or dinner with a salad. Strive for at least four bowls per week.

SUPER FOOD Cereal

Healthy, filling and ready to eat, high-fibre cereal is the perfect weight-loss food any time of day. Studies show it can rein in your appetite and work as a clever, low-kilojoule 'meal replacement' at lunch or dinner.

Instead of thinking of that cereal in the pantry as breakfast food, see it in a new light – as a snack, quick lunch or even the centrepiece of a healthy dinner. In a US study of 109 overweight women and men, those who ate cereal with fruit and fat-free milk for breakfast and either lunch or dinner cut 2688 kilojoules from their total daily energy intake. Another survey found that women who had cereal several times a week weighed 4 kilograms less than those who generally bypassed it.

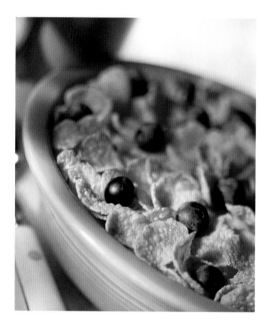

The key is picking the right cereal – one with at least 3 grams of fibre per serving. More is even better: Some cereals pack 6 to 11 grams per serving. When 60 women and men had high-fibre porridge for breakfast instead of low-fibre cornflakes, they ate 30 per cent fewer kilojoules at lunch, according to researchers from the New York Obesity Research Center at St. Luke's–Roosevelt Hospital. The appetite-control factor seems to be all that satisfying fibre, which helps you stay full for longer.

It's also important to look for cereals with low sugar content. That way, you'll control kilojoules and stay off the blood-sugar roller coaster that leads to mid-morning munchies and food cravings. (A British study found that eating sugary cereal actually led to overeating at lunch.)

Health bonus: Another US study found that participants who ate wholegrain cereals every day were 17 per cent less likely to die over the next several years from any cause, and 20 per cent less likely to die from cardiovascular disease, than those who rarely or never ate those cereals.

Keep it interesting: Mix it up – the smart way. *ChangeOne* suggests setting aside an extra 5 to 10 minutes on your next shopping trip to explore the cereal aisle. Make sure to take your reading glasses so you can compare the fibre and sugar content of various brands. (You'll find this important data on the Nutrition Facts label on the side or back of the box.) And remember to look up high and down low; the healthy cereals are often relegated to inconvenient spots on the shelves.

Get this much: Make cereal your breakfast default – have a bowl any morning you don't have the time or desire to prepare something fancier. If controlling portions is a challenge at lunch or dinner, we recommend having cereal once in a while instead. Set a goal of eating at least five bowls of high-fibre cereal a week.

SUPER FOOD Seafood

Prawns grilled with pineapple and red capsicums. Poached oysters on a bed of freshly sautéed spinach. A gorgeous salmon fillet dressed up with yogurt-dill sauce. If there's a glamour food on your list of sensible, weight-pampering edibles, it should be seafood, no doubt about it.

Low in kilojoules, high in flavour, loaded with satisfying protein and packed with nutrients (including zinc and omega-3 fatty acids), seafood can control your appetite without clogging your arteries with bad fats. Even better, seafood can feel like a splurge – a lifesaver when you're faced with challenges to sensible eating, such as navigating a party buffet or ordering at a restaurant. So get the prawns – 110 grams has just 500 kilojoules.

Or go for the salmon. An 85-gram piece has just 840 kilojoules and more than a half day's quota of omega-3 fatty acids. Go ahead, enjoy the grilled scallops! One hundred and ten grams has just 635 kilojoules and delivers omega-3's and lots of vitamin B_{12}.

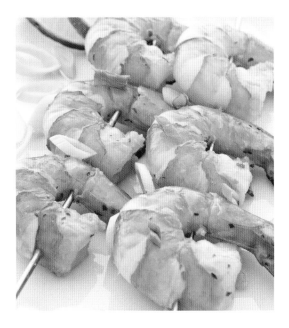

Want proof that seafood is a smart choice for dieters? In a four-month Australian study, fish was shown to help volunteers lose weight and reduce the risk of heart disease and diabetes.

Health bonus: The good fats in seafood protect your heart by helping blood to flow smoothly. B vitamins help to lower levels of homocysteine, a compound in the blood associated with clogged arteries and heart attack, and may also protect against colon cancer.

Keep it interesting: Check out the single-serving foil packs of salmon and prawns in the canned fish section of your supermarket. And don't overlook canned salmon – it's an inexpensive, widely available form of wild salmon that's great in a quiche. Or mix it with low-fat mayonnaise to make salmon salad. Other ways to expand your seafood habit include having a bowl of steamed New Zealand or Tasmanian mussels once or twice a week, a grilled fish fillet every Tuesday evening and an occasional bowl of pasta topped with scallops sautéed with vegetables, olive oil and wine.

Get this much: Try for at least two fish meals per week. That should be easy: a tuna sandwich for lunch one day, sautéed prawns for dinner another day and you're there.

SUPER FOOD Chicken

This consistent favourite earned a gold star as a *ChangeOne* superfood for purely pragmatic reasons: There's no high-protein, low-fat weight-loss food that's more convenient.

True, chicken earns top marks in almost every weight-loss plan in existence – low carb or high carb, low fat or high protein – and it's no wonder. A roasted, skinless breast weighs in with just 500 to 590 kilojoules and is packed with all the satisfaction of protein and less than half the fat of a trimmed, top-grade T-bone steak. But how satisfying is chicken? When French researchers gave either a high-protein chicken snack or a high-carb rice pudding snack to some volunteers, the carb group got hungry as quickly as another group of volunteers who had no snack. But the chicken snackers reported feeling full for nearly an hour longer than all the others.

We believe that any protein-rich, low-fat food will help you stay satisfied longer, but here's why we love chicken. You can find it, ready to eat, virtually everywhere. Need a snack on the road? Pull up to the drive-through window for a grilled chicken sandwich, no sauce. Toss the bun and eat the chicken for a hunger-stopping 670-kilojoule snack. Need a quick dinner? Go for grilled chicken (on a bun or, even better, on a salad) at your local fast-food outlet. Planning menus for a busy week? Grab pre-cooked chicken breast slices or quick-cooking boneless, skinless breasts at the supermarket. And stock up on those smoked chicken breasts from the supermarket, which are great on bread, in a salad or in soup.

One warning you are already familiar with is to avoid eating the skin, which is absolutely loaded with kilojoules.

Health bonus: Chicken is packed with B vitamins, important for energy production and heart health.

Keep it interesting: Chicken's mild flavour makes it a blank canvas for culinary adventure. Top with chopped coriander, a squirt of lime juice and a dollop of reduced-fat sour cream; barbecue in teriyaki sauce; cut into small cubes and mix with chopped garlic, basil and balsamic vinegar or with tarragon, grapes and low-fat mayonnaise. Yum!

Get this much: Hungry? Think chicken. There's no reason not to have it several times a week.

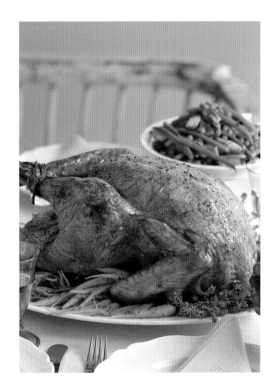

SUPER FOOD Yogurt

Most dairy products can help you to slim down faster if you're on a low-kilojoule program like *ChangeOne.* But only one can be part of breakfast or dessert, a vegetable dip or a base for a sauce, or the main ingredient in a drink. We're talking about versatile, hardworking yogurt – and it's better than ever.

Yogurt is a powerhouse full of calcium and protein, factors that may help explain studies showing that dairy foods can turbo-charge your weight-loss efforts. But unlike milk or cheese, yogurt's smooth, pudding-like consistency allows it to go places other dairy products fear to tread. You can blend fat-free yogurt with fruit and ice for a low-kilojoule smoothie; freeze it in the tub, then whirl it in a food processor with fresh or frozen fruit for an intensely flavoured dessert; or mix it with herbs and lemon juice to make a dressing or dip. You can also drain out the liquid to create a cheese-like spread that tastes great on bagels.

Buy yogurt plain rather than flavoured and in large containers rather than in small tubs. Flavoured yogurts are very high in

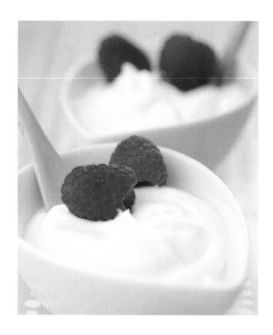

sugar and kilojoules; buying plain yogurt and adding a teaspoon of fruit jam – and perhaps some nuts, sultanas or high-fibre cereal – is almost always healthier.

Health bonus: Look for yogurt that contains live, active cultures. These probiotics – the name scientists use for beneficial bacteria – can help digestion and may fight infection.

Keep it interesting: Layer yogurt, fresh fruit and muesli in wine glasses or dessert cups for a healthy dessert. Or add a fruity liqueur, such as Amaretto, to yogurt for a simple yet wonderful sauce for cakes or fresh fruit.

Have this much: Work yogurt into your meals several times a week. Have some every day if you don't like milk or are lactose intolerant. (Enzymes in yogurt convert milk sugars into a digestible form that's perfect for you.)

SUPER FOOD 10 Beans

Whether black or pinto, kidney or cannellini, beans may seem too starchy or too heavy in carbohydrates to get top billing as superfoods. But these morsels have what weight-loss experts call satiety power. Thanks to their blend of fibre and protein, beans keep your blood sugar low and steady. Eating beans will help you to feel full longer and avoid blood sugar swings that lead to impulse buys at a vending machine or snack bar.

In fact, no other natural, ready-to-eat food has more fibre than beans. Here's the bottom line: a cup of black beans, kidney beans, peas (actually members of the bean, or legume, family), or even baked beans delivers 15 to 17 grams of fibre – half of your daily needs. And all that fibre, plus protein, means that beans are ranked low on the glycemic index (GI) – a measure of a food's impact on blood sugar.

Low-GI foods are weight-loss heroes because they raise blood sugar levels only slightly. A growing number of studies show that building your meals around low-glycemic choices can help you to lose weight faster and more easily – without feeling so tired or hungry. That means you'll be more likely to stick with your plan longer and have the energy to get up and get active – another key component of success on the *ChangeOne* plan.

Health bonus: Beans contain two kinds of fibre: insoluble, which helps your gastrointestinal system eliminate waste products more quickly; and soluble, which forms a gel in your intestines that helps lower levels of 'bad' LDL cholesterol by whisking cholesterol out of your body. Research shows that eating a cup of beans per day can reduce cholesterol by up to 10 per cent in just six weeks.

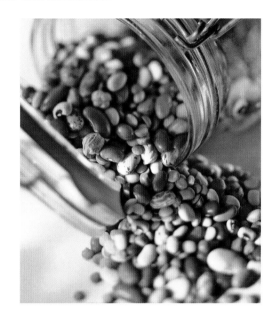

Keep it interesting: Use beans in place of meat in soups and on salads. Toss together a quick lunch salad with rinsed, canned beans (½ cup is enough), fat-free dressing and chopped vegetables. Experiment with bean salads – as simple as white beans with olive oil, red wine vinegar and parsley, or as bold as black beans with Eastern spices and chillies. The variations are endless.

Get this much: Aim to include beans as part of a meal five times a week.

ChangeOne superfoods

Just to recap, here are the 10 superfoods to choose for easier weight loss, to keep you feeling satisfied longer, increase your metabolism and help you to reduce your overall kilojoule intake.

- Water
- Eggs
- Nuts
- Salad
- Soup
- Cereal
- Seafood
- Chicken
- Yogurt
- Beans

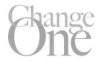

Keeping
on track

By now you're hitting your stride. You're dropping the weight. The success feels great.

Still, as almost any successful slimmer will tell you, it's crucially important to keep track. The pressures that surround us to eat, eat, eat don't go away. Serve sizes have a way of creeping up again. Plans to go for a walk or to the gym can fall by the wayside. And the weight has a way of sneaking back on.

This week you'll devise your own 'first-alert' program to sound an alarm if you begin to get off track.

We're not suggesting that you measure every bowl of cereal or serve of pasta for the rest of your life. But staying alert to how you're feeling, what you're doing and how much you're eating will have a huge payoff in terms of weight, health and self-confidence.

Schedule a regular check-up

With the end of the 12-week program just around the corner, it's time to take a moment to celebrate how far you've come. If you're like some of our *ChangeOne* volunteers, you may have already reached your target weight. Now it's time to make the transition from a diet that contains fewer kilojoules than you need to one that balances the kilojoules you take in with those you expend.

If you began *ChangeOne* hoping to lose a significant amount of weight, you may still have some kilograms to go. There's nothing wrong with that. Slow and steady is the best kind of progress to make.

Wherever you are on the path towards your desired weight, start planning ahead. Almost any diet program will help you to lose weight during the first few months. That's the easy part. If you've slimmed before, you know that the real trick is maintaining weight loss – which requires turning the healthy changes you've made into lifelong habits.

Sadly, that's where most diet plans falter. We've already mentioned one pitfall. Call it the on/off trap. People go on a diet to lose weight and go off it once they've shed the kilograms. And unfortunately, that means going right back to the way they were eating before. You know how the story ends. Before long, the numbers on the scales are right back where they started.

There's another pitfall – one that's probably more common. As people near their desired weight, they begin to ease up a little. They stop paying as much attention to portion sizes. They splurge a little more often on rich desserts. They eat an extra snack. Nothing dramatic. But if they're not watching, all those little nibbles can add up to a kilo here, a kilo there. Before they know it, they've regained a chunk of the weight they had worked so hard to lose.

Regaining a couple of kilos shouldn't be a big deal. You already know what it takes to lose them. But losing ground can spell real trouble, for several reasons. If you begin to gain weight again, it's natural to assume that the diet isn't working and to abandon it completely. Worse, it's easy to

Almost any diet will help you to lose weight in the short term; the trick is maintaining the weight loss for good.

If your weight is holding steady, get on with your life. Forget about being on a diet for a while.

begin to blame yourself, to begin replaying all kinds of negative messages in your head. 'I'm a failure.' 'I'll never be able to lose the weight and keep it off.' 'I'm destined to be fat.' Losing weight only to gain it back can also make you reluctant to try again. And if you do try again, you might feel discouraged from the start.

Thanks to the careful work you've already put in, this is far less likely to happen to you than it is for people on fad diets. You've learned that eating can be a pleasure, not something you have to fear. You've seen that you can lose weight and keep it off eating regular food that you actually like to eat. You've discovered on *ChangeOne* that you can eat sensible serves without feeling hungry. Along the way, you've seen which changes have made the biggest difference for you and your weight-loss goals.

Now, all it takes to ensure that weight creep doesn't happen is keeping a watchful eye not only on your weight but also on how your clothes are fitting, how you feel, how much exercise you're getting and what's on the menu.

The *ChangeOne* first-alert program

Starting this week, you'll take a few minutes once a week to do a quick self check-up. Record your weight. Estimate how much physical activity you were able to fit in. Rate your overall mood. And jot down any issues or problems you may be dealing with. That's all. To make your weekly check-ups even easier, we've included a *ChangeOne* Progress log on page 347, which will allow you to track four weeks of check-ups. At the end of these four weeks, chart how your weight has changed on the simple graph at the bottom of the form.

We're not suggesting you fill in weight-monitoring forms for the rest of your life. We do recommend logging your progress report for the next two months. If your weight is holding steady and you're comfortable with how things are going, tuck the form away in a drawer and get on with your life. Celebrate your success. Forget about dieting for a while.

But don't forget to pay attention. Weigh yourself at least once a week. Keep track of how your clothes feel or where you notch your belt. Be alert to your moods. If you notice a change for the worse – if your favourite trousers feel a bit snug, or you've added more than a kilo, or you're going through a rocky period at home – take a copy of the progress report and start filling it in weekly.

Remember, most people's weight goes up or down a little, week by week. You probably already know how much yours normally varies. If your weight creeps up by more than 2 kilograms from your desired weight, it's time to take some action. Don't panic. You haven't failed. And don't even think of giving up. You already know exactly what it takes to lose weight. You've done it before and you can do it again.

Add up your activity

Keeping track of exercise isn't as easy as watching kilos on the bathroom scales. True, if you go to a gym, it's easy to write on the calendar each time you go and how long you spend. But if your exercise consists of doing everyday physical activities – taking the stairs, walking from the far end of the car park, doing a circuit round the block during the advertisements on TV – keeping track can be trickier.

One approach is to fill out an activity log, adding up the time you spend every day. (Remember, we've included one for you on page 346.) Your goal should be to add up at least 30 minutes of moderately intense activity daily.

Another simple strategy, which many people come to love, is to use a pedometer to measure your activity. Pedometers are devices about the size of a pager that can be attached to your belt or waistband. The device automatically records your every step by means of a mechanical pendulum that moves back and forth with each step you take.

The simplest devices, the ones that just count steps, are the most economical buy. Pedometers can also compute the distance you've covered, and some models can estimate how many kilojoules you've burned. A basic pedometer will be reasonably cheap (around $30) and can be found at most sporting goods shops, or you can buy one online. See page 261 for more on pedometers.

Using a pedometer

For the first few days, wear the pedometer but go about your usual day. At the end of each day, jot down how many steps you took. This number will serve as your baseline. Then set your first goal for increasing the amount of walking you do. Without doing anything but going about your daily business, you're likely to take about 3000 steps. Doing

A pedometer is easy to use, inexpensive and invaluable for keeping track of daily activity.

roughly 15 minutes of walking, stair climbing and other basic activities will add about 2000 steps. The optimum goal for weight maintenance is around 12,000 to 15,000 steps a day.

Not quite there yet? Don't worry. Scale up your weekly goals gradually. Start by aiming for 7000 steps one week, for example, and the next week, increase your goal to 9000 steps. Like many people, you may find that using a pedometer will give you a little push when you need it. From time to time, check to see how many steps you've taken. If you're barely up to 2000 steps when lunch time rolls round, it's time to consider a brisk walk after you eat. If you've finished dinner and are still falling short on steps, take a walk.

If you decide to use a pedometer, include the average number of steps you take on your progress log. That way you'll see your increasing activity at a glance.

Monitor your moods

While you're keeping tabs on your weight, how your clothes feel and how much exercise you get, also be alert to how you feel – happy, sad, enthusiastic, discouraged, busy, bored, really keen, whatever. You'll find a place on the progress log to record what your overall moods were like during the previous week.

Staying in touch with the way you feel is important for several reasons that you probably already recognise. For a lot of people, stress, boredom, loneliness or feeling a bit down are triggers for eating. If you're among such emotional eaters, keeping tabs on your mental state will help you to recognise patterns. You may see that the times your weight tends to creep back up again are times when you're bored.

The solution could be as simple as making a list of three or four things to do when you're feeling that way that don't involve eating. Let's say that stress at work is your downfall; every time you start ticking the 'stressed out' box on your progress report, you can almost be sure your weight will start to climb. Simply recognising that familiar pattern can help you to change it – by finding healthier ways than eating to deal with stress, for instance, or by increasing the time you spend exercising.

Like many people, you may discover that by paying attention to your moods, you begin to notice early warning signs of trouble. You realise that you're beginning to feel worn down by stress before you become completely frazzled. You notice the first signs of feeling blue. That awareness can help you to remedy the situation before you find yourself in a deep slump. Get together with friends. Schedule time to do something you really love. Set aside extra time for exercise, which is a proven mood-booster. Treat yourself to something special. Turn your attention back to healthy eating as a way to avoid overeating when you're feeling discouraged or down.

The truth is, everyone feels down now and then. And sometimes, there's a perfectly good reason for it. Money problems. Relationship difficulties. A bad day at work. But some people find their moods dragged down again and again when there's no good reason, except for a feeling of low self-esteem. Given the emphasis our society places on being thin, it's not surprising that many people who struggle with their weight end up having a negative image of their bodies. The problem is compounded by a tendency on the part of many people to think that being overweight is the result of a lack of willpower. It's not that at all. It's the result of a complicated mix of factors, from genes and family eating patterns to body type and psychology.

So here's another reason for monitoring your moods: if your mental state tends to sour because you have feelings of low self-esteem, take time to remind yourself of how far you've come in making healthful changes. Remember that not all of us are magazine-cover models. Healthy bodies vary tremendously in terms of size and shape. Don't get into the trap of wanting the 'perfect' body. Concentrate, instead, on achieving a healthy, reasonable weight for who you are.

Easier said than done? Of course it is. Sometimes feelings of low self-esteem reach all the way back into childhood, making them very hard to change on your own. Feeling sad or hopeless can be no more than a passing emotion for some people, but for others it can be a symptom of clinical depression. If you find yourself struggling without success against feelings of sadness, hopelessness or low self-esteem, talk to your doctor or a counsellor. There is a proven link between depression and weight gain. And studies show that treating depression can help people get down to a healthy weight.

Forget the 'perfect' body myth; focus on a healthy, smart weight that suits you.

Taking action

If you notice your weight beginning to climb – or your clothes or belts beginning to feel tight – search for the reason. You may know exactly why you're gaining weight. Stress at work, perhaps, or weeks of holiday party-going. Maybe you've just stopped being as strict as you were before about keeping serves under control. The notes you've jotted down should tell you a lot. To do more in-depth troubleshooting, fill in the diagnostic checklist below.

Once you've focused on the specific problem, take action. Just don't try to change everything all at once. That's what *ChangeOne* is all about: focusing on one thing at a time.

Having trouble with a specific meal? Check back to the first four weeks of *ChangeOne* for advice on how to take control of breakfast, lunch, dinner or snacks. Eating when you're not really hungry? Make a conscious effort to stop and ask yourself whether you're actually hungry, or just responding to an emotional or environmental cue. If you're

Diagnostic checklist

When the first-alert warning bell rings, use this checklist to identify the sources of trouble. ☺ A smile means you're doing just fine. ☺ A neutral expression means you're holding your own. ☹ A frown – well, you know what that means. After you're done, look over the categories that scored a frown. These are the areas on which to focus your troubleshooting efforts.

	☺	☺	☹	FOR HELP:
Breakfast				Page 24
Lunch				Page 40
Snacks				Page 60
Dinner				Page 84
Eating out				Page 110
Stress relief				Page 182
Resisting pressures to eat				Page 131
Emotional eating				Page 68
Environmental cues				Page 64
Self-esteem				Page 217
Stopping when I'm satisfied				Page 86
Motivation				Page 174

not genuinely hungry, distract yourself by doing something else – take a walk, phone a friend or help yourself to a bit of sugar-free gum. Feeling just plain overwhelmed? Your best bet may be that tried-and-true jumpstart for any weight-loss plan: the food diary. Keep one for a week. Even if you make no other change, chances are you'll see progress on the scales.

Keeping track is so important that we urge you to set aside a particular time each week to conduct your *ChangeOne* check-up. Use whatever day and time works best for you. Just try to stick to it. Put a reminder on your calendar. Post your weekly check-up form on the refrigerator or beside your desk – wherever it's easy to find. If you have a tendency to misplace pieces of paper, record your weight and activity level in a couple of places – in a notebook or on your phone or computer, for instance. That way you'll have a back-up. And if all is going well, then you'll have several reminders to tell yourself, 'Congratulations! Be proud!' By learning the *ChangeOne* way to lose weight, you have changed yourself in untold wonderful ways.

Changes ahead: *ChangeOne*...for life!

Next week is devoted to making sure that eating remains the pleasure it's meant to be. We're going to invite you to shake things up a little – to try something new in the kitchen or at your favourite restaurant. Treat yourself to something special. Have a blast – you deserve it. Over these past 11 weeks you've made some important changes. You've worked hard. Next week is your chance to celebrate those changes and to look ahead at how to make them last a lifetime.

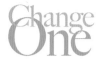

ChangeOne ...for life!

It's celebration time. Put down the book for a moment, take a deep breath and let out a victory yell.

Congratulations! You've reached week 12, the end of the formal *ChangeOne* program. Over the past three months you've done something remarkable. You've redirected your life. You've changed the way you eat. More importantly, you've proved to yourself that you are in control of your life and your eating habits. You've learned that small steps in the right direction can add up to a giant leap forward.

So in this final week, have fun. We want you to be playful with food. At least twice, try a new combination or flavour you've never had before.

Why? Because the enemy of weight loss is boredom. Eat the same way all the time, under tight restrictions, and you'll soon rebel. And if *ChangeOne* is about anything, it's about a love and respect for good food.

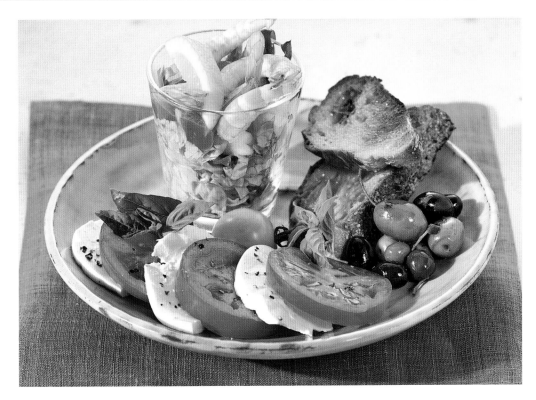

Satisfying starters

Little dishes let you enjoy a diversity of flavours and textures as well as cuisines. Plus it's a fun and social way to eat. Here is an Italian approach, with other ideas.

ANTIPASTO DINNER

100 g cooked peeled king or tiger prawns (4 to 6) on shredded lettuce (unlimited) topped with 1 tablespoon tomato and chilli relish or salsa (1 salad-dressing cap)

25 g mozzarella cheese (coaster), sliced, interleaved with sliced tomatoes (unlimited), sprinkled with fresh basil leaves and balsamic vinegar

10 herbed olives

1 slice crusty bread

1694 kJ, 405 kcal, 37 g protein, 11 g fat (4 g sat fat), 185 mg cholesterol, 35 g carbohydrate (8 g sugars), 5 g fibre, 1403 mg sodium

Reward yourself

Give yourself a big pat on the back, but don't stop there. Reward yourself with something special. Make it a complete extravagance, if you want – a weekend away or a night on the town. Or choose something that reinforces your changes, your results and the new you: running shoes, a new bicycle, a series of yoga classes or an appealing cookbook.

Why make so much of rewarding yourself? Because too often we tend to be aware of when we've fallen short while taking our progress for granted. Even people who have lost weight and made healthy changes in the way they live may think they've failed – unless they celebrate their successes.

Acknowledging a job well done also serves as a way to mark those milestones we talked about before – the small steps you take that add up to a giant leap forward. Unless you celebrate them, you may not even be aware of how far you've come. And when we say celebrate your victories, we mean all of them. Some of your successes are easy to recognise. Eating a healthier breakfast, for instance. Or taming runaway snacks. But other positive changes may be more subtle, though more important: discovering that you can decide on a plan of action and stick to it; gaining self-confidence; banishing a negative voice that used to sound in your head; learning that you can slip for a day or two and get yourself back on track.

Small steps? Yes. But each one makes an important difference. This week take a little time to think about the obvious and not-so-obvious ways you've changed over the past 12 weeks. Give yourself kudos for every positive step you've taken.

Isn't it the people around us who are supposed to give us a pat on the back when we've done something wonderful? Of course it is. And maybe you're lucky enough to have someone who does give you accolades for what you've accomplished. Still, it's important to give yourself kudos too. As helpful as other people can be, changing for the better is up to you and you alone. You have to be your own best friend. By giving yourself rewards, you also reinforce positive self-messages – a powerful antidote against those discouraging words that can sometimes repeat in your ears.

> Pat yourself on the back. Why? Because too often we emphasise our failures over our successes.

Trust your instincts

Yes, you'll celebrate your success this week. But – and no surprise here – we've included a lesson for the long haul. Relax. It's a lesson you'll love.

First, a question: what's the toughest challenge slimmers face when it comes to keeping the weight off? When we asked our *ChangeOne* volunteers at the beginning of the program, many of them listed things like 'snacks', 'hunger' and 'a sweet tooth'. Most people starting a diet think that the hardest part will be resisting temptation. In fact, as we mentioned at the start, the biggest pitfall slimmers face over the long haul is something more basic: boredom.

People often give up on a diet because it gets tiresome. They grow weary of counting kilojoules or consulting long lists of foods they should or shouldn't eat. They rebel against the rules that most diets include.

We've made sure *ChangeOne* doesn't include a lot of strict rules, banned foods, complex theories and other guidelines that tie you up. A healthy diet, after all, is about eating sensible servings of tasty and (mostly) nutritious food. You can eat just about anything, but if your choice is rich in kilojoules, you'll have to watch serve size. It's that simple.

But even with the varied *ChangeOne* menus, you could be feeling restless. So this week shake things up a little. Prepare something you haven't eaten before. Get creative in the kitchen and concoct a dish of your own inspiration. Treat yourself to a meal at a restaurant that you've been eager to try. Forget the *ChangeOne* meal plans for a whole day. In fact, take a whole week off, if you want. Imagine that you're taking the stabilisers off and going for a solo spin after 12 weeks of learning how to keep your balance. This week, let the principles of *ChangeOne* guide you as you venture out on your own.

To get started, turn the page for a party of festive ideas; then go to page 226 for more eating adventures.

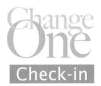

Check-in

Think back to where you were when you started *ChangeOne*. Write a list of the positive changes you've made since then. Put a star beside the changes that have had the biggest impact on how you look and feel. And then, as we suggested back in Week 11, put the list away, out of sight and out of mind. But remember where you put it. If, in the coming months, you find yourself getting off track, look back at it. You'll find listed there the changes that work best for you. Zero in on them and chances are you'll be able to take control of your weight again.

Taco party

Tacos migrated from Mexico and are one of the most popular dishes in the USA. They're enjoyed in Australia and New Zealand, too. A taco party is a lot of fun. Set out a buffet of oven-warmed tortillas, vegetables, low-fat cheese and hot grilled or fried meats or beans; everyone creates their own taco. A serve is two tacos, filled as below.

How to build a taco:

1. Line your plate with a small corn or flour tortilla (wrap).

2. Top with a golf ball-size serve of cooked lean minced beef, minced or shredded poultry, or refried beans (see below) or drained canned kidney beans.

3. Add 2 tablespoons (2 thumbs) grated reduced-fat cheese, guacamole and/or sliced olives.

4. Cover with vegetables – chopped tomatoes, diced red and green capsicums, shredded lettuce, sliced red onion, chopped green chillies (all unlimited) – and some mild or spicy salsa.

5. Fold over and eat.

For flour tortilla and beef taco: 888 kJ, 212 kcal, 20 g protein, 10 g fat (5 g sat fat), 44 mg cholesterol, 11 g carbohydrate (6 g sugars), 3 g fibre, 353 mg sodium

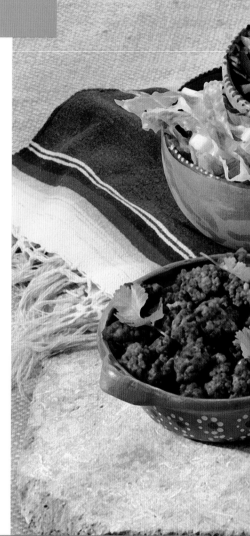

TIPS ON CHEESE

Mexican 'queso fresco' is a soft white cheese with a mild flavour. Mild cheddar is a good substitute. Tilsit-, gouda- or edam-style cheeses are also good in tacos. To save kilojoules, look for reduced-fat varieties of cheese, and when grating use the fine holes. Chilling the cheese well before grating helps to prevent it from falling apart. To save time, you can grate a large quantity of cheese and then freeze; it doesn't need to be thawed if you are going to heat it in a savoury crumble or sauce.

ABOUT REFRIED BEANS

Traditional Mexican refried beans, 'frijoles refritos', are made by frying onion and sometimes garlic in lard, then adding cooked pinto beans and mashing. Make your own lower-fat, lower-kilojoule version by cooking a chopped onion, and an optional crushed clove of garlic, in a non-stick frying pan with 1 teaspoon of olive oil and a splash of chicken or vegetable stock until the onion is soft. Add a 400 g can of pinto or other beans, drained and rinsed, and 1 teaspoon ground cumin, and mash the beans as they heat. Season with salt and pepper to taste.

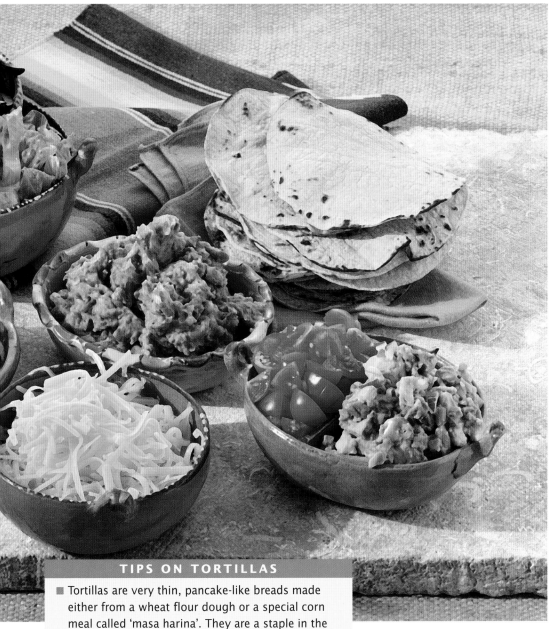

TIPS ON TORTILLAS

■ Tortillas are very thin, pancake-like breads made either from a wheat flour dough or a special corn meal called 'masa harina'. They are a staple in the Central American diet.

■ Corn tortillas have fewer kilojoules than flour tortillas because they are made with no added fat. And corn tortillas can deliver another bonus: when they're made with lime, a calcium compound, they can provide some of this important mineral.

■ Crisp taco shells, which can be bought in most supermarkets, are corn tortillas that are folded over in half and usually fried. This gives them about double the kilojoule count of a soft tortilla.

HEALTH TIP

Keep your total serve of cheese, guacamole and olives to no more than 4 tablespoons. While they add great flavour and texture to tacos, all are high in fat and kilojoules.

Try something new

How you shake things up this week is up to you. If you've been sitting down to cereal every morning, see how a yogurt parfait appeals. If you've been packing a sandwich, take yourself out for lunch this week. If you've been following the *ChangeOne* dinner meal plans scrupulously, pull a couple of cookbooks down from your kitchen shelf and try out a few new recipes. Do a *ChangeOne* makeover of an old family standard. Give a big dinner party. Take the family out for a lavish meal. Splurge on a dessert you haven't had for a while. Visit the local farmer's market or greengrocer and take home something you've never tasted before.

Giving yourself a little freedom doesn't mean putting your progress at risk. Last week you set up a first-alert system that will warn you if you get off track. Trust it. And trust your instincts to guide you. Gaining the confidence to make healthy choices is one of the measures of lasting success.

Not sure how to add some excitement to your menu? Here are a few suggestions.

Make your own salad bar
For dinner one night this week, put together a salad bar and invite everyone to create their own salads. Include at least two vegetables that may not usually be on the menu – artichoke hearts, beetroot or radicchio, for instance. Warm up a loaf of crusty wholegrain bread. For dessert scoop up a selection of colourful sorbets topped with berries.

Give a taco party
Tacos are a terrific way to serve up lots of vegetables – tomatoes, lettuce, capsicums and onions – and provide a balanced meal all in one. Put out the components and let

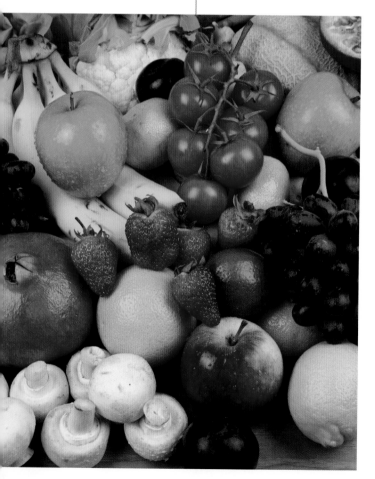

Colourful vegetables and fruits add pleasure to your plate. Look out for unusual varieties in specialist shops or markets and experiment with new recipes and flavour combinations.

everyone make up their own. Help yourself to as much salsa as you want and don't forget to dab on some guacamole, or even a little reduced-fat sour cream if you like. Look back to pages 224 to 225 for more ideas.

Slim down an old family friend

Choose a favourite casserole or bake, a pasta dish or pilaf, and give it a boost by adding an extra serve of vegetables. Broccoli is terrific in a fish pie. Chickpeas make a great addition to spaghetti with tomato sauce. A good helping of green capsicums can liven up, and lighten up, a bowl of chilli con carne. If fish fingers are a family favourite, serve them with a fresh tomato and onion salsa for added zest. If it reassures you, use a kilojoule counter to add up the precise number of kilojoules in your adapted meal.

Order a feast of starters and side dishes

Choose a restaurant with a wide range of good starters and vegetable accompaniments and have a feast. Share the dishes with your companions and you can order practically every small dish on the menu without having to worry about serve sizes. Start with only as many dishes as there are people at the table. If you're still hungry, order more. Steer clear of fried foods, of course, and make sure the selection includes plenty of vegetables.

Go fish

Chances are your local fishmonger features at least a few kinds of fish you haven't tried. Be adventurous and cook something that's new for you – fresh sardines, king prawns or swordfish, for instance. Choose a recipe that involves baking or grilling, not frying. There are many low-kilojoule ways to give fish a burst of exotic flavour. For example, many supermarkets now offer spices that create the 'blackened' flavour of American Cajun cooking. A scattering of capers can also turn a plain piece of fish into something special. And spicy salsas are also terrific on fish.

Bake bread

As a special treat, take the time this weekend to bake your own loaf of bread. If you don't have a bread machine, consider investing in one. They make bread-making simple and easy. Pop the ingredients in, and then run a couple of errands.

Try some exotic foods and find out how delicious they are.

New ways with tuna

Most tuna sandwiches are dripping with mayonnaise. But why settle for such a high-fat, ordinary-tasting treatment? In this alternative version, lemon juice, natural yogurt and dijon mustard add moisture and a great tangy flavour.

VARIATIONS

■ For Italian tuna filling, replace the yogurt and mayonnaise with fat-free Italian dressing.

■ For Indian tuna filling, add 1 tsp curry powder and 2 tbsp sultanas.

■ For a Mexican tuna filling, replace the gherkin and mustard with 2 tbsp salsa.

TUNA SALAD SANDWICH

Serves 2

1 can (about 200 g) tuna in water or brine, drained
1 tablespoon lemon juice
1 tablespoon natural yogurt or yogurt cheese (see page 31)
1 tablespoon low-fat mayonnaise
1 tablespoon finely diced gherkin
1 teaspoon dijon mustard
1 tablespoon finely chopped onion
4 slices wholemeal bread
lettuce and sliced tomato

1. Place the tuna in a small bowl and add the lemon juice, yogurt, mayonnaise, gherkin, mustard and onion. Mix well.

2. Line 2 bread slices with lettuce and tomato. Top each with half of the tuna mixture. Top with the other slices of bread.

Per sandwich: 1029 kJ, 246 kcal, 26 g protein, 5 g fat (2 g sat fat), 46 mg cholesterol, 23 g carbohydrate (4 g sugars), 4 g fibre, 832 mg sodium

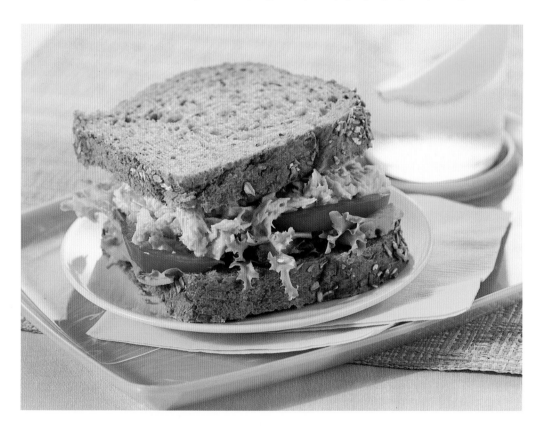

By the time you're back, the house will be filled with the delicious aroma of freshly baked bread. Choose recipes that include wholemeal flour and, even better, whole grains, such as oats.

Have a pizza extravaganza

Most supermarkets sell ready-made pizza bases that make preparing a home-made pizza fast and easy. Get your family or friends together for a make-it-yourself pizza party. A few tips: include at least two vegetable toppings. Use grated cheese rather than slices and you'll get more coverage with less cheese. For even more flavour, try smoked mozzarella instead of plain.

Make a new acquaintance

It's easy to get into a rut, especially when you go shopping. This week look a little more closely at things you've been overlooking in the greengrocer's and take home a vegetable you haven't tried before. More and more supermarkets carry once-exotic leafy greens like radicchio and Swiss chard. Have you tried bulb fennel? It's delicious roasted. What about fresh artichokes? Or grilled parsnips? If these vegetables are new to you, you're missing out on some of the world's great taste treats. This week, add a new vegetable to your repertoire.

Create your own signature pasta

No other food is as versatile as pasta. It comes in a wide range of shapes and colours, from familiar spaghetti to fun shapes like wagon wheels, bow ties, shells, corkscrews, tubes and ears. And the ingredients that show up in pasta sauces are virtually limitless – from prawns or chicken to olives, artichokes, basil, diced ripe tomatoes, broad beans, tuna, onion, capers, mushrooms, cauliflower, broccoli, parmesan... you get the idea. Put on your chef's hat this week and create your own pasta masterpiece.

Pasta shapes and sauces

Everyone knows spaghetti goes with tomato-based sauces, but what about other noodles? In general, the lighter and more delicate the pasta is, the lighter its sauce should be. Thicker or textured pastas go best with heavier and chunkier sauces. Here are some pairings of pasta shapes and sauces.

- Angel hair (thin spaghetti): light sauces.
- Conchigliette (shells): cheese-flavoured sauces, and also good in soups.
- Farfalle (bow ties): chunky sauces.
- Fettuccine (ribbons): creamy sauces, tomato-based sauces.
- Fusilli (twisted spaghetti), ravioli (stuffed pillows), rotelle (spirals): chunky, tomato-based sauces.
- Macaroni (elbows), ziti and penne (hollow tubes): meat sauces.
- Tortellini (small stuffed dumplings): tomato-based sauces.

The food diary revisited

We've touted the virtues of keeping a food diary more than once. It's a great way to see exactly what you eat and to spot patterns that may be scuttling your efforts to lose weight, such as skipping breakfast or going overboard on snacks. From time to time while you're slimming, filling out a food diary for a day or two is also an effective way to make sure you're still on track.

As you strike out on your own this week, consider keeping a food diary for at least a couple of days. Don't let the diary stop you being adventurous. Use the form on page 345 to record what you eat – that's all. When the week is done, you can look back at the form to see how you did setting out on your own. Check on how the number of low-kilojoule dishes compared to the number of higher-kilojoule treats. Do a quick count of the average servings of vegetables. Use what you learn from the food diary to fine-tune your food choices over the coming weeks. If you noticed yourself falling short on foods from the greengrocer, for instance, make a point of including a salad at dinner or a piece of fruit with lunch.

Travel the world

A rich variety of ethnic restaurants, from Italian and French to Indian and Chinese, and the increasing availability of ingredients from round the world, have created interest in the cuisines of different countries. This week, sample a cuisine you haven't tried before, or at least one you don't eat very often. If you're an avid home cook, try preparing something from a cuisine you've never explored before. Search your library or local bookshop for a cookery book that specialises in a particular cuisine. Chances are you'll discover a world of new and exciting ingredients and tastes.

Find a new move

While you're shaking things up this week in the food department, do the same for exercise. The goal is simple: find something fun to do that you haven't done before, something that involves being active. Take the plunge at the local swimming pool. Go for a ramble in a nearby park. Take the kids boating. Go power-walking around the park. If you haven't given the *ChangeOne* fitness routine from pages 278–295 a try, do it this week. And make it fun.

Don't hide behind the excuse that you don't like being active. Don't tell us that you don't like strolling in a beautiful park, playing ball with the kids, walking past the shop windows in a shopping centre or bicycling in some attractive area. It's this kind of activity that makes life worth living.

Strike a balance

ChangeOne is based on the simple principle that, to lose weight, you have to take in fewer kilojoules than you burn. To maintain your weight, you have to balance kilojoules in and kilojoules out.

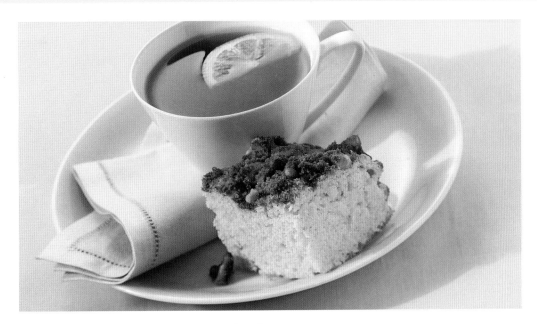

Cake for breakfast

Instead of croissants, brioche, Danish pastries and other high-kilojoule indulgences, try this lightened version of a moist, crumble-topped cake to start the day.

STREUSEL CAKE

Serves 16

¼ cup (50 g) soft light brown sugar
2 tablespoons chopped walnuts
1 teaspoon ground cinnamon
2 cups (280 g) plus 2 tablespoons
self-raising flour
60 g unsalted butter, melted
⅔ cup (130 g) caster sugar
½ teaspoon salt
1 egg
1 cup (250 ml) buttermilk
1 teaspoon grated lemon zest

1. Preheat the oven to 200°C. Spray a 23 cm square baking tin with cooking spray.

2. In small bowl combine the brown sugar, walnuts, cinnamon and 2 tablespoons flour. Add 1 tablespoon of the melted butter to the walnut mixture and stir until crumbly.

3. In large bowl stir together the remaining flour, the caster sugar and salt. Make a well in the centre. Add the egg, buttermilk, lemon zest and remaining melted butter. Stir until just combined.

4. Scrape the mixture into the prepared tin. Sprinkle evenly with the walnut topping. Bake for 40 minutes or until a skewer inserted in the centre of the cake comes out clean.

5. Allow to cool, then cut into 16 squares. A serve is 1 square. Wrap leftovers in foil and freeze for up to 1 month.

Per serving: 641 kJ, 153 kcal, 3 g protein, 5 g fat (2 g sat fat), 23 mg cholesterol, 25 g carbohydrate (12 g sugars), <1 g fibre, 250 mg sodium

VARIATIONS

Choose one of the following.

■ Add some chopped mixed dried fruit.

■ Fold in 4 tablespoons chocolate chips.

■ Divide the mixture in half, and stir 4 tablespoons cocoa powder into one half. Drop the mixture into the tin in spoonfuls, alternating plain and chocolate. Swirl with a knife to create a marbled pattern.

That notion of striking a balance is a powerful one and worth keeping in mind as you move forward. As far as diet goes, there are many ways to build that healthy balance. One is to watch every bite you eat. Another, more relaxed way, is to be aware of what you eat throughout the day, balancing a little indulgence here with a little restraint there. If you treat yourself to a sumptuous lunch with friends, for instance, go light on dinner and try to fit in extra exercise. If there's a big birthday dinner planned in the evening, go easy on snacks and have a simple lunch.

As you've probably learned by now, one day of overdoing it on food doesn't mean the end of your diet. Cut back on serve sizes for the next day or two and you'll be able to regain your balance. Even a week of overdoing it, it turns out, won't bring your diet crashing down. Naturally, people worry about the holiday season at the end of the year, when every occasion seems to centre around food. The reality is that you can enjoy yourself over the holidays without much danger of putting on a lot of weight.

It used to be held as a gospel truth that people typically gained 2–2.5 kilograms during the Christmas holiday period. Not true, according to a research study conducted by the American National Institutes of Health. They tracked 200 men and women from late September to early March (autumn to early spring in the northern hemisphere) using weight and other health measurements. The average weight gain was about half a kilo. And it turns out that that extra half a kilo may have had less to do with eating than with exercise. People who said they weren't physically active during the six months of the study typically gained about 750 grams. Those who stayed active throughout the cold winter months actually lost weight in this period.

No, we're not advising you to throw caution to the wind when holidays or special occasions come around.

Top 10 *ChangeOne* weight-loss tactics

This week, as you set out on your own to enjoy what you've achieved, let these simple but powerful directives of *ChangeOne* be your guide.

1. Eat breakfast every day – and include at least one serve of fruit.
2. Favour foods with plenty of fibre.
3. Help yourself to two serves of vegetables at lunch.
4. Keep an eye on serve sizes. If it looks oversized, divide it in half.
5. Eat slowly, savouring every bite.
6. Stop when you're satisfied.
7. Reach for a snack if you're genuinely hungry.
8. Drink plenty of water during the day, including a glass (1 cup/250 ml) at each meal.
9. Help yourself to two serves of vegetables at dinner.
10. Stay active!

It's still important to make smart choices. Our point is that even a couple of weeks of eating more than usual isn't enough to topple your healthy diet. Become extra active, and you can counterbalance the extra food you eat. Even if you do gain weight, it's not likely to be that much. When you return to your healthier habits as the holidays end, you'll regain your balance and steadily lose any weight you might have put on.

Keep your perspective

There's one more way in which keeping your balance is important as you set off from here. You've already heard about the pitfalls of all-or-nothing thinking. It's the tendency to think that a diet is working as long as you're losing weight, and that it has failed the moment you hit a plateau or gain a bit. It's the tendency of some people to think, the moment they slip up, 'I'm a failure'. All-or-nothing thinking doesn't acknowledge anything in between and is nothing more than a skewed perspective.

One thing we hope the *ChangeOne* approach has given you is a more balanced perspective on what it takes to lose weight and keep it off. It's not an all-or-nothing proposition. It's about the choices you make every day. If you go overboard on serves one day, you have the next to restore your balance. If your weight stays on a plateau for a while, so be it. You haven't failed. The diet hasn't failed. You can give yourself a little break and then make another change or two when you feel ready. If you gain a few kilos when things at work or home are stressful, don't worry. You know what it takes to lose it again. The only way to fail is to decide that you've failed – and to give up.

Keep that in mind as you relax this week and move into the weeks ahead, and you'll be just fine. You've got what it takes to do almost anything you want. Just take it a step at a time. Keep your spirits up and your resolution firm. Stay positive. Have as much fun as you can. If you hit a rocky patch, go easy on yourself. Set your sights on a new goal. Figure out the best ways to get there. And then go for it.

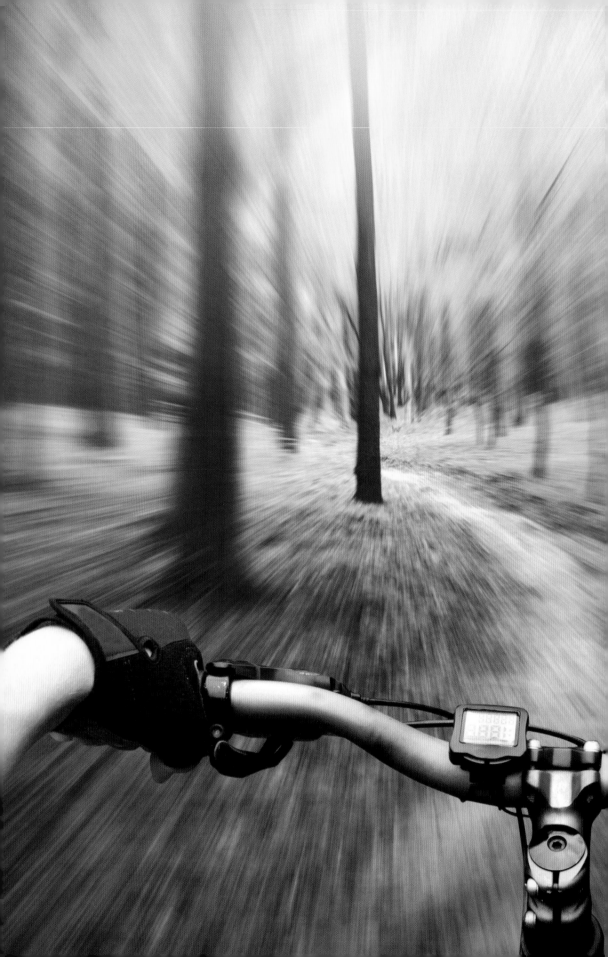

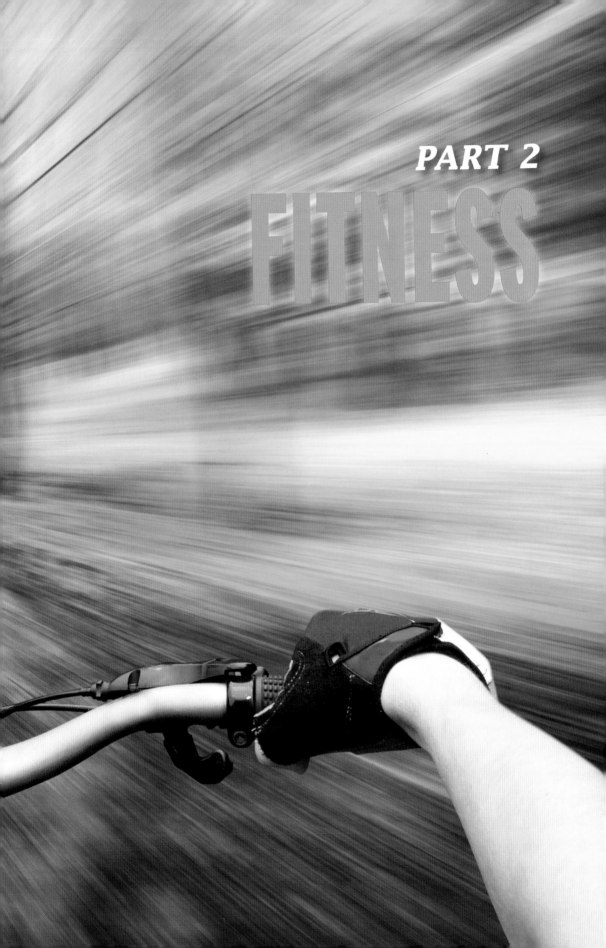

PART 2

FITNESS

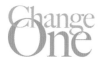

The truth about fitness

Consider the strange history of Product X. By all rights, it should be a huge success. Everybody needs it, and most have tried it – over and over again. Yet 8 in 10 people say that they simply can't use Product X, no matter how hard they try.

In the business world, X's spectacular failure would be blamed on the product, not the customers. But what if we told you that Product X is actually *exercise*? Surprised? Don't be. We firmly believe that a big reason 80 per cent of us have given up on exercise is the sweaty, competitive, numbers-driven, 'no pain, no gain', testosterone-pumped definition of exercise that the fitness industry has pushed upon us.

The *ChangeOne* approach to fitness is 100 per cent natural, fun and easy. Try it, and you'll never look at exercise the same way again.

It doesn't have to be any harder than that. In this chapter, you'll learn to forget about athletes, supermodels, sports drink advertisements and national gymnasium chains.

Traditional fitness:
for fitness fanatics only

There's a good reason why most exercise routines – and most gyms – make you feel as if you've suddenly, inexplicably signed up for high-school football or time-travelled back to PE class with your school's most notorious drill sergeant as a teacher. The fact is, most exercise programs are based on the old sports-team model of getting into shape. Lots of grunting and perspiration ... lifting heavy weights until your muscles shake ... pushing your body hard and then even harder still ... constantly measuring results and striving for improvements that can be expressed in numbers ... workouts that involve counting repetitions and watching the clock and constantly checking your heart rate ... competition, with others and yourself ... odd clothing you'd never wear on the street ... routines that must be performed in special places – certainly not at home with the kids, with a friend or while you do the dishes! Anything less, this model asserts, just isn't fitness.

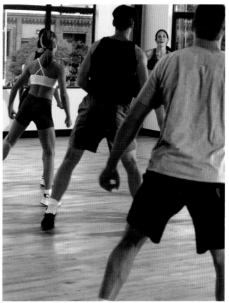

This approach may assure victory for professional sports people – and it's a good fit for a small percentage of athletically inclined women and men, but for most of us, it's beyond useless. It hurts, it's boring and time-consuming, and it's also punishing. Whatever the reason, it's just the wrong approach.

But if you want to exercise – to lose weight, get healthier, boost your energy or any other reason – it has long been the only 'official' way. Even governments have joined the bandwagon, putting forth an official standard for fitness based entirely on formal exercise sessions and all types of measurements and exertion thresholds.

So you try it. You sweat and grunt – and eventually, you stop. And you probably feel pretty guilty about it, too.

Millions of Australians and New Zealanders join gyms every year. But only approximately one in five keep going to the gym for more than a month or two. (There go hundreds of dollars, lost to an unused gym membership.) Sound familiar? If it does, take heart, because you're not alone.

Casual wins

If your workplace allows you to come to work dressed casually, take advantage of it – you just might lose more weight. When US researchers checked the activity levels of 53 men and women who wore pedometers to work, they found that the number of steps they took – and kilojoules they burned – increased significantly on casual days.

Study participants took an average of 491 (or 8 per cent) more steps on casual days. Over the course of a year, that could translate into burning an extra 26,250 kilojoules – and help you lose (or offset the gain of) nearly 1 kg.

What's more, two-thirds of Australians and over half of New Zealanders are not physically active enough, despite the fact that we know full well that activity is crucial to weight loss and improved cardiovascular health. So why aren't we out there exercising? A recent poll in the US found that 40 per cent of Americans say they don't have enough time, 20 per cent say they get enough exercise at work or at home (we think those people are on to something!), 15 per cent can't exercise due to health problems, 12 per cent say exercise is boring, 10 per cent believe they're too old, 9 per cent think exercise isn't necessary and 7 per cent are too tired. The picture is much the same in Australia and New Zealand.

The usual reaction from fitness experts is a resounding 'Get over it! Get out there! Go! Go! Go!'

So you go, go, go for a while ... and then stop again. Perhaps you start feeling as if you have failed at fitness – as if you maybe don't have a natural-born right to a toned, healthy, happy body. Which, of course, everyone does, within the limits of individual body shape and the genes you've inherited. Because the truth is, fitness has failed you.

Natural exercise

ChangeOne advocates that now is not the time for a new gung-ho attitude towards fitness, but rather a completely new definition of fitness in order to keep up with modern trends.

Stroll into a summer morning, alive with the sounds of birdsong and the scents of blooming flowers. Slowly strengthen and stretch your muscles until you feel as lithe as a Siamese cat. Park as far from the supermarket as possible and smile as you walk to get your shopping trolley – you've just added some secret, kilojoule-burning activity to your day. Swim, sail, garden or play with the kids this weekend, secure in the knowledge that simply enjoying yourself under the clear, blue skies is good for your mind, body and spirit. For most of us, being active is not about pain, it's about pleasure.

Change One Quiz

Your fitness attitude

How do you define fitness, and is that definition helping or hurting you? To find out, answer these questions as honestly as you can and keep a record of your answers.

1. **If there were a gym within a short walking distance from where I live, I would:**
   a. Still not join; I just don't like gyms.
   b. Probably join, but not use it much. Who has time?
   c. Be there all the time.

2. **I find that doing the same exercise routine over and over again is:**
   a. Boring, of course.
   b. Okay for a short time, but then I try to vary things.
   c. The proper approach; practice makes perfect, after all.

3. **In high school, PE was:**
   a. My least favourite class.
   b. Occasionally fun, particularly when we were doing a sport or activity I liked.
   c. One of the classes I looked forwards to most.

4. **I have played on this many organised sports teams in my life:**
   a. Very few, if any, unless you count neighbourhood footy games.
   b. A fair number over the years, but never very competitively.
   c. Loads, and some were highly competitive.

5. **My favourite vigorous activity is:**
   a. Gardening or fixing up my house.
   b. Hiking, cruising on a bike or some other outdoor pastime.
   c. Running, working out with weights or playing a high-intensity sport.

6. **My attitude toward sweating is:**
   a. It's a miserable feeling that I try to avoid.
   b. I don't mind it on occasion when I'm outdoors and in the right clothes.
   c. I love it – it means I'm being active, healthy and alive.

7. **We keep the following in our home for strengthening exercises:**
   a. Nothing really, unless you count a lawnmower or hammer.
   b. A few dumbbells or other basic exercise tools.
   c. A weight-lifting bench, a barbell set and more.

8. **When I see world-class weightlifters competing on television, I think:**
   a. What a waste of a person's life.
   b. Definitely not for me, but I respect their achievements.
   c. If only I could get to the gym more ...

9. **When I'm on a bicycle, I like to:**
   a. Chitchat, look at the world around me and make frequent stops.
   b. Have a mildly strenuous but mostly pleasant ride to a nearby destination.
   c. Put my head down and go, go, go.

10. **When I see a TV ad for a sports drink that features overachieving athletes, I think:**
    a. This is revolting!
    b. Clever marketing, but not for me.
    c. I've gotta try that!

Turn to next page to continue quiz.

11. My idea of a good time in a swimming pool is:

a. Dozing while lying on an inflated mattress.
b. Playing games in the shallow end with the kids.
c. Swimming laps, having races and making up competitions.

12. I know the following statistics about my fitness level:

a. Not a thing, but ask me about the footy.
b. I know my basic medical numbers – my weight, pulse rate, Body Mass Index – but not much else.
c. A lot; I monitor things like my daily step count, heart rate, maximum weight levels I can lift and more.

Quiz score

Give yourself 1 point for (a.) answers, 2 points for (b.) answers, and 3 points for (c.) answers. Tally up your score and check below to find out where your fitness attitude falls.

12–15 Anti-exercise. Not only don't you exercise much, you have a negative attitude about fitness. You sorely need a new, more positive mind-set. The *ChangeOne* approach is perfect for you, since it will slowly get you moving in easy, fun ways that won't intrude much on your everyday life.

16–22 Apathetic. You aren't anti-exercise, but you probably don't think about it much and don't worry about getting it into your life. *ChangeOne* will help you see why exercise is important to health and weight, and show you that getting the amount you need won't require much effort at all.

23–28 Healthy. You understand the benefits of active living and probably enjoy the great outdoors, but you aren't committed to formal exercise regimens. *ChangeOne* is great for you in that it will inject a little routine into your efforts, making sure you get all the fun and movement you need on a daily basis for health and weight loss.

29–36 Athletic. You are quite comfortable in the world of exercise and sports and enjoy the rigours and benefits of formal workout routines. *ChangeOne* is still very useful to you, though, because it will broaden your perspective on fitness and show you how to integrate movement into your entire day.

Welcome to *ChangeOne* Fitness! We feel that physical activity is far too important to leave to traditional sports-based workouts alone. We have a new, more natural way to help you get the benefits of physical activity, without the need to work out like a professional sportsperson.

But first, let us not deny that exercise is crucial for health – and a healthy weight. After all, activity is *the* most effective way to boost your metabolism (so your body burns more kilojoules all day and night, even while you sleep). Regular exercise turns that flabby fat into sleek and shapely muscle. It burns kilojoules, helping you to lose weight and, more importantly, keep it off. It boosts energy, improves your overall attitude and, when done properly, is much more fun than watching weeknight television.

ChangeOne Fitness lets you get all the benefits of exercise in just half an hour a day, plus about 2 hours of fun time on the weekend. The components of our plan are:

A brisk daily walk Your target is 20 minutes a day – long enough to kick your body's fat-burning power into action, yet short enough to fit into your lunch break or to be an after-dinner activity. This is the fat-blasting part of the plan.

More daily activity You'll discover dozens of ways to add extra steps and movements to your day – from parking at the far end of the car park to washing the dishes by hand – and see how they can add up to a significant kilojoule burn. This part of the plan helps you replace activity that's slowly been erased from daily life over the past 60 years – one of the reasons why Australians and New Zealanders weigh more now than in the past.

Outdoor fun Clear your Saturday morning or Sunday afternoon schedule, because we want to see you having fun in nature for 2 hours a week. Get the kids outdoors for touch football; rake up the leaves, then have a barbecue; take a hike; go to the beach. What you choose to do is up to you. We just know that moving and having fun out in sunshine, fresh air and natural surroundings is happiness defined. You'll feel more alive – and ready to get out there again soon!

Muscles aren't fat!

Lots of fitness experts warn that if you stop exercising, your muscles will 'become' fat. That's not true. Inactivity allows muscles to shrink, leaving room for larger fat deposits, but the cellular make-up of your muscles themselves doesn't change. The good news is that you don't have to join a gym to hold on to muscle. Vigorous everyday activities, from walking the dog to sweeping the porch or cutting the lawn with a push mower instead of a petrol mower, are usually enough to maintain muscle density.

Strengthening and stretching Just 10 minutes a day will help you to build sleek, high-metabolism muscle. You'll lose fat faster, keep it off more easily and get strong and confident. And our *ChangeOne* stretches will pamper your body, relieving aches and pains and helping to build flexibility. This component helps to protect and rebuild muscle lost to ageing and to reduced-kilojoule eating, and it can help to prevent you from getting stuck on a weight-loss plateau.

Smarter fitness

Don't be put off by the snobbery of the weight room at the gym or the confidence of the regulars in aerobics or Zumba classes. You can take the *ChangeOne* Fitness plan seriously because it's amazingly effective. Research proves the benefits.

- **Slow and steady means better results** Moderation burns more kilojoules, according to research. When they compared the fitness levels of people who participated in moderate physical activity, such as walking and cycling, with those who exercised vigorously, they found that those who exercised vigorously for short periods were actually more inactive for the rest of the day. In contrast, the moderate exercisers tended to be more active overall.

- **A lean, sexy figure** You'll replace fat with muscle in just 10 minutes a day. Don't worry about bulking up; you won't on our fitness plan. In fact, it'll be the opposite. Muscle tissue takes up much less space than fat tissue, and our exercises are gentle in their nature, meaning they create lean, not bulky, muscles.

- **An energy boost** We're bowled over by the number of studies showing that simple, easy activities supercharge your energy level. For example, one study found that a 10-minute walk gives you more energy than eating a chocolate bar, because exercise increases levels of an energy-boosting hormone. Other studies show that people who begin exercise programs greatly increase their physical activity around the clock and also are more likely to take up new hobbies and pursuits.

Be a better lover

One of the most exciting, though least discussed, benefits of physical activity is that it pays big dividends in bed. Studies show that exercise can:
- Help you to feel more sexually desirable and experience greater levels of satisfaction.
- Cut the risk of impotence.
- Boost circulation for better potency and orgasms.
- Cut stress and boost your spirits so you'll be in the mood.

ChangeOne versus traditional exercise programs

Here's how *ChangeOne* helps you to overcome the most daunting exercise roadblocks, and how traditional exercise programs handle the same issues.

ROADBLOCK: I don't have time.
Traditional approach: Make time! Fitness is important!
ChangeOne **approach:** Do everyday activities and super-short routines.

ROADBLOCK: It hurts!
Traditional approach: No pain, no gain.
ChangeOne **approach:** You may feel a little sore, but fitness should *never* hurt.

ROADBLOCK: I'm too tired.
Traditional approach: Do it anyway.
ChangeOne **approach:** Just do a little – you'll be energised!

ROADBLOCK: It's boring.
Traditional approach: Keep doing the same routines; just change the exercises.
ChangeOne **approach:** Choose activities you like.

ROADBLOCK: I'm not in the mood.
Traditional approach: Do it anyway.
ChangeOne **approach:** Not ready for walking just yet? Try doing some a little light gardening instead.

- **Efficient weight loss** Combining *ChangeOne* Fitness with our winning diet plan guarantees faster, easier weight loss. You need more proof? When 24 overweight women walked three times a week and followed a reduced-kilojoule diet similar to *ChangeOne*, they lost 8 per cent of their body weight – and their body fat fell by an amazing 15 per cent, meaning they had replaced flabby fat with lean, kilojoule-burning muscle. Wow – that's amazing!

- **Staying skinny for life** By increasing the amount of muscle in your body, our 10-minutes-a-day strengthening plan also revs up your metabolism. That means your body burns more kilojoules around the clock, no matter what you are doing!

- **More energy burn without exercising** Sixty years ago, Australians and New Zealanders burned approximately 2950 more kilojoules per day than we do today – not by running marathons but through daily activities that we've engineered out of our lives, from rolling down car windows by hand to washing the dishes. We'll show you how to put activity back into your days – and burn hundreds of kilojoules more than you could in a formal exercise program. In fact, adding 'lifestyle activity' keeps weight off more successfully than formal exercise classes, according to US researchers who compared the body weights of women in a step aerobics class with those who simply fit more activity into each day.

■ **Natural happiness** It's hard to believe, but we often spend around 20 to 23 hours per day being inactive – in the car, at work, watching television, eating meals, sleeping. We'll show you how to get outdoors, have fun and once again feel the happiness that comes from time spent in fresh air and sunshine amid flowers and trees.

■ **A graceful, ache-free body** Each of our *ChangeOne* strengthening routines ends with some refreshing stretches. These are more than feel-good moves (although stretching can help you relax, both physically and mentally). Including stretching will make your muscles more flexible and increase your range of motion.

Getting started

Choose to
stand rather
than sit
and to walk
rather than
stand.

As you can see, *ChangeOne* Fitness isn't about formal exercise sessions done a few times a week. It's part of a total lifestyle program, meaning that it's part of each and every day. It's choosing to stand rather than sit and to walk rather than stand. It's about bounding up stairs with energy at every opportunity, rather than taking the escalator or lift and leaning sleepily against the mirrored walls inside. It's about starting the morning with a 10-minute, in-your-pyjamas workout that revs you up for the rest of the day rather than staring blankly at the morning news while the coffee brews. It's about getting outdoors in the evening rather than watching nature shows on TV. None of that requires workout clothes, a gym membership, a personal trainer or sports drinks.

Like the *ChangeOne* approach to eating, this change in your approach to fitness is best achieved by taking one small step at a time. We haven't broken down this section into a 12-week plan, because one such program is enough to follow. But you know what to do – first, focus on walking, because it's the easiest way to start out. Once that becomes a regular habit, try to increase your time outdoors. When that's working, take on the daily 10-minute workout, and so on. Along the way, whenever you have a chance to be up and moving, take that chance and capitalise on it!

Most people think that exercise makes you tired, but the opposite is true – the more you get, the less tired you feel. If you've been reading the *ChangeOne* Success Stories, you've probably noticed how almost every person has mentioned that the combination of more exercise and less weight has made them more energised – so stop using 'I don't have the energy' as an excuse for not getting up and moving. The moment you can overcome the urge to sit, you will begin a wonderful journey back to the energy and weight you so desire.

One important thing to remember is that if you're over the age 40 and have had a sedentary lifestyle, or you have a chronic health condition, talk with your doctor before starting the *ChangeOne* program. He or she may want to check you out to make sure everything is in working order, and will probably advise you to start out easy but definitely to start exercising. That's because easy fitness can help a wide range of conditions from diabetes to asthma.

Read through the pages ahead and get started! You'll discover that *ChangeOne* Fitness will bring a surprising amount of fun and relaxation into your life. And your weight-loss efforts will go so much more easily!

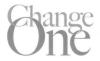

Get ready for action

A mystic once said that every journey begins with a single step. This is literally true with *ChangeOne* Fitness, which begins with nothing more complicated than walking. But before you take that first step towards fitness, take the *ChangeOne* quiz on the next page.

We'll show you how to use your answers to create an active lifestyle that you'll love, full of pleasure, energy and easy moves that are guaranteed to get results.

As you start your *ChangeOne* Fitness journey, you may remember past exercise attempts that fizzled, plans that sounded great but just didn't fit into your life, activities that seemed promising but were in reality no fun at all. This journey will be different – we promise – because you'll tailor it to suit your fitness level, your personality and even your secret hopes and dreams.

Change One Quiz

What's your starting point?

1. **On a typical Saturday afternoon, I'm:**
   a. Watching sport on TV or otherwise deepening the depression in my chair.
   b. Working in the garden, playing golf or doing something else active.
   c. Watching the kids' soccer or netball game or driving around to do a few errands.

2. **If I walked briskly for 15 minutes, I would feel:**
   a. Invigorated and ready for another lap.
   b. A little pooped, but still able to hold a conversation.
   c. Like someone knocked the wind out of me.

3. **I would rate my strength as:**
   a. Not what it used to be; the grocery bags seem to weigh a tonne, and I think twice before picking up children.
   b. Pretty good; I could lift a bag of potting mix or carry luggage.
   c. Embarrassing; when I get out of a chair, I have to push off using the armrests.

4. **My attitude about exercise is:**
   a. Ugh! I get flashbacks to high school PE classes.
   b. It's a waste of storage space; my house is jammed with dusty exercise bikes, treadmills and thigh slimmers.
   c. Once I get going, I know it will feel good.

5. **I enjoy physical activity most when it's:**
   a. Playful; if I'm feeling the wind in my hair, moving to my favourite songs or throwing a ball with my kids, I'm happy.
   b. Practical; if it gets the house cleaned, or the car washed, I'll do it.
   c. Barely noticeable; I'd rather sneak it in while socialising or watching TV.
   d. Competitive; nothing motivates me like winning.

6. **When I was a kid, I loved:**
   a. Competition; whether it was backyard cricket, tennis or touch football, I was in on the action.
   b. Adventure; I liked to explore, climb trees, swim, skate and walk on stilts.
   c. Fantasy and fairy wings; I loved to dance, create and pretend.

7. **My average day is:**
   a. Fairly leisurely, with plenty of holes in my schedule.
   b. Sometimes hectic, but I usually take a break for lunch.
   c. Crazy; once the day gets going, there's no time to stop.

8. **My biggest fear about exercising is:**
   a. It will tire me out.
   b. I'll get big and bulky.
   c. I won't be able to do it.

9. **My top-secret wish about exercising is:**
   a. That I'll be able to eat everything I want.
   b. That I'll spot-reduce my tummy, waist, hips or thighs.
   c. That I'll look and feel like I did about 10 years ago.

Quiz score

As we're sure you figured out, there are no right or wrong answers. But to help interpret your answers, the rest of this chapter offers advice and guidance based on each of these nine questions. Armed with this information, you'll be in a much better position to get moving, *ChangeOne* style.

Set aside your doubts

What is stopping you from starting up a daily walk? From turning off the television and going outside? From trying a little stretching? Some of it might be lack of knowledge, but for most of us, the obstacles are things like lack of time, or fear, or ingrained habits and daily patterns that don't include exercise. The following tips will help convince you that it's time to reject all those internal arguments against exercise and finally get started.

1 **Weekends too busy for fun?**
Fix your schedule – and your attitude.

More everyday movement, more outdoor fun – those are the simple tenets behind *ChangeOne* Fitness. Saturdays are the perfect times to be outside, having a good time. So make a commitment to it: From 10 o'clock to midday, it's fun time. Or 3 to 5 o'clock in the afternoon; whenever works. If you spend your Saturdays doing errands and small jobs, learn to get these tasks done on weekday evenings. If you're a sports watcher, either learn to record broadcasts to watch later or set a goal. For each hour spent watching a game, spend an hour outside being active. If you're at a child's sporting event, get up, walk around and be playful while you cheer. Your children are having fun on this beautiful Saturday and so should you! You'll find more ideas for getting active throughout the following chapters.

2 **Not ready for vigorous walking?**
Start slow and smart.

The key to successful exercise, for *every* fitness level, is to exert yourself based entirely on your current capabilities, and from there, progress slowly but steadily. If you plunge into some crazy exercise regimen, the odds are high that you'll throw in the towel in no time. Remember, exercise is never an all-or-nothing proposition. With *ChangeOne* Fitness, it's simply about adding more movement to the life you're already leading.

Whether you are an experienced, super-fit walker or a first-time fitness walker coming off a long period of sedentary living, your exertion level is the same. Walk at a speed and for a distance at which you feel you are breathing a little heavily, but you can still hold a conversation. Whether you reach that point during a slow 10-minute stroll or an arm-churning, hour-long power walk, it's the right pace for you.

From there, slowly build up the length and intensity of your activities. If you're already fit, look for ways to take things up a notch. This approach isn't wimpy, it's smart. In a US study of 78 inactive people, those who set small, doable exercise targets (in this case, adding just a bit more walking to their days) were three times more likely to stick with it than superambitious types who started with Everest-size goals.

You probably don't need to check with your doctor before beginning our gentle fitness program. However, if you take medication for high blood pressure or a heart condition; feel extremely breathless or dizzy after a little activity; develop pain or pressure in your chest, neck, shoulder or arm after exercising; or have a bone or joint problem or a chronic medical condition such as diabetes, do consult your doctor first.

3 Consider yourself too stiff or too weak for muscle-strengthening exercises?
Start easy and give it a few weeks.

ChangeOne Fitness isn't about achieving someone else's idea of acceptable strength. You are accountable only to yourself. Don't be hard on yourself if you have become out of shape – as we said in the last chapter, 60 per cent of Australians and New Zealanders are in the same position, thanks partly to a fitness industry gone haywire. Just start easy and progress slowly.

Remember, too, that muscle strength and flexibility naturally diminish as we get older. When we don't exercise, the results start to show themselves in everyday ways: big and little aches, trouble bending and stretching, a harder time picking up a full bag of groceries or 2 litres of milk. *ChangeOne* Fitness will help you gradually reverse that decline with our daily 10-minute stretching and strengthening program. After a few weeks, you'll begin to discover a sleeker, fitter, stronger you, minus the aches and pains. The bonus is that having more muscle mass means your body burns more kilojoules, so it will become easier to lose weight and keep it off. But reject the old philosophy of 'no pain, no gain'. If an exercise hurts, skip it. If you're very sore afterwards, take it easier next time.

4 Had too many bad experiences with fitness?
Think enjoyment, not punishment.

Forget about that whistle-blowing PE teacher, those get-fit-quick gimmicks and those overexuberant aerobics classes you tried, and failed at, years ago. *ChangeOne* Fitness is based on a new definition of exercise: fitting fun, pleasure and natural movement into every day. That translates to gardening, playing with the kids, walking the dog and catching up with a friend as you stroll through a gorgeous summer morning, and it all counts! We also promise that you'll never have to wear skin-tight gym gear or do push-ups.

You'll get hooked on enjoying movement, and you'll see results. In a four-year study of 124 overweight women and men, US National Institutes of Health researchers discovered that people who tried fitting short periods of exercise into their days or getting half an hour of 'lifestyle activity', such as gardening, heavy cleaning or walking the dog daily, lost as much weight as those who signed up for a traditional aerobics class – and they were more likely to still be fit a year later.

5 Have unique exercise likes and dislikes?
Work with your personality.

Just as our tastes in spouses, friends and pasta sauces aren't all the same, neither are our activity likes and dislikes. With *ChangeOne* Fitness, the idea is to move your body more, no matter how you do that. If you enjoy group fitness classes, go for it. If the idea of bouncing or bending in front of 12 other people mortifies you, go for a bike ride instead. Need to see concrete results to feel good? You'll discover how to turn everyday jobs into energy-burning mini-routines. You can also find ways to add a higher purpose to your activities, such as walking to raise money for your favourite charity.

If you're a true television addict, get your exercise by dusting off that treadmill-turned-coathanger and walking while you watch, or do the 10-minute exercise routines starting on page 278. (We still want you to turn off the television occasionally and get outside, though.) Or get a mobile phone with a headset and move while you talk. The point is that fitness shouldn't be work, but it should work for you.

6 Forgotten the pleasures of active fun?
Return to your childhood.

The key to succeeding in business is also the key to succeeding at exercise: do what you love. If you're not sure what that is anymore, then try doing what you used to love as a child. That could mean bike rides, basketball, dancing, tennis or merely walking along a beach.

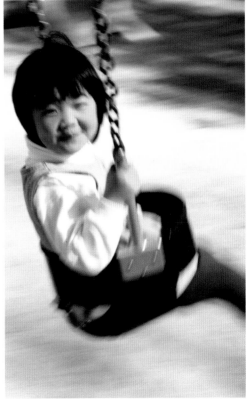

Recapturing childhood joy adds excitement and enthusiasm to your new active lifestyle. If you loved the competition and camaraderie of team sports, look for an amateur team to join. Are you an explorer at heart? Discover new worlds by joining a local kayaking or canoeing club, or planning an adventure holiday with a hiking or walking group. Have the soul of an artist? Express yourself by learning how to salsa or belly dance. The bottom line is get in touch with what makes you tick, and you'll never run out of batteries.

7 Don't have time in your day for exercise?
Start by finding just a few minutes here and there.

Fitness, particularly the *ChangeOne* Fitness approach, can work with any schedule. If you're the type who can take a break, relax for a few minutes and then get back to work, you may find that short bursts of activity are perfect for you. (How about a brisk stroll around the office parking lot?) If there's no time to stop once you get going, fit in a 20-minute walk in the morning, before the craziness begins. You'll be energised for the day and have a sense of accomplishment before you've even turned on your computer or started your first task. And if the day just never stops, consider using that lovely, golden hour after dinner for a stroll around the neighbourhood – imagine you're taking an old-fashioned Italian *passeggiata*, or evening stroll – or an hour of gardening.

Still struggling? Then you need to analyse your time more carefully. What is it that's taking up 16 hours of waking time a day? Is there television time that can be sacrificed or half a lunch or dinner hour? Can you hold one-on-one discussions at work while walking? Is there a way to alter your commute times so you aren't in the car during peak-hour traffic? All you need to start is 10 minutes a day for our strengthening and stretching program, along with moments here and there for brisk walking. Make it a priority, and you will succeed in finding the time.

8 Intimidated by the prospect of daily exercise?
We understand, but you can overcome it.

When the US American Council on Exercise asked 1500 certified personal trainers to name the top fitness myths, three answers to question 8 topped the list. Afraid you'll be tired? The truth is that activity boosts energy in several ways. It cuts stress, improves sleep and helps your body better use the oxygen, blood glucose and fat it burns for energy. Will you bulk up? Only if you embark on a Schwarzenegger-style bodybuilding routine. (And if that's what you want, you're reading the wrong book!) Afraid you won't be able to keep up or won't have the time? *ChangeOne* Fitness is meant to work with your schedule, your personality and your personal fitness level. You'll never ever feel as if you can't do it. That's a promise.

9 Worried that you might fail?
Be realistic with your expectations.

It's better to have modest hopes and be pleasantly surprised by your progress than to have high hopes and lose heart when they don't pan out. Unless you run marathons, you won't be able to eat with wild abandon – but you will be able to indulge occasionally without seeing the results on your behind, belly or thighs. That's because exercising burns more kilojoules than sitting still, and it increases your metabolism slightly.

Can a fitness routine magically shrink one body part? Probably not. Expect to look sleeker all over as you firm up your flab and trim body fat. Doing extra tummy, hip or leg exercises could make muscles in those areas tighter more quickly, but it can't banish fat selectively.

Exercising her way to success

Although she wasn't an avid exerciser before she started *ChangeOne*, Donna Westog has made physical activity part of her daily routine. The results have been spectacular.

'The weight just fell off me,' she says. Already down 21 kg, she's well on her way to her goal of 57 kg.

Being active has made an enormous difference for Donna. 'If you expect to lose weight and become healthier – get moving! I make sure I get some form of exercise or physical activity every day of the week. Since I began *ChangeOne*, I've only missed a total of seven days.'

Donna's latest toy is a shiny new treadmill. 'I just love it!' she says. 'I still walk outside whenever possible, but with the treadmill, I am now working towards running instead of walking, and am training to do a 5 km run. This is something I never, ever dreamed of doing before *ChangeOne*. I have a marathon-running brother who is hoping someday I'll join him. We'll see!'

The portion-control tips have also been extremely helpful to Donna. 'I have discovered how much food I *don't* have to give up as long as I am watchful of portions,' she says.

Donna confesses that she can't take all the credit for her success with *ChangeOne*. She gets a lot of encouragement from friends. 'I never

Donna Westog lost more than 21 kg by getting some form of physical activity every day of the week.

could have got this far without their support,' she says.

She advises people on *ChangeOne* to be patient. 'Just change one thing at a time, and you will become a healthier person – and thinner, too! Your extra weight did *not* come on overnight – don't expect it to come off that quickly. So many think that the kilos will magically disappear! It takes a lot of hard work and discipline, but this plan is really great.'

Nine tips for fitness success

For every 10 people who begin a fitness program, as many as 7 will drop out in less than six months. Here are ways to help you from contributing to the drop-out statistics.

Start slowly

1 The *ChangeOne* philosophy is the same whether you apply it to healthy eating or to fitness. Make just one small change at a time. That's the best way to guarantee that the changes you make will become permanent. So while we hope you ultimately adopt all of the *ChangeOne* Fitness tenets, focus on one at a time. Even then, start slowly. Remember, you are making changes that should last the rest of your life. Don't try to rush them.

Avoid boredom

3 It's among the top reasons people drop out of exercise regimens; after all, who wants to be bored? It's up to you to keep things fresh. Vary your walking route or work in new activities to keep your routine fun and different. Do your usual walk in reverse, go cycling next week instead of walking, stop and investigate outdoor places or try activities that have always piqued your interest.

Surround yourself with support

2 Some people can stay more committed if they have a regular fitness partner. In one US study that tracked 309 people for two years, those who had a support group lost 30 per cent more weight than those who dieted alone. If you can find someone who shares your enthusiasm and exercises at the same pace and for the same length of time as you do, you'll be more likely to stick with your plan – and have fun along the way. Remember to think beyond just close friends, co-workers and family members. An online group, a hiking club or a gym or exercise class may offer just the support you're looking for. Most importantly, end up with an arrangement that helps you to succeed. If you're a loner, having a partner could hurt, but having someone cheering you on might help. Be true to your personality.

Dress for success

4 There's no reason to spend any money on specialised workout clothes to do the exercises in the *ChangeOne* Fitness program. Comfortable pants or shorts and a top made from breathable material such as cotton will do just fine. In fact, you don't even need to change your clothes for most *ChangeOne* Fitness activities. But if you do, make sure they are clothes you love to be in. Clothing should motivate you, not embarrass or irritate you.

Fuel up

5 Nothing takes the pleasure out of an activity more than running out of energy. Too little water or food beforehand can make that happen, so make sure you're hydrated and not hungry before you start out. If you think you'll be exerting yourself, have a large glass of water and a healthy snack 30 minutes before starting. If you're active for more than 30 minutes, make sure you drink more water every 15 to 20 minutes.

Adopt a new attitude

6 It's okay to be a bit selfish about your exercise time. Schedule it, commit to it and protect it by gently reminding intruders – including your spouse and children – that sorry, you're busy doing something important and that exercise is a priority you'll be sticking with. Do the same at work. Don't let peer pressure force you to eat lunch with the usual gang when you've planned to be outside walking. And don't feel guilty. In fact, be proud of your new priorities. You may not realise it, but you're being a role model for your friends and family, and perhaps some of them will soon follow in your footsteps.

Celebrate fitness success

7 Of course, you're paying attention to your weight-loss achievements. Ultimately, that's what *ChangeOne* is for. But as you progress down the fitness path, you're probably going to want to monitor progress directly related to the exercise. Consider keeping an exercise journal to note your personal observations, and think about monitoring your energy levels, body measurements, sleep patterns or sports performance – anything that would improve as a direct result of your new exercise patterns. When you show improvement, as you inevitably will, don't forget to reward yourself!

Work with – not against – your body

8 Elsewhere in this chapter, we talk about respecting your personal likes and dislikes when it comes to choosing activities. You also need to respect your unique physical limitations. For example, if a physical condition makes it difficult for you to walk, there are many other wonderful ways to keep moving for 20 minutes, whether swimming or using a rowing machine or merely doing calisthenics in a chair. Similarly, chronic conditions such as arthritis or back pain can limit your mobility. Respect that, and find movements you can do and enjoy. What's crucial is that you don't use physical limitations as an excuse not to get moving.

Just as important, play to your physical strengths. If you have strong legs, bushwalking or cycling will suit you. If you have strong arms, there are plenty of sports, such as tennis and softball, that are great for you. Are you naturally graceful? Sign up for a dance class. With *ChangeOne*, it's not the specific activity that matters; just that you are active. Feel free to improvise as required for your unique needs.

Stay motivated

9 Goals, treats, inspiration, fun and lots of positive self-coaching can help you to stick with your new fitness plan. There are many ways to do this. Get a portable music player and load it with upbeat music so you can have fun listening whenever you're on the go; create an inspiration wall from a family notice board or cork board to display logs of your improving health statistics, photos of you as you slim down and other motivating photos or quotes; constantly keep up the positive self-talk ('I can do it!') and ban negative self-talk ('I can't do it'); and give yourself nice rewards (a book, a movie, earrings) for reaching small thresholds, such as five consecutive days of walking or getting through the entire strengthening sequence for the first time.

Get walking

Stride along on a sunny morning alive with birdsong. Take a lap around the shopping mall before hitting the clearance sales. Walk to the neighbourhood post office instead of dropping a letter in a nearby post box. Opportunities to walk are endless, and that's exactly the point.

Walking is the most natural, intuitive and practical form of exercise. Besides getting you from point A to point B, it burns kilojoules, boosts energy, improves mood, wards off food cravings and helps keep you slim. That's why walking is at the heart of *ChangeOne* Fitness.

Our goals for you? Fit more kilojoule-blasting steps into your daily routine, and take a dedicated 20-minute brisk walk every day.

In this chapter, we'll prove to you that this simple strategy (no gym memberships, no equipment, no fancy moves, no huge time commitment required) is the most powerful way to lose weight and feel great – for life.

What's your walking quotient?

1. **My thinking about walking is:**
   a. It's a slow but cheap mode of transportation. Full stop.
   b. It's probably good for you, but certainly not serious exercise.
   c. It's a legitimate form of exercise I should do more of.
   d. It's great exercise, plus a wonderful source of relaxation and pleasure.

2. **If the weather's nice, I might walk for this long:**
   a. 1 minute – the time it takes to get from my car to the supermarket entrance.
   b. 5 minutes – the time it takes to find a nice bench in the park.
   c. 20 minutes – a relaxed stroll in the sun is a rare but pleasant treat.
   d. 30 minutes or more – I jump at every chance to be outside and moving.

3. **My usual walking shoes are:**
   a. Fuzzy slippers or old socks; that's all you need for strolling around the house.
   b. My everyday work shoes; who has time to change shoes for a little walking?
   c. Sandals, clogs or thongs; feet like sunshine, too.
   d. Dedicated sneakers or hiking shoes; 'sturdy' and 'supportive' are the operative words.

4. **My favourite parking spot is:**
   a. I don't know; I shop online.
   b. Right up front; I'll circle the parking lot endlessly until a great space opens up.
   c. Relatively near; I don't obsess over getting close and don't mind a bit of extra walking.
   d. The furthest parking space; this gives me a chance to get in one more brisk stroll.

5. **I stash my walking shoes:**
   a. Um, don't you walk in *all* your shoes?
   b. When last glimpsed, my circa 1980 Dunlop volleys were buried at the back of my shoe cupboard.
   c. Relatively new, well-fitting joggers are prominently arrayed with my other shoes.
   d. I keep dedicated walking shoes in the car, at work and by the front door.

Quiz score

We were pretty obvious with this one – for each question, the answers go from worst to best. Here are some of the underlying messages of each question.

1. Walking is for real. As you'll read shortly, study after study shows the substantial, measurable benefits of regular walking to your health, weight and mental wellbeing.

2. Walking is a pleasure. It's a simple, convenient, fun way to add exercise to your life and an effective way to lose weight.

3. If the jogger fits, wear it. Your feet were made for walking, and your shoes should be, too. Studies show you're likely to walk more during the day if you're wearing comfortable shoes.

4. We're talking about a lifestyle, not fitness quotas. *ChangeOne* Fitness is a philosophy as much as a plan. Any chance you see to fit a few more steps into your day – such as parking your car in no man's land – you should grab.

5. Ready, set, go. You'll know you're in the *ChangeOne* Fitness mind-set when you're ready to walk, stroll or play outside at a moment's notice.

Walking your way to weight loss

A growing stack of research shows that if you want to lose weight, combining a sensible eating plan with exercise such as walking is far smarter than just cutting kilojoules. It also tames the dreaded 'jiggles', helping you look and feel firmer.

One example of this strategy's power comes from a study where researchers asked 24 overweight, inactive women to begin walking three times a week (one day on a treadmill in the lab for 30 to 45 minutes, and two days on their own for any length of time they wanted) and to cut 1050 kilojoules per day from their diets, following an eating plan based closely on the nutritional guidelines of *ChangeOne*. After six months, the volunteers had lost 8 per cent of their body weight – about a 6.5 kilogram reduction for an 82 kilogram woman. Total body fat fell by 15 per cent, meaning each woman shaved off about 12 kilograms of fat and replaced half of it with muscle. And they all felt stronger because their aerobic capacity – a measure of the lungs' ability to take in oxygen – increased by 8 per cent. The bottom line is that thanks to the diet-plus-walking strategy, these women were slimmer, fitter and had more stamina.

The benefits of walking are many. It can help you:

Burn fat Blasting fat requires using your body's biggest muscle groups – those in your buttocks and legs – rhythmically, briskly and consistently for at least 20 minutes at a time. (That's exactly why we ask you to dedicate yourself to a brisk 20-minute walk every day.) During an aerobic workout such as walking, your muscle cells first burn sugar stored as a fuel called glycogen; after about 15 minutes, your cells turn to fat as their primary power source.

Trim stubborn stomach fat Walkers lost significant abdominal fat – the stubborn fat that can be toughest to lose (and the kind that raises your risk of diabetes and heart disease) in one research study.

Make your 'skinny jeans' your everyday jeans, for good Adding just 2000 steps a day to your regular activities – that's just 15 minutes of walking – could mean you'll never gain another

Help!

'My knees and shins hurt after a walk. What can I do?'

First, make sure you've picked a walking surface that's kind to your body, one that's firm but not too hard. Avoid concrete, the hardest walking surface of them all. Best to walk on are grass, wood-chip paths, dirt paths, or a regular running track. Next, be sure that you're also doing the *ChangeOne* strengthening/ stretching program to build the muscles around your knees. Increase your time and speed gradually. And be sure that your walking shoes have flexible soles.

gram, according to top weight-loss experts from the Center for Human Nutrition at the University of Colorado Health Sciences Center in the USA.

Have energy to burn Many research studies have found that exercise makes people feel more energetic. Even better news is that just a short walk is all it takes! A recent study looked at people who reported persistent fatigue. One group rested for six weeks, while the others either did a leisurely walk or a fast hill-walk. Both of the exercise groups reported improved energy levels compared to the resting group.

Turn on your happy switch Can you walk your way to happiness? Absolutely. In fact, US psychologists at Duke University have found that walking relieves mild-to-moderate depression better than drugs do.

Brisk walking basics

If you're new to walking or haven't hit the pavement for a while, or if your doctor – or your body – tells you to start slowly, we recommend beginning with baby steps. Walk for 10 minutes at a comfortable pace and gradually, over the next few weeks, build up to the full 20 minutes. *Then* pick up the pace. If you already walk regularly or are reasonably fit, go for 20 minutes most days a week right away. (Of course, if you find that you are enjoying walking, there's no harm in going longer.)

Perfect timing We recommend walking in the early morning, before your day starts. This strategy guarantees that you'll fit in your walk and will add a relaxed, energetic glow to everything else you do. If midday or evenings are better for you, or if your best time changes from day to day, that's fine, too. Just try to identify your walk time the night before so you can build it into your day. Keep walking shoes and socks in your office or your car (or on your feet) so you can get out when the getting's good.

Best places Feed your soul, feast your eyes and breathe clean, sweet air by choosing the prettiest streets in your neighbourhood or the nicest nearby parks or tracks. Avoid walking along busy highways or in parking lots. It's no fun being assaulted by traffic noise, and bus fumes can be harmful for your health.

Walk this way Everybody knows how to walk, right? Yes… and no. Just as we don't always sit the right way, we don't always walk the right way. When they're walking for fitness,

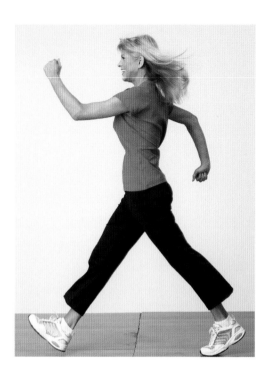

people sometimes do funny things. They flap their elbows like they're doing the chicken dance or march with stiff arms; they take super-elongated strides or lean forward as if heading into a cyclone.

The best walking style is natural and free, but not lazy. Stand up straight, tuck in your tummy, relax your shoulders and look forward, keeping your gaze about 6 metres ahead rather than down in front of you. (If you're walking on an uneven surface, look down, of course!)

The right pace? Simply aim to walk briskly – at the speed you'd reach if you were about 10 minutes late for an appointment. You should be breathing a little hard but still be able to carry on a conversation in full sentences. This easy 'talk test' works as well as a heart monitor for making sure you get to, and stay in, the best kilojoule-burning, fitness-building zone. If you're breathing normally, pick up the pace a bit.

Boost the kilojoule burn Once you're comfortable with your 20-minute brisk walk, you can burn even more kilojoules by adding a few fast-paced intervals. Here's how. Walk at your usual speed for 3 to 5 minutes, then walk even more briskly for 1 to 2 minutes. To pick up the pace, take short, quick steps. (Most people try to walk faster by elongating their strides, but this actually slows you down and can lead to joint and shin injuries.) Bend your arms at 90 degrees and pump them quickly. After your fast-walking interval, resume your usual brisk pace for 3 to 4 minutes, then pick it up again for 1 to 2 minutes. Do this several times during your walk. Boosting the intensity intermittently can increase the kilojoule burn by 60 per cent.

Stepping up your steps

Researchers estimate that Australians and New Zealanders today burn around half as many kilojoules a day as we did a half century ago – in part, because we don't walk to the supermarket, the bus stop, school, the movies or doing housework as our parents did. In addition to a dedicated

20-minute walk every day, we want you to fight 21st-century sitting disease by adding steps back into your life. They *do* add up. 'I park my car as far away from the entrance as possible,' one *ChangeOne* participant says. 'The steps add up eventually. At work, I add 250 steps to my day just by parking in the space furthest away.' How can you fit more steps into your day?

Volunteer on the home front Walk to the letterbox to get the mail. Instead of sending your partner or kids to bring in the laundry or let the dog out, see these tasks as a chance for some extra steps. While you're watching television, march in place during a 30-minute program, use your treadmill or walk around the house during the ads. Don't chat on the phone while you're sitting in a lounge-room chair – take calls on a cordless phone or mobile phone and walk while you talk.

Make every step count

Can a tiny plastic gadget that costs as little as $30 help you to walk more and lose weight? You can count on it. Pedometers are scarcely larger than a box of matches and clip unobtrusively to your belt or waistband. They count each step you take, and some also track the kilometres travelled and kilojoules burned. For many people, simply knowing that the number on the readout is increasing with every step inspires them to take more steps. 'The pedometer is a wonderful, motivational tool. I love mine,' says one *ChangeOne* participant.

Experts recommend aiming for an ultimate goal of 10,000 steps a day for weight loss and fitness. We recommend a more modest goal of adding 5000 steps (including those you accumulate on your new daily 20-minute walk) to whatever you're doing now.

Those 5000 steps add up to a real weight-loss advantage, according to a US study of 179 women and men.

They all followed a *ChangeOne*-type diet, and for 40 weeks, they either went to the gym four times a week, did calisthenics at home or simply tried to increase their daily steps by 5000. At the end, the steppers lost as much weight as the others and kept it off just as easily.

How to get there: First, wear your pedometer on a typical day *before* you begin the walking program and note how many steps you walk. Watch how that number increases as you begin the *ChangeOne* Fitness walking plan. Basic, everyday activities such as taking out the rubbish and picking up the mail use about 100 steps per minute. So does strolling at a lively yet relaxed pace while shopping at the supermarket or growers' market. Rushing to a meeting or appointment tallies about 130 steps per minute. Walking 1.5 km takes about 2000 steps. We estimate the *ChangeOne* 20-minute fitness walk will add around 2500 steps to your day.

Step it up at work Get off the bus a stop or two early and walk the rest of the way. Choose the entrance furthest away from your work space, then park as far away from it as possible. Take a walking break every half an hour at work and head to the water cooler or bathroom furthest from your desk. Go to a co-worker's desk when you have a question instead of always using email or the phone; you may find that you even improve your working relationships.

Get out of the car, up from your seat or off the stadium seats Running errands? See which ones you can do by walking from home. For others, park in a central location and walk to as many shops as possible. Circle the field during kids' sporting events. Take a walk instead of waiting in the car or the hall during play practices, piano lessons and so on. Stuck at the airport? Take a good walk around the terminal and skip the moving walkways.

Keep it interesting

Stay motivated, enjoy your walks more and walk in all weather with these tips.

Pair up with a buddy Sometimes the lure of inertia is irresistible, but if you have a walking date to keep, you're much more likely to make it past the threshold of your front door. If you don't have a friend who wants to walk with you, find a walking partner by asking around your neighbourhood or at work (for lunchtime walks) or by posting a notice at your church, gym or community centre.

Get a gadget Invest in an iPod or a portable CD player with earphones and walk to your favourite tunes. Upbeat songs can help you maintain a faster pace. Or catch up on your reading with audiobooks. Another idea is to equip your mobile phone with a headset, hit the road and phone your mum or your best friend for an uninterrupted chat.

Outsmart the seasons If the mail carrier can deliver mail in any weather, you can walk in any weather, as long as you're dressed for it. But if you live in a climate that's often too hot or too cold for comfort, consider investing in a treadmill. A word of advice: try before you buy. Features to think about include the deck size (a longer walking surface feels less cramped than a short one, but make sure your chosen machine will fit the space available in your home), shock absorption (thicker belts, floating decks and special shock absorbers decrease the wear and tear on your legs and feet but also raise the price), and the range of speeds and incline levels. (Most walkers will be fine with a top speed of 8 to 9.5 kilometres per hour, but consider a wide incline range so you can vary your walks and add a bigger challenge.)

Try an indoor track – with cash registers Shopping centres can be a great venue for walking when the weather's bad. You could also easily walk for 20 minutes in a big general department store. 'I began walking five times a week at the local shopping centre about three months ago,' reports one *ChangeOne* walker. 'I walk along the interior walls and through one or two of the larger shops. I wasn't going to look at the scales that often, but when my co-workers kept asking me if I was losing weight, I checked, and I'd lost the first 5 kilograms easily – plus some centimetres, as my pants became baggy.'

Be inspired Once a week, find and walk in a special new spot such as a lovely neighbourhood across town, a pretty coastal walk or a bushwalking track. Feel at one with nature and yourself by focusing on your breathing and your steps. Or repeat a soothing word or phrase as you walk. (Or pretend you're seeing everything around you for the very first time.) Soak up the year-round beauty of nature and enjoy it even more with inspirational quotes from a book of quotes. Check the newspaper or online for local nature hikes and bushwalks, or walking tours of local homes, gardens and historic spots.

Give back Plan to participate in a fund-raising charity walk as soon as the opportunity presents itself. Many are 5 kilometres long. You'll stay motivated as you 'train' on your daily walks and help support a worthy cause such as breast cancer research or preventing birth defects.

ChangeOne shoe tips

The only equipment you really need is a good pair of walking shoes. Finding them is a cinch – just be sure they're comfortable. You shouldn't need to 'break them in'. When shopping for shoes:

- Wear the socks you plan to walk in, not thicker or thinner ones.
- Look for flat shoes (your heel and the ball of your foot should be at about the same level) with lots of toe room.
- Do the twist test. A good walking shoe should be flexible enough to accommodate your foot's natural heel-to-toe roll. If the shoe doesn't bend at the ball of the foot, and you can't twist the sole from side to side, it's too stiff.
- Reserve these shoes for walking to extend their life. Experts recommend that you replace walking shoes every 800 km – about every 10 months on the *ChangeOne* Fitness program.

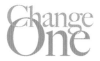

Get outdoors

'The world is mud-luscious and puddle-wonderful,' wrote the poet e.e. cummings. If you can't remember the last time you splashed in – or at least walked around – a fine, fat mud puddle, you've come to the right chapter.

In these pages, you'll be inspired to reconnect with the outdoors and with your own sense of playfulness and fun.

If life doesn't afford you much time for outdoor fun, we'll show you how working in the garden and even home maintenance projects can count towards your *ChangeOne* Fitness goal of spending at least 2 hours a week outdoors. Why 2 hours? We want you to break away from that indoor disease – the sitting, snacking, sedentary lifestyle that packs on kilos, zaps energy levels and leaves you choosing between an endless round of little household jobs and watching endless television series and reality shows. It's time to live a little – and we think getting outside is an essential component of a happy, healthy life.

Outsmart indoor disease

If you're plopped on a bed, sofa or chair right now, surrounded by four walls and a ceiling, you're taking part in Australia and New Zealand's number 1 *anti*-activity – indoor disease. It's the biggest reason why more and more of us are overweight and under-energetic. This housebound, car-bound, office-bound lifestyle claims at least 20 to 23 hours out of the days of most adults in both countries. Shocked? Check out this sobering arithmetic: add up 2 hours for cooking and eating meals; 1–2 hours sitting in the car, bus or train while commuting; another 7–9 hours on the job (or working at home); 3 hours of watching TV and 7 hours of snoozing. Not much time left for activity, much less for going outside, is there?

The *ChangeOne* response? Turn off the TV, push the footstool away from the couch, lace up your shoes and get outdoors for a minimum of 2 hours of fun a week. What you do once you land on the other side of the front door is up to you. Follow your bliss. Of course, ahead in this chapter, you'll find dozens of ideas for backyard fun, practical house and garden projects, and short jaunts and longer trips in the wide, beautiful, natural world. But we believe that even enjoying your morning coffee or an after-work cool drink on the verandah counts, because the more you get outside, the more likely it is that you'll stay out – strolling across the lawn to check out the first roses blooming or the last summer tomato, walking next door to chat with a neighbour, or playing cricket with the kids or fetch with the dog. (Or finally fixing up that bit of guttering.)

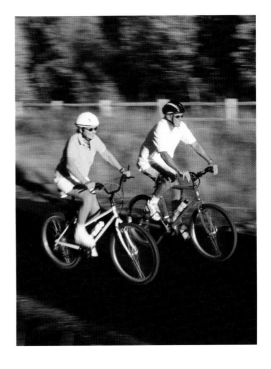

Your mission is simple. Get outdoors and trust that nature will take its course. Your personal happiness index will go up, stress and fatigue will begin to melt away, and you'll find yourself inventing excuses to get back out there in the sunshine and fresh air again very soon. Even better, you may find that the more time you spend outside, the faster the kilos will fall away.

Personal benefits

Need hard facts about the benefits of living outside the big box called home? You'll:

■ **Cash in on extracurricular weight loss** Watching 30 minutes of TV burns a piddling 155 kilojoules. In contrast, 30 minutes spent painting the house will work off 840 kJ; gardening uses 195 kJ; a fast-paced footy game works off 1345 kJ; washing the car, 750 kJ; and mowing the lawn, 795 kJ – if you rake up afterwards, you'll sweat off 835 kJ. In winter, stacking firewood burns 1010 kJ.

■ **Multiply your happiness** Looking at flowers eases depression, according to US psychologists, who tested the moods of 100 women and men in the presence and absence of colourful flowers. Meanwhile, exposure to sunlight lifted depression in another study. No surprise there – most of us have heard (and know instinctively) about sunlight's power to lift winter depression. Yet the researchers also found that we don't always act on what we know. When they issued sunlight meters to the study's volunteers to measure their exposure to sunlight over two days, they found that most got just an hour of exposure, and some had none at all.

■ **Feel pleasure, have fun** Kick off your shoes, taste a sun-ripened strawberry, smell the autumn leaves. Every little kid delays coming indoors as long as possible after a day in the open air, and that kid is still inside you. Nature is gloriously romantic. The poet Kahlil Gibran said, 'Forget not that the earth delights to feel your bare feet and the winds long to play with your hair.' Or, as one *ChangeOne* participant told us, 'Whenever I garden, I forget time, aches or even to eat! I would sooner be outside than doing almost anything else!'

■ **Spend plenty of quality time with the family** In one eye-opening survey of 500 families in the United States, kids confided that they spend hardly any meaningful time with their parents – by which they meant doing something fun together. (Parents thought they spent lots of quality time teaching their kids how to do things.) The situation is much the same in Australia and New Zealand. We think getting outdoors together will bring you closer to your children and create a lasting, deeper bond.

Change One Quiz

Are you an indoor or outdoor person?

Answer each of the following true-or-false questions as honestly as you can.

1. **I can swim and like to do so.**
   ☐ True   ☐ False

2. **If I were invited to play in an easygoing softball game, I'd probably say yes.**
   ☐ True   ☐ False

3. **Sunsets, wildflowers and mountaintop views make me very, very happy.**
   ☐ True   ☐ False

4. **I'd rather grow my own tomatoes than buy them.**
   ☐ True   ☐ False

5. **I understand why people are attracted to the game of golf.**
   ☐ True   ☐ False

6. **When I see a well-equipped playground, the kid inside me wants to stop and play.**
   ☐ True   ☐ False

7. **I'd rather read a book in a hammock than on a couch.**
   ☐ True   ☐ False

8. **I'd rather take an evening stroll than watch the evening news.**
   ☐ True   ☐ False

9. **At least one pair of shoes in my cupboard has dried mud caked to the bottom.**
   ☐ True   ☐ False

10. **I have my own bicycle, and it's ready for riding.**
    ☐ True   ☐ False

11. **I can identify at least three constellations in the night sky.**
    ☐ True   ☐ False

12. **I can identify at least five different types of bird where I live.**
    ☐ True   ☐ False

Quiz score

Tally up your 'true' answers. Here's how to rate your score.

9–12: You are clearly a person who loves the outdoors! Now that you know that being outdoors is part of the active, healthy-weight lifestyle, you should be motivated to get out even more often.

5–8: You enjoy the outdoors, but being outside probably isn't an integral part of your life. Find outdoor activities you particularly enjoy and pursue them as much as you can.

In time, you'll broaden your activities and become far more passionate about your time in the big outdoors.

1–4: Modern living has clearly got the best of you. The time has come to reconnect with your childhood spirit and to relearn the joys of cool breezes, soft grass and outdoor play. Try to do your walks outdoors, and slowly find interests that get you out of the living room, out of the shops, out of the car and into nature.

■ **Build self-esteem** People who spend lots of time outdoors tend to be doers, not watchers. Not only are they physically stronger than their sedentary counterparts, they also often have lots of self-confidence as well. They are often leaner and healthier, thanks to all the activity they do, and they frequently have more positive attitudes about life as well. Sure, we admit these are stereotypes, and there are plenty of exceptions. But think about people you know who are passionate about the outdoors. Are we very far from the truth?

Get ready

As a kid, your wardrobe was probably sharply divided between 'good' clothes, 'school' clothes and grungy, the-dirtier-the-better 'play' clothes. We'd like you to revive the play clothes category so you're prepared, at a moment's notice, to get out in the sunshine (or moonlight). Here's how.

■ Gather into one drawer or onto one shelf your oldest, machine-washable T-shirts (long- and short-sleeved), shorts and jeans; a cotton jumper or hoodie; comfy socks that can get dirty; and for women, a supportive bra you won't mind sweating in.

■ Keep outdoor shoes and a brimmed hat by the front door. Store sunscreen and insect repellent. If you don't like chemical repellents, try one with lemon eucalyptus essential oil. According to those who use the natural alternative regularly, it's just as good as commercial preparations for repelling mosquitoes.

■ Put on your outdoor clothes when you get home from work or first thing on weekend mornings when you don't have to go anywhere.

■ Resurrect the toy box. Stock it with things you might enjoy playing with, such as practice golf balls and a 9-iron, a Frisbee, a skipping rope, a fishing rod (practice casting into a bucket), a 10-pin bowling set, quoits or even a painting set. If you have children, grandchildren or neighbourhood children who visit, include a football or soccer ball, chalk for drawing hopscotch squares on the concrete and perhaps even a hula hoop. You'll always be ready to play at a moment's notice.

Plan it, then do it

If your excuse for not getting outdoors is lack of time, then you need to reclaim your weekends – and that bit of time between dinner and sunset – by wielding your pen and your calendar. Here's how.

Use weeknights more effectively

Why do so many of us spend our weekends shopping, cleaning and cooking? Not only are the shops most crowded then, but we sacrifice our days off to tasks that are easily and more efficiently done during the week. Assign weekend tasks to particular evenings of the week. For example, do your grocery shopping on Monday night, spend Tuesday night cooking dinners for the rest of the week and designate Thursday night for vacuuming. Your goal is to wake up on Saturday with as few mandatory tasks as possible.

Spread out the work Do you know what the perfect gardening schedule is? Fifteen minutes of work, first thing every single morning. Do that, and we guarantee your garden will never be in better shape – and your body will thank you for it, too. Saving up all the backyard work for intense, hours-long sessions is not only tough on your muscles, patience and schedule, it isn't great for the flowers, either! Instead, create a daily routine of planting, weeding, feeding and watering one small area at a time. Over time, you and your garden will flourish. The same holds true for housework, by the way – 15 minutes a day may make your house less cluttered and cleaner than ever!

Schedule, schedule, schedule Does the following conversation sound familiar?

'What do you want to do today?'

'Uh, I don't know. What do *you* want to do?'

'I don't know, either. I asked you first!'

If your family regularly gets into this kind of cycle of indecision come weekend mornings, it's time to break out of it. The method: during the previous week, be specific in your

Help!

'I just don't like being outdoors. I'm bothered by insects, find it unpleasant to wear sunscreen and don't enjoy sweating. What can I do?'

Ease into it by creating a comfortable 'outdoor room' that is strictly for your relaxation. Your space should have a few comfortable folding chairs, a chaise longue or a picnic table with padded benches or dining chairs.

To deal with the insects, cover up as best you can with long-sleeved clothing, which will discourage biting insects. Also get citronella candles or a mozzie zapper to discourage flying insects.

Put on a wide-brimmed hat for protection from sun and glare. Make yourself some tea and put it in a sealed cup or travel mug. Then settle into your outdoor room with something fun to read and see what happens. We bet you'll discover the sounds of birds and wind to be relaxing and the breeze refreshing. In time, you'll come around to the pleasures of outdoor activity.

planning for the upcoming weekend. Don't just suggest a nature walk on Sunday afternoon. Pick a time and place. Think through what you'll need and what preparations or reservations will be required. Having a set agenda and being prepared is the best way to avoid inactivity due to indecision.

Say no to excuses

When the temperature's a pleasant 25 degrees, the humidity's a perfect 50 per cent, the sun's shining and it's Saturday afternoon with absolutely nothing else on your agenda, you don't need too many extra enticements to get you out the door. In less than perfect conditions, however, it's sometimes tough to get going. Here's how to get motivated when time's running short, the weather's challenging or the great indoors is pulling you towards the couch.

If you've got just a few minutes Pour your coffee into a travel mug with a lid and wander into the backyard or down the street. Grab garden shears and create a bouquet for the table or pinch off all those past-their-prime blooms in your border garden. Pull out a tennis racquet, golf club or cricket bat and practise your stroke for a few moments. Crunch through the autumn leaves or rake the front yard. If you have only a little time to spare at work, walk to a place 5 minutes from your office for lunch, then walk back. Or head over to a playground for 10 minutes of silliness with a friend. Keep a Frisbee and a ball in the car boot for some quick fun.

If you're with the kids Go out for miniature golf; stay home for badminton, backyard cricket or football; bounce on a trampoline; or teach them your favourite old street games – skipping rope, elastics, French cricket or tug-of-war. (An hour of playing tip burns more than 1250 kilojoules, too!) Dust off your bike and take a ride. Go bushwalking in a park or reserve with a simple set of trails and let the kids be in charge of the map – an experience that builds confidence. Play every sport in the book – soccer, touch football, cricket; the good news is that most kids will get more exercise and have more fun in vigorous backyard play than in an organised league, where less skilled athletes often meet with discouragement. Or try an old-fashioned favourite: family backyard work interspersed with fun, silly breaks.

1001 things to do

If you put your mind to it, we're sure there's no shortage of things you'd enjoy doing outside. But few of us bother to put our minds to it. We say, just do it! Once you list ideas, pick a few of the best and schedule them. Here are some to get you started.

If you prefer activities with practical results, inspect your home's exterior and garden and list jobs that would make you feel better once they're completed. Repaint the letterbox post, hang a window box, move the garbage bins to a different storage location, paint the back steps.

If you love sports or solo activities, join a hiking club or scour the newspaper for a top-level sports group. Or spend an evening at a sports shop buying a bat and ball, a tennis racquet, a cricket bat or roller skates – equipment for whatever you once enjoyed. It's time to revive the activities of your youth!

If you love wandering in nature, pick a park, mountain, beach or lake that's close enough for you to take advantage of visiting regularly. Find a map and check if there's an admission fee. Also consider cultivating an interest in birds. Bird-watching is a very popular hobby, thanks to the wonderful diversity of colours, shapes, songs and personalities among Australian and New Zealand birds.

If you're social, schedule and plan fun outdoor events. If you have kids, consider water parks, cycling tracks, playgrounds, pools and zoos. If you don't have children, have barbecues, parties and hikes or go to outdoor craft shows or music festivals. Or combine an outdoor activity with a treat. Fix up the backyard, then have the neighbours over for a sunset barbecue. Invite your guests to play old-fashioned, grown-up lawn games. Bocce or croquet, anyone?

If it's cold out Dress in layers. For example, put on a moisture-wicking T-shirt, a woollen base layer, a fleece jumper and a wind jacket; for your bottom half, start with thermal underwear or tights or pantihose, then wool pants and finally waterproof rain or snow pants if you live in a very cold area. The same goes for your feet – moisture-wicking socks, then wool socks, then waterproof boots. Cover your head and ears effectively, then completely forget about the temperature. If you live in a snowy area or are holidaying near the slopes, go sledding or skating. Rent cross-country skis and take a Saturday afternoon ski class at a local park or sports shop, then ski until sunset.

If it's raining Wear waterproof outer clothes, grab the umbrella and walk! Enjoy the sights and sounds of the city or country during a shower. It's surprisingly fun and sensual.

If it's windy Fly a kite! Any type will do, but for a great upper-body workout, use a stunt kite. Don't have a kite? Then just walk into the wind. It's fun, silly and strenuous, and you'll never feel more awake.

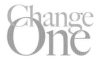

Get stronger

Once, building muscle was the nearly exclusive domain of big, sweaty guys working out in smelly gyms filled with the sounds of grunts and clanging iron. Their ultimate goal: cartoonish, overpumped, muscle-man physiques.

One notable exception is Marilyn Monroe. This blonde bombshell reportedly performed muscle-toning exercises several times a week and credited her curves to her strength-training routine. She had the right idea. Muscles are far too important to leave to the bodybuilders. There is compelling research that shows that a short, easy, fun strengthening and stretching routine won't leave you with Popeye-style arms. Instead, you'll look and feel more like Marilyn (or if you're a guy, a young Kirk Douglas) – lean, sexy and strong.

In this chapter, you'll discover three 10-minute routines that harness the amazing weight-loss power locked inside your muscles.

This gentle strengthening and stretching will tone your body, boost your energy levels and help you burn more kilojoules around the clock.

What Marilyn knew

Left to their own devices, your muscles begin to diminish in size and strength in your thirties or forties. At first, the change is so gradual that you may barely detect it. You may weigh the same but you somehow look rounder, puffier – or your favourite jeans may no longer zip shut.

What's happening? As long, lean muscle mass shrinks, puffy, blobby fat moves in. Then weight gain accelerates. Muscle is metabolically active; that is, it uses up kilojoules even when at rest. Each 500 grams of muscle burns about 125 to 200 kilojoules per day. Fat, in contrast, burns next to none. So when you replace muscle with fat, your metabolism slows down, and you begin gaining weight even if your diet and exercise habits haven't changed. It may seem like nothing, but after the age of 35 or so, you lose 150 to 225 grams of muscle each year – a loss that could eventually add up to an extra 1250 to 1900 kilojoules a day that your metabolism isn't burning off! The result is that weight begins to climb. This metabolic decline hits women harder than men, probably because men have more muscle mass to begin with.

Trying to lose those extra kilos just by cutting kilojoules can backfire or prove to be amazingly difficult. Why? Because your metabolism is already running slowly, eating less only further reduces your muscle mass.

That's where the *ChangeOne* Fitness strengthening/stretching plan comes in.

You'll use resistance, in this case your own body weight and sometimes small dumbbells, to put a little healthy stress on the muscles in your upper and lower body and at your core – the key muscles of your abdomen and back. During resistance exercise, muscle fibres actually experience microscopic tears; as they heal, they grow denser and larger. You'll also stretch so your muscles and joints become more limber.

Help!

'Strength training is supposed to hurt, right? How else could it build my muscles? The trouble is, I don't want to do exercise that causes pain.'

'No pain, no gain' is an outdated myth perpetuated by competitive muscle builders and athletes. Strength training should never cause you pain. Research shows that a gentle routine can alleviate backaches, fibromyalgia and arthritis pain, and chronic neck discomfort.

As you get started with this routine, note that your muscles may feel a *bit* sore for a few days, and you may feel a little tired. That's normal. It's quite likely that your muscles haven't been used in these ways for a long time. Imagine that they are being awakened after a long slumber. But if you're exhausted, your joints are sore or your muscles feel like they're cramped or pulled, you're overdoing it and need to go easier on yourself. Proceed slowly, with fewer repetitions of each exercise to start, and build up from there.

What you get is more muscle, less fat and the ability to move with youthful ease and grace. Since muscle takes up less space than fat, you look trimmer even if you don't lose any weight. In fact, some people actually gain a little weight when they begin strength training because they're building muscle – and muscle weighs more than fat. But they also notice that their clothes fit more loosely, or they even drop a dress size or two. Over time, weight loss speeds up as the extra muscle burns more kilojoules all day long.

Five big benefits of strengthening and stretching

The bottom line is that a little strength training is a girl's (and guy's) best friend. It's motivating. As one *ChangeOne* participant says, 'Just feeling my muscles as I move the rest of the day reminds me that I am working on being healthy, and it makes me think twice before sabotaging it all with a bad "treat".' Here's a rundown of what's in it for you.

A firmer, more shapely figure Muscle is smooth, lean, hard and small; fat is lumpy, flabby, soft and big. Experts say that compared to 500 grams of fat, 500 grams of muscle takes up about 22 per cent less space. In one US study of 40 postmenopausal women aged between 50 and 70, those who performed easy strength-training exercises for about 80 minutes a week were significantly leaner and trimmer than those who didn't do the exercises.

A metabolic tune-up In another US study, women and men who strength-trained three times a week for six months gained 2 kilograms of lean muscle, lost 2.75 kilograms of fat, and increased their metabolisms by 12 per cent. Their bodies burned an extra 965 kilojoules per day, even on days when they weren't working out.

More energy and a more active life These researchers noticed something interesting about the women who strength-trained in their study. They increased their activity levels by 25 per cent. In the year after the study ended, non-exercisers grew less active, but the muscle-strengthening group was on to new things. One woman went whitewater rafting with her family; another moved 3.5 tons of topsoil, one load at a time, in a wheelbarrow as she spruced up her garden; others took up in-line skating, mountain biking and ballroom dancing. One woman even outscored the study's lead researcher at bowling. The study authors suspect that added strength (the women were eventually as strong as or stronger than their own daughters) made all these activities easy to do.

Better posture; more everyday power By doing a routine that targets all areas of your body, you will improve your posture, and handling heavy stuff – from grocery bags loaded with canned goods to toddlers to heavy furniture – will be a breeze.

A more limber, graceful, ache-free body Each of our *ChangeOne* strengthening routines ends with a couple of refreshing stretches. These are more than just feel-good moves

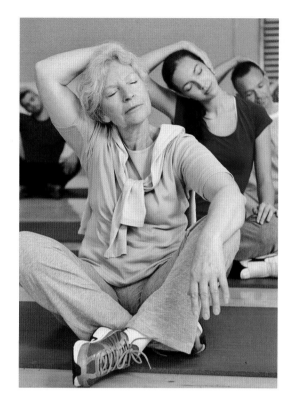

(although stretching can help you relax, physically and mentally). While strength training contracts and flexes your muscles, stretching lengthens them, increasing your flexibility and range of motion and improving blood flow to your muscles. This means more oxygen and blood sugar for nourishment and more efficient whisking-away of waste products. 'Each morning before I get dressed for the day, I do gentle stretching exercises,' notes a *ChangeOne* participant. 'What a difference for stiff joints! The flexibility lasts for quite a while.'

Get ready, get set, go!

Some strength-training programs require serious equipment. Not *ChangeOne*. Our routines are just as effective and much more convenient. In total, we ask you to have two light dumbbells, a chair, a towel, a step and a wall. These routines are designed for the home, although you can do them while travelling, either using a bag or briefcase in place of the dumbbell or just doing the movements without a weight but with your muscles tensed.

For even more convenience, we've broken the program into three 10-minute routines – an upper-body routine, a lower-body routine and a core routine (the core being the back, abdomen and hips). Do one routine each and every day. We recommend that you do it first thing in the morning, but for those who are night owls, in the evening or before bed is fine, too. The important thing is to do it – don't skip a day! If you don't like the idea of an 'exercise period', just think of it as a quick household task, like moving the laundry from the washing machine to the dryer. That's what one *ChangeOne* participant does to get herself going. 'It's easier to say to myself, "It's just 10 minutes." It doesn't seem so hard mentally to fit in that way when I really don't feel like exercising.'

Now let's be honest. At first, some of these exercises will feel a little awkward. Some will be more challenging than others. Constantly remind yourself that this is not a contest or a race or a program you'll be tested on. You are doing this for *you*, at your rate of speed, at your rate of progress. If you're struggling with a few of the moves, that's fine. Make the movement a little smaller or do it without the hand weight. If merely getting onto and off the floor is challenging, fine; start by just getting down onto the floor and then back up again, skipping the exercise for now. We're sure that in time, you will not only be able to get through each routine comfortably but will also enjoy them immensely. Here are some tips.

- **Don't fixate on time** At first, you may want a little longer rest period between movements, or you may choose to do fewer repetitions of each exercise. What's important is that you learn to do the routines correctly. Over time, you'll become more efficient.
- **Do the exercises slowly** Count 2 to 4 seconds as you perform the first half of each exercise and another 2 to 4 as you do the second half. That way your muscles work

Check-in

We've asked you to fit four kinds of physical activity into your week: Walking, strengthening and stretching, outdoor fun, and extra everyday movements. Have you found time for all four – and does it feel relatively easy? Or has fitness become a source of stress? If so, go back to basics – with a twist. Start with fitting extra steps and movements into your everyday life. After a week or so, add 20 minutes of brisk walking a day. Once that's a regular part of your life, find time for 10 minutes of strengthening and stretching. You'll be feeling great – and ready to look for some outdoor fun.

harder. Take time to perform each exercise slowly and correctly so that you get the best results.

- **Breathe well** Inhale before you begin each move so you can exhale during the first part (usually the more strenuous part of the exercise) and inhale during the second part.

- **Remember to rotate the routines** A key component of strength training is giving your muscles a day or two to rest, heal and grow. By rotating through our three routines, you'll exercise each major muscle group at least twice a week, which is exactly the right amount. Never repeat the same routine two days in a row.

- **Try to do the exercises in the order listed** It's a sensible progression. Most importantly, though, always stretch after strengthening. Experts agree that it's best to stretch muscles when they're warm, not at the start of your routine when they're cold and tight.

- **As with the exercises, do the stretches slowly and deliberately** Hold each one for 10 to 30 seconds, as indicated. Move smoothly – never bounce or jerk your muscles. Inhale before you start, then exhale going into the stretch and inhale again as you release it. Breathe slowly to encourage relaxation. Never stretch to the point of pain. You may feel slight discomfort, but anything more means it's time to back off.

■ **Equipment needed** Two light dumbbells, one chair

The upper-body ROUTINE

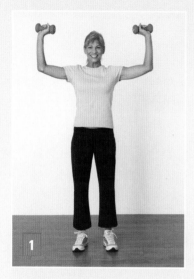

1

■ **EXERCISE ONE**

Cross-over chest squeeze

1 Stand holding a light dumbbell in each hand. Bend your arms to 90-degree angles and hold them out to your sides so your upper arms are parallel to the floor with your palms facing forwards.

2 Squeezing your chest muscles, move your elbows towards each other until they're about shoulder-width apart. Return to the starting position. Slowly do 8 to 12 repetitions.

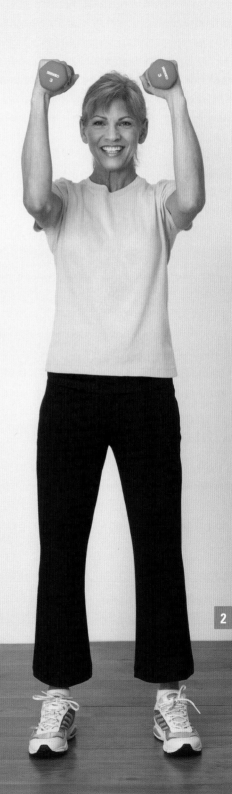

2

Pec pull

1 Holding a dumbbell in your left hand, stand with your right leg one huge step in front of your left, with your back heel lifted off the floor. Rest your right hand on your right thigh for support and lean forward slightly. Hold your left arm across your chest so your palm faces back.

2 Keeping your elbow bent, move it out to the side until your upper arm is extended even with your shoulder. Pause, then return to the starting position. After doing 8 to 12 repetitions, swap sides and repeat the exercise with your other arm.

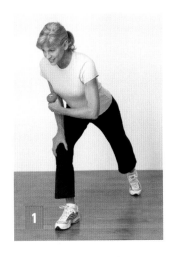

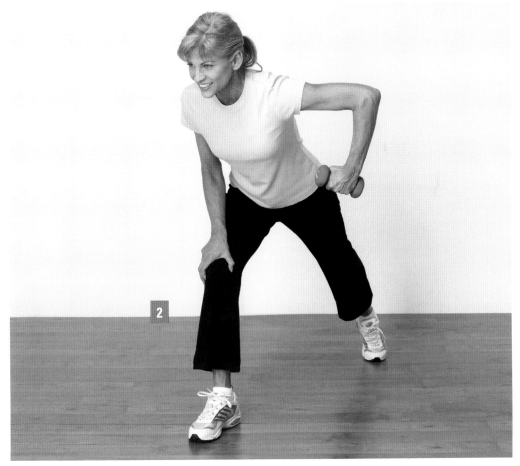

The upper-body *Routine continued*

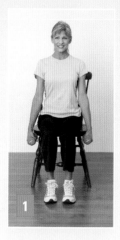

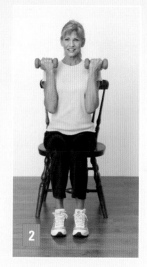

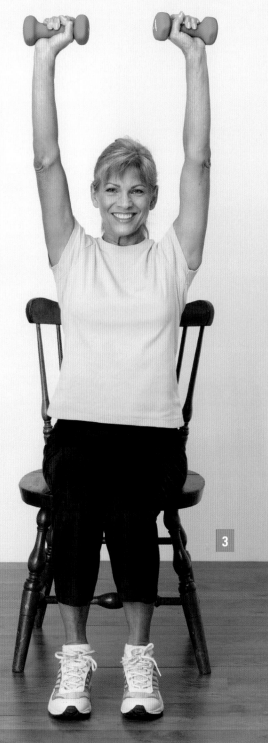

■ EXERCISE THREE

Curl and press

1 Sit on a chair (preferably one without arms) with your feet flat on the floor. Hold a light dumbbell in each hand with your arms extended down at your sides.

2 Keeping your upper body stable, bend your elbows and curl the weights up towards your shoulders.

3 Immediately rotate your wrists so your palms are facing away from you and press the weights overhead. Pause, then reverse the move, lowering the weights to your shoulders, rotating your palms in toward your body, and lowering the weights back down to your sides. Do 8 to 12 repetitions.

■ EXERCISE FOUR
Triceps kickback

1 Grasp a dumbbell in your left hand and place your right knee and hand on a chair seat so your back is parallel to the floor. Hold your left elbow at your side so your arm is bent at a 90-degree angle and your forearm is perpendicular to the floor.

2 Extend your elbow and move your hand backwards until your forearm is parallel to the floor. Pause, then lower to the starting position. Complete 8 to 12 repetitions, then switch sides.

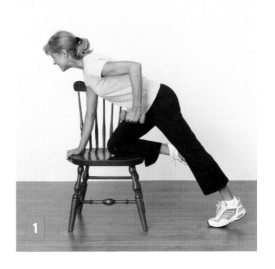

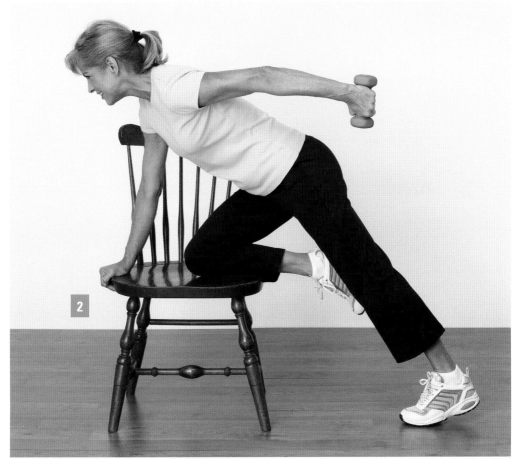

The upper-body *Routine continued*

■ STRETCH ONE
Rag doll

1 Sit on the edge of a chair with your knees spread slightly and your feet directly below your knees.

2 Slump your body forward over your legs so your chest rests on or above your knees and your arms hang down. Wrap your arms under your knees and press your back up towards the ceiling. Hold this position for 20 to 30 seconds.

■ STRETCH TWO
De-hunch

1 Sit on the edge of a chair with your legs spread and your pelvis tilted slightly forwards. Lift your chest and squeeze your shoulder blades together and down away from your ears.

2 Extend your arms at 45-degree angles from your body and reach slightly behind you with your palms facing forward. Hold for 10 seconds, then relax for a few seconds. Repeat 3 times.

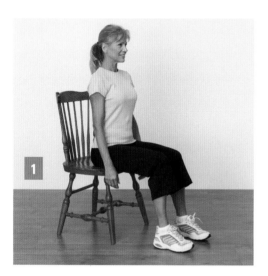

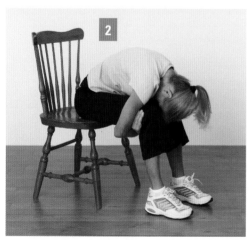

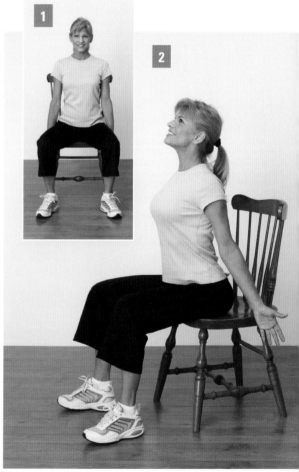

■ STRETCH THREE
Hand press

1 Sit on a chair with your feet flat on the floor. Press your palms together in front of your chest so your elbows are pointed out to the sides.

2 Keeping your hands pressed together, drop them down and slightly towards your body until you feel a stretch in your wrists and forearms. Hold for 20 seconds.

■ STRETCH FOUR
Sit and reach

1 Sit tall in a chair with your feet flat on the floor. Place your right hand on your left upper arm.

2 Twist to the right and grasp the back of the chair seat with your left hand, bringing your chin over your right shoulder as you turn. Hold for 15 seconds, then switch sides.

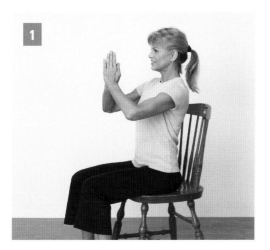

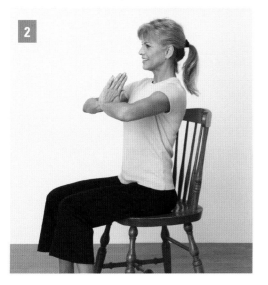

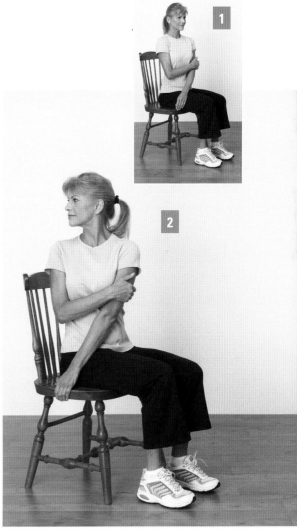

■ **Equipment needed** One light dumbbell, one chair, staircase or exercise step, wall

The lower-body ROUTINE

■ **EXERCISE ONE**
Lawnmower pull

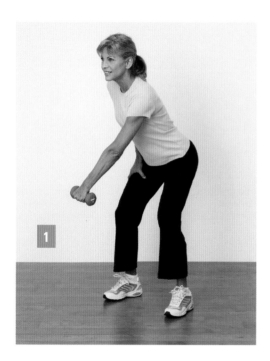

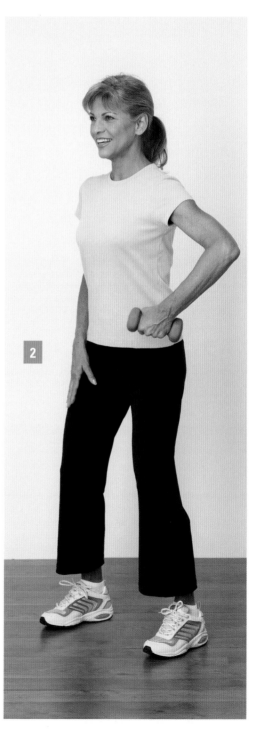

1 Stand with your feet hip-width apart, holding a light dumbbell in your left hand. Squat slightly until your legs are bent at about 45 degrees and place your right hand on your right thigh for support. Reach across your body with your left arm, holding the dumbbell in front of your right knee.

2 In one smooth motion, pull your arm back across your body (as though pulling a lawnmower cord) and stand up slightly, though not fully. Squat back down and repeat 5 times, slowly and carefully. Then switch sides.

■ EXERCISE TWO
Chair taps

1 Stand tall, facing a chair, with your feet about hip-width apart and your hands on your hips. (You can place one hand on a wall for balance if you need to.)

2 Keeping your abdominal muscles tensed to support your back, lift your right foot and tap the seat of the chair with your toes. Return to the starting position. Repeat 10 times, then switch sides.

■ EXERCISE THREE
Heel drop

1 Stand on the bottom step of a flight of stairs, or, if you have one, an exercise step. Lightly grasp the banister, or place your hand on a wall if using a step, for support. Bend your right leg and place the toes of your left foot on the edge of the step.

2 Let your left heel drop as far as comfortably possible. Press into the ball of your left foot and raise yourself onto your toes. Pause, then return to the starting position. Repeat 8 to 12 times, then switch legs.

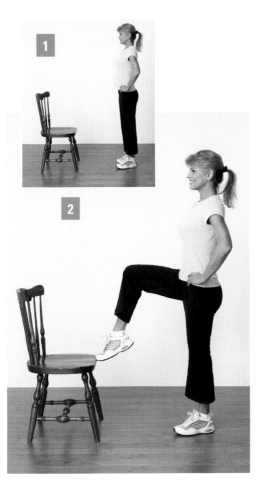

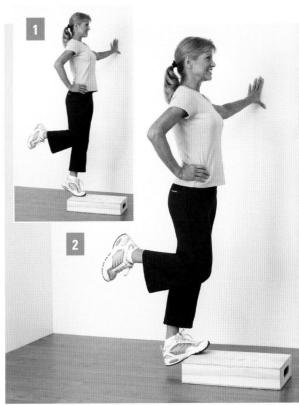

The lower-body *Routine continued*

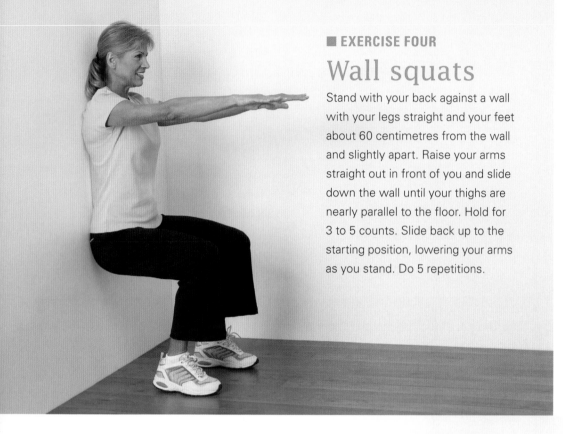

■ EXERCISE FOUR

Wall squats

Stand with your back against a wall with your legs straight and your feet about 60 centimetres from the wall and slightly apart. Raise your arms straight out in front of you and slide down the wall until your thighs are nearly parallel to the floor. Hold for 3 to 5 counts. Slide back up to the starting position, lowering your arms as you stand. Do 5 repetitions.

■ EXERCISE FIVE

Seated leg lift

Sit on the floor with your legs extended in front of you, your back straight and your feet flexed. Place your hands on your lap or on the floor behind you for support. Keeping your foot flexed, tighten your left thigh and slowly raise your left heel off the floor. Pause, then slowly return to the starting position. Complete 8 to 12 repetitions, then switch legs.

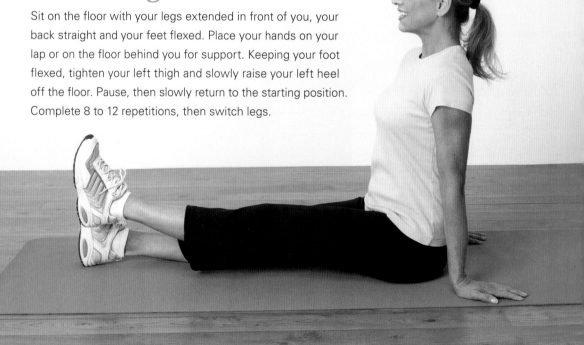

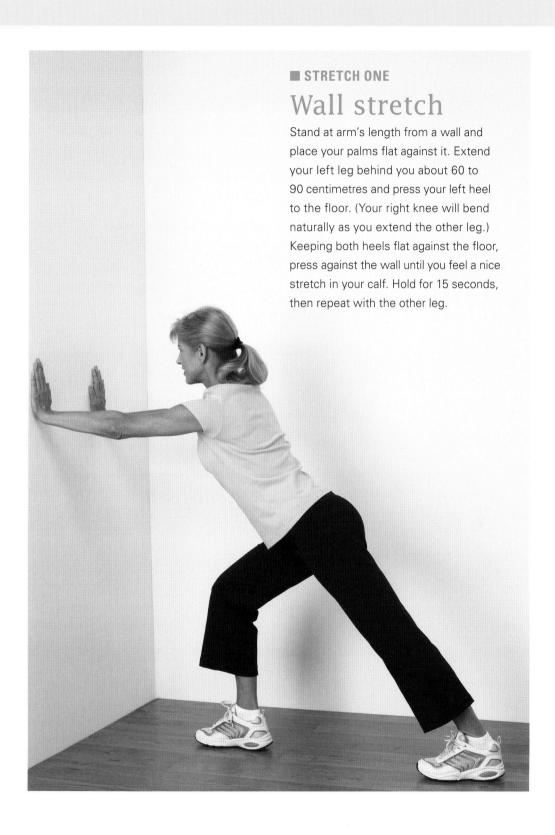

■ STRETCH ONE

Wall stretch

Stand at arm's length from a wall and place your palms flat against it. Extend your left leg behind you about 60 to 90 centimetres and press your left heel to the floor. (Your right knee will bend naturally as you extend the other leg.) Keeping both heels flat against the floor, press against the wall until you feel a nice stretch in your calf. Hold for 15 seconds, then repeat with the other leg.

The lower-body *Routine continued*

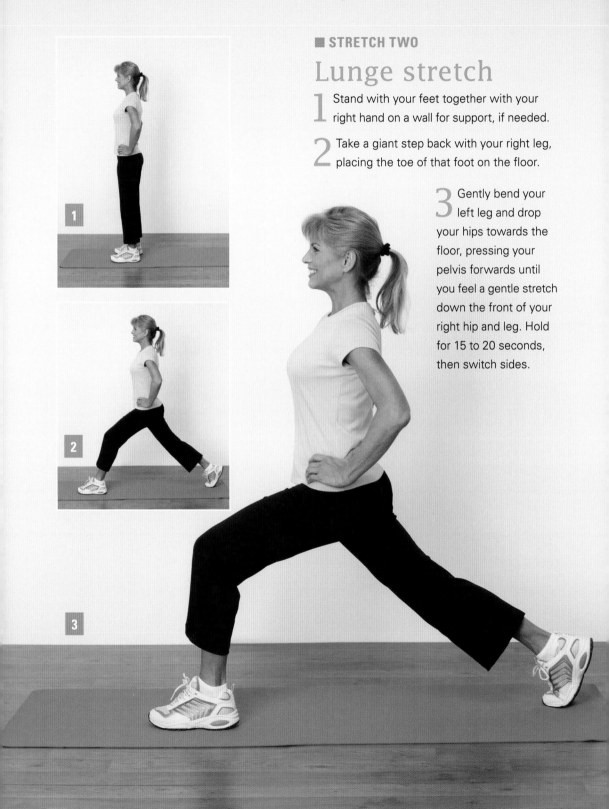

■ **STRETCH TWO**

Lunge stretch

1 Stand with your feet together with your right hand on a wall for support, if needed.

2 Take a giant step back with your right leg, placing the toe of that foot on the floor.

3 Gently bend your left leg and drop your hips towards the floor, pressing your pelvis forwards until you feel a gentle stretch down the front of your right hip and leg. Hold for 15 to 20 seconds, then switch sides.

■ STRETCH THREE
Butterfly

Sit on the floor with your back straight, your knees bent and the soles of your feet touching so your knees fall out to the sides. Grasp your ankles with your hands. Keeping your back straight (don't hunch over), gently bend forward from the hips as you press your knees down towards the floor as far as comfortably possible. Hold for 20 to 30 seconds.

■ STRETCH FOUR
Standing hamstring stretch

1 Standing upright, place your left heel about 30 centimetres in front of you and point your toes up. Place your hands on your right thigh for support.

2 Bending your right knee, gently bend forwards from the hips, pressing your weight back until you feel a stretch in the back of your left leg. Hold for 15 seconds, then switch legs.

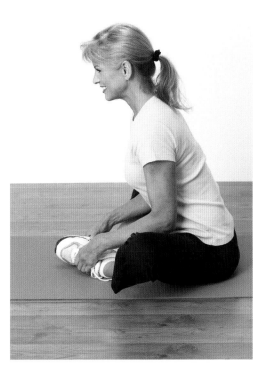

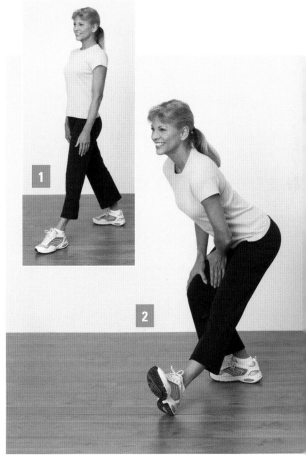

■ **Equipment needed** Floor mat or soft carpet

The core-body ROUTINE

■ **EXERCISE ONE**

Knee drop

1 Lie on your back with your knees bent, feet on the floor, arms straight out to the sides and hands resting on the floor, palms down.

2 Lift your legs so your knees are above your hips and your lower legs are parallel to the floor.

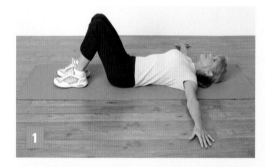

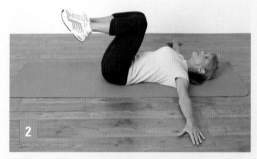

3 Contract your stomach muscles and drop both knees to the left as far as comfortably possible while keeping both shoulders on the floor. Pause, then return to the starting position. Repeat to the other side. That's 1 repetition. Alternate for a complete set of 10 repetitions.

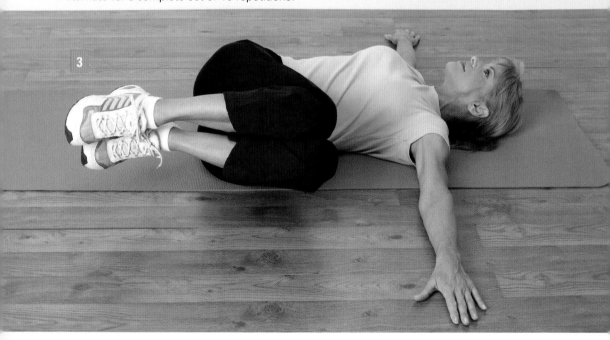

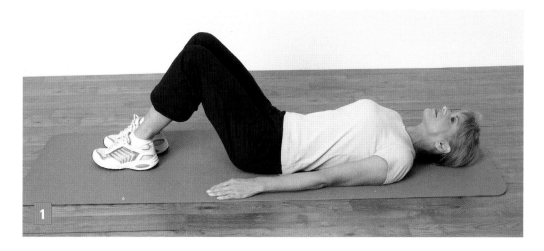

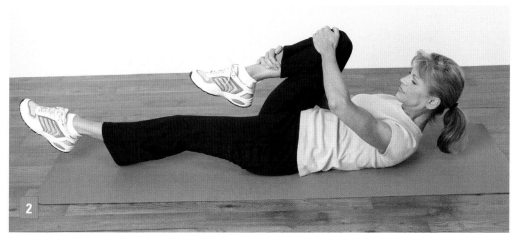

■ EXERCISE TWO

Single-leg stretch

1 Despite the name, this is a strengthening exercise. Lie on your back with your knees bent at about 45 degrees to your spine and your head on the mat.

2 Tuck your chin to your chest and place your right hand on your right ankle and your left hand on your right knee. Lift your left leg about 10 centimetres off the floor and pull your right knee towards your chest. Keeping your abdominals tight, switch sides, pulling your left knee towards your chest and lifting your right leg. Alternate 10 times for 1 set.

The core body *Routine continued*

■ EXERCISE THREE
Standing side crunch

1 Stand with your feet hip-width apart and your left foot pointed slightly out to the side. Place your right hand on your hip and extend your left arm straight overhead.

2 Lift your left knee up and out to the side at waist height as you move your left elbow down to meet your knee. Repeat 10 times, then switch sides.

■ EXERCISE FOUR
Standing crossover

1 Stand with your feet shoulder-width apart. Bend your arms at right angles and hold them out to each side with your upper arms parallel to the floor and your palms facing forwards.

2 Contract your stomach muscles and pull your left knee and right elbow towards each other. Pause, then return to the starting position. Perform 8 to 12 repetitions, then switch sides.

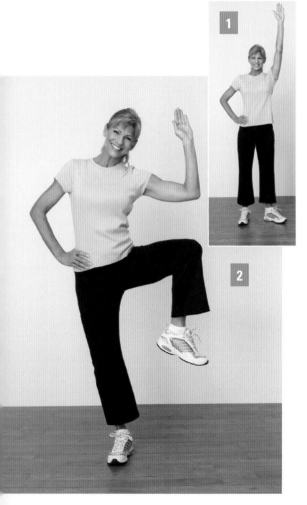

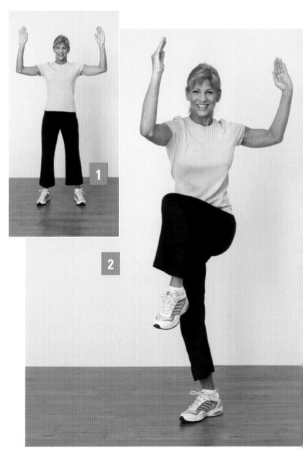

Cat stretch

1 Kneel on all fours with your hands directly below your shoulders and your knees directly below your hips. Pull your abdominal muscles in, drop your head and press your back up, rounding it towards the ceiling.

2 Hold for 15 seconds, then raise your head and drop your belly towards the floor, arching your back in the opposite direction. Hold for 15 seconds.

Spinal twist

1 Kneel on all fours with your hands directly below your shoulders and your knees directly below your hips.

2 Extend your right arm under and across your body (your left arm will bend slightly) until your right shoulder is near or on the floor. Hold for 15 seconds, then switch sides.

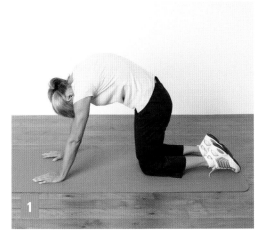

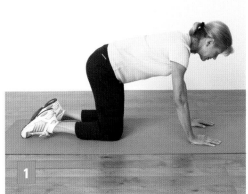

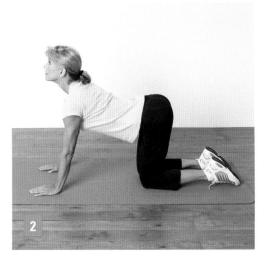

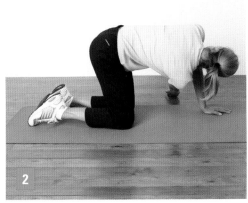

The core body *Routine continued*

■ STRETCH THREE
Lower-back stretch

1 Lie on your back with your legs straight, then bend your knees towards your chest.

2 Clasp your right hand behind your right knee and your left hand behind your left knee and pull gently. Hold for 30 seconds.

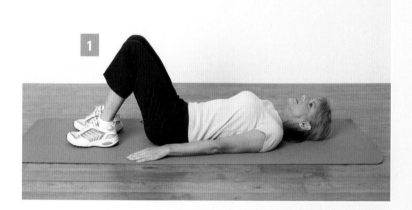

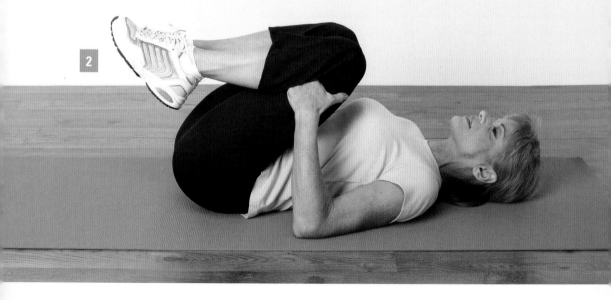

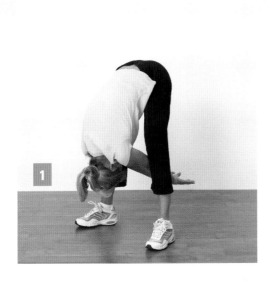

Bend and reach

1 Stand with your feet shoulder-width apart. Contract your stomach muscles and bend forwards at the hips and knees, reaching your hands between your knees, if possible.

2 Pause, then use your hips to straighten up, extending your arms overhead and slightly behind you. Hold for 10 seconds, then repeat. (If you have back pain, skip the first part of this stretch and simply stretch overhead.)

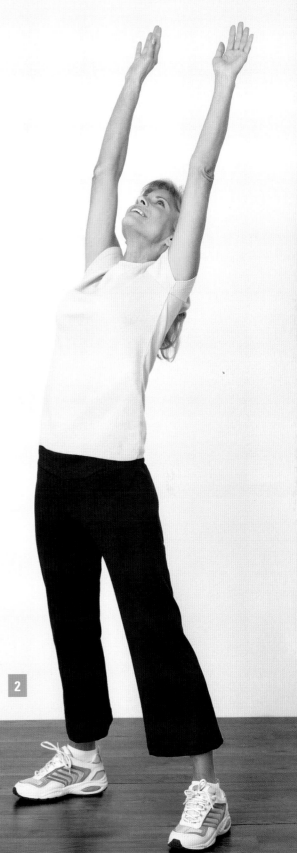

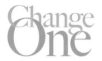
Get active

Move more, weigh less. That adage is so simple, so obvious, such a 'Duh, I already knew that' statement that it barely seems worth repeating. That is, until you consider that when US scientists at the Mayo Clinic compared the minute-by-minute activity levels of overweight and skinny 'couch potatoes', they discovered that the lean people were actually on their feet, moving around, for 152 more minutes every day than the others.

'Kilojoules burned in everyday activities are far, far more important in obesity than we previously imagined,' the lead researcher noted. This discovery inspired him to attach his computer to a low-speed treadmill and stash his telephone in a desk drawer so he would move more during the work day.

Now it's your turn. In the pages ahead, we'll help you find easy, fun, habit-forming ways to add more activity to your day.

You'll be surprised at how a little pacing, fidgeting and walking can contribute to lasting weight loss.

Change One Quiz

Does daily activity *really* matter?

For each question, choose True or False.

1. Sometimes the only difference between overweight and thin is the amount of 'lifestyle activity' a person gets – standing, moving or even twiddling your thumbs or flipping your hair out of the way.

☐ True   ☐ False

2. Communicating with co-workers in person – by walking to their desk or office – rather than via email or phone could, over time, save you two dress sizes.

☐ True   ☐ False

3. Little 'extra activities' – beating the cake batter by hand, parking in spot furthest away from the supermarket, scrubbing the floor by hand – can help you keep weight off better than a formal exercise routine can.

☐ True   ☐ False

4. The reason people were thinner 50 years ago isn't just that they ate less. They moved more – so much more that few needed formal exercise programs to stay thin.

☐ True   ☐ False

5. Walking up stairs can burn more energy faster than setting out on a fitness walk.

☐ True   ☐ False

6. You could find a babysitter for the kids while you workout, but you can burn just as many kilojoules, and work your muscles just as hard, if you do some gardening with your family and then play a game of catch or footy.

☐ True   ☐ False

7. The following are great pieces of exercise equipment: a cast-iron frying pan, a kitchen cleaver, a push lawnmower, a hose and a bucket of sudsy water to wash the car.

☐ True   ☐ False

8. Even small amounts of activity can boost your energy quotient because movement sends more oxygen- and glucose-rich blood to your brain and muscles.

☐ True   ☐ False

9. Who needs barbells? If you have a dog, you have a built-in arm-strengthening friend living at your house. Just find a rope and start your workout!

☐ True   ☐ False

Quiz score

The answer to each question is an emphatic 'True'. Lifestyle activity is a big part of the *ChangeOne* Fitness approach because it's both effective and versatile. It works all your muscle groups, it's easy to fit into your day, it requires no special clothes or equipment and it usually requires just slight adjustments to whatever you're doing now. Lifestyle activity also burns more kilojoules than you might think – in one study, it kept weight off better than step aerobics!

Motionless in Australia and New Zealand

Ever wonder why people in 1950s-era photos look so slim? Most of them (except a few notables) weren't pumping iron, training for a local 5-kilometre race or dashing to the gym for a Pilates class. The truth is, everyday life was packed with hundreds of activities that added up to a big energy burn.

Among them, doing the laundry often meant using a hand-cranked wringer to squeeze excess water out of the wash (most machines didn't have automatic spin cycles); drying it meant hauling baskets of heavy, wet clothes, sheets and towels outside to hang on the line; car windows opened only if you rolled them down; and the only way to tune in to the radio was to get off the couch, cross the room and turn the knob to switch channels. Corner shops were commonplace, making it convenient to walk over for milk or an ice-cream – and most families had just one car, so daytime errands were often performed on foot. At work, communicating with co-workers required walking to their desks, and sending a message outside the company meant typing a letter on a manual typewriter, often with stiff keys that only responded to very muscular banging. The kids played outside, so parents would wander out, too, to talk with the neighbours. Few families owned electric or ride-on lawnmowers, so cutting the grass entailed pushing a heavy mower around.

Now, fast forward to the 21st century – the era of the motionless Australian and New Zealander.

Thanks to modern technology, we've engineered so many old-fashioned 'inconveniences' out of our lives that we burn an astonishing 2950 *fewer* kilojoules a day now. You can now bank online, and buy a hamburger, grab a cappuccino, purchase a six-pack of beer and even (in some places) pick up prescriptions at a drive-through. Remote controls operate our TVs and DVD players; at the push of a button (a movement that burns next to no energy) you can wash the dishes, shop online, roll up your car window, heat dinner in the microwave (no preparation required either), or email your neighbour. And many modern vacuum cleaners and lawnmowers are self-propelled.

As the number of TV channels grows, seemingly daily, we're glued to the tube for hours each day – entering a trancelike

Modern conveniences help us burn 2950 fewer kilojoules a day.

state that US researchers at Harvard University say requires even fewer kilojoules than reading a magazine, sewing or playing a board game.

Trouble? You bet. Even if you add more dedicated exercise time to your day, you still won't compensate for all that inactivity. And this round-the-clock inaction only perpetuates itself. After all, inactivity leads to feeling lethargic. When you're feeling lethargic and low on energy, the last thing you want to do is get up and do something, so you feel more lethargic, and ... well, you see how this leads to more couch time and even less activity.

The answer is to rediscover the joys of an active lifestyle – defined here as a daily routine in which you embrace as much movement as possible, whenever possible. It means standing and pacing while on the phone, opting for the stairs rather than the lift, stretching your muscles while standing in line, and getting on your feet whenever possible.

ChangeOne Fitness will help you engineer activity back into your day in clever, enjoyable ways that add up to a significant, slimming kilojoule burn. It's your insurance policy against weight gain – and a strategy that top weight-loss researchers say is proven to work. Combine a more active lifestyle with 10 minutes of daily strengthening/stretching moves and a daily walk, and you will be well on your way to a leaner, healthier, more energised you.

Getting active has multiple bonuses, too. Among them are:

- **No need to leave home** If you're taking care of the kids or staying home with an elderly or ill loved one, it's not easy finding time to take a walk or head out to the gym. But washing the car, scrubbing a floor, putting on a silly CD and dancing around the living room, or weeding an overgrown flower bed are all possible.

- **Instant gratification that's doubled** Finish one of our recommended 'get active' activities, and you'll burn an extra 420 to 1250 kilojoules and have something to show for it: clean, organised cupboards, a shiny kitchen floor, a beautiful flower bed or a bunch of smiling, happy kids (who have been dancing or running around with you)!

Rules of active living

1. Never sit when you can stand.
2. Never stand when you can walk.
3. Always have some part of your body in motion.
4. Carry things more often and further.
5. Use your feet for transportation whenever possible.

Help!

'I'm too tired after work to move more! What can I do?'

We'll assume that you are watching television in the evening. We recommend that you do a little bit of exercise at every ad break or every 10 minutes of viewing. (We won't let channel flipping be an excuse not to do this!) At first, limit yourself to stretching. Roll your ankles in circles, clockwise and then anti-clockwise. Then draw big imaginary letters with your big toes; spell out your full name. Sit up straight, raise your arms over your head, clasp your hands and reach higher to stretch your shoulders.

Feeling more ambitious? Increase the exertion level during the ads. Walk around the house; do sit-ups; or assign each character in your favourite show an exercise, then do that move 10 times during the ad break after the character first appears. Also do jobs during the ads. Emptying wastebaskets, vacuuming a room, putting on a load of washing or cleaning a dish that's been soaking in the sink can all add up to plenty of kilojoule-burning activity every hour. When you're finished, your home will shine – and you will have saved hundreds of kilojoules by not snacking.

Watching TV with the kids? Announce a new rule: everybody dances for the length of the ad breaks.

■ A guaranteed energy boost

Moving more helps to cut stress and improves the flow of blood – and oxygen and blood glucose – to your muscles and brain. That can only be a good thing.

It really works!

Researchers have long known that fitting more titbits of activity into every hour of the day can help you lose weight as effectively as formal exercise – and may even be better for keeping it off.

When 40 overweight women in the US either followed a low-kilojoule diet and added step aerobics classes three times a week or tried to squeeze more lifestyle activity into every day, both groups lost about 7 kilograms after 16 weeks. After one year, the aerobics group had regained about 1.5 kilograms, but the lifestyle group had put on less than 115 grams.

When scientists assigned 235 overweight women and men to either two years of formal exercise or a plan of stepped-up daily activity, both groups got fitter – and the lifestyle group lost more body fat.

At the world-renowned Mayo Clinic in the USA, one research team not only measured the daily activities of lean and overweight study volunteers (with the participants wearing specially wired undergarments). They also put both groups on diets so the overweight people would slim down and the lean people would gain weight. The result was that even at their new weights, naturally active people moved around more and naturally sedentary people remained more motionless. The take-home lesson? If you tend to sit around, you'll have to resolve to get out of your seat more frequently.

That's where we come in. The rest of this chapter will give you dozens of ways to do just that.

At home: slimming jobs

How would you like to burn 1050 kilojoules in an hour, maybe more, and have a sparkling clean house afterwards? You can if you see the hidden activity opportunity in housework. You'll also use most, if not all, of your major muscle groups – in your arms, legs, torso and back. Here are some ways to maximise the burn.

Don't just wait; do something Instead of pausing while the microwave heats something or waiting for the washer or dryer to finish a cycle, do squats or push-ups against a wall or just march in place. Walk around the first or second floor of your house or jog lightly in place.

Get a Chinese cleaver These big knives, favoured by many chefs, weigh more than almost any other kitchen knife, and therefore, you'll burn more kilojoules every time you wield one instead of a puny vegetable knife.

Cook as if it's 1914 Chop vegetables by hand instead of in the food processor, whip eggs with a fork or whisk, mix cake batter with a big spoon instead of the mixer, dig out your manual can-opener and get rid of the electric model and, if you have time, wash and dry the dishes by hand. Use a cast-iron frying pan – it's heavy! And you'll get a bonus workout if you store it in a low cupboard and lift the pan up to the stove every time you use it.

Make more trips Stop fretting about making extra trips up and down the stairs and view them as your real-world Stairmaster routine. Skip the laundry chute and carry the clothes down to the laundry in a basket. On weekends, consider resurrecting the lost art of drying clothes on a clothesline; your sheets will smell like sunshine and fresh air. Volunteer to take the rubbish out or empty the car after a holiday.

That's amazing!

Just 10 minutes of doing an everyday activity may burn more kilojoules than you'd expect.

Activity	Kilojoules burned*
Walking downstairs	330–465
Walking upstairs	850–1210
Making beds	195–275
Washing windows	200–290
Dusting	130–185
Washing floors	220–315
Gardening	175–250
Weeding	285–410
Using a push lawnmower	220–310
Preparing a meal	195–275
Washing or dressing	155–220
Shovelling earth	375–550
Painting a house	170–230
Chopping firewood	350–510
Repairing a car	180–250
Caring for babies or toddlers	170–265
Playing the piano	135–200
Electrical work/plumbing	190–275

*Kilojoule range is for weights of 80–115 kg.

Scrub it Washing floors by hand – the very old-fashioned way, on your knees – works your arm, back and abdominal muscles. Just be sure to keep your tummy muscles tight so they help to support your back.

Chew gum while you're working The simple act of moving your jaws uses about 45 kilojoules per hour.

Bake bread once a week Kneading dough is soothing and works muscles in your arms and shoulders. And it tastes divine.

Outdoors: the whittle-your-waist work party

Here are some more ways to use the great outdoors as your personal gym.

Rake leaves You'll burn 210 extra kilojoules per half an hour when you rake by hand rather than using a leaf blower.

Skip the carwash Wash your car by hand. You'll save money by not going to the car wash and burn up to 1175 kilojoules in an hour. Why not vacuum the carpets and upholstery, wash the plastic trim on the insides of the doors and do the insides of the windows, too?

Sweep the steps Since you're not using the leaf blower, haul out the broom to clear your steps. Wouldn't it be nice to give them a scrubbing, too? Got an extra 15 minutes? How about washing down the front door and the doorsill while you're at it.

Trim the old-fashioned way Leave the electric edger and trimmer in the garage and grab your old hand tools. Use thick foam or an old carpet square to cushion your knees.

Resurrect the push lawnmower Revive the sound of past summers: the whisk-whisk-whisk of a muscle-powered push lawnmower. Buy one and consider it an investment in a piece of exercise equipment, or rehabilitate the old one stashed way down the back of the garage.

Automatic activity

When the phone rings ... talk standing up and move around your house.

When sitting at a desk ... tap your toes, bounce your knee and do leg lifts.

When standing in line ... stand on your heels and lift your toes as high as they can go.

When washing dishes ... repeatedly rise onto your toes.

When bored ... put your palms together in front of your chest and push them into each other as hard as you can.

When using a laptop ... put it on a high benchtop and stand up to work.

While watching TV ... walk in place.

While waiting at a red light ... fully stretch your legs, arms and neck.

ChangeOne Success Stories

Choosing to be healthy

It's hard to imagine how, as a mother of four, Cindy Bonsteel finds the time to exercise and make healthy meals. But, thanks to *ChangeOne* and her hard work and determination, she's already lost 50 kilograms and is well on her way to her ultimate weight-loss goal.

'My husband and I have been married for 18½ years and have four beautiful children who are 17, 14, 3 and 2 years old,' she says. 'I had decided that I needed time to put me first, and by doing that, I have become healthier and now have more energy for the children and my husband.'

Even with the demands of caring for her large family, Cindy still finds time to exercise. 'I started to do step aerobics in the afternoons when my little ones were sleeping,' she says. 'As I got more healthy and lost more weight, I started to add kilometres to my walks, and now I am power walking. Three days a week, I go an hour early to pick up my 3-year-old at his pre-school, and I do my walk there. We purchased a strength-training machine, so I do strength training three or four days a week with that, and I also use it while the kids are asleep, which is handy for me.'

Her entire family has picked up on her new healthy habits. 'The family likes *ChangeOne* meals, and they don't have any problem adjusting to that,' she says. 'We also have plenty of fresh fruits and nuts on hand to snack on.'

She recommends that people who are just starting on *ChangeOne* stick with

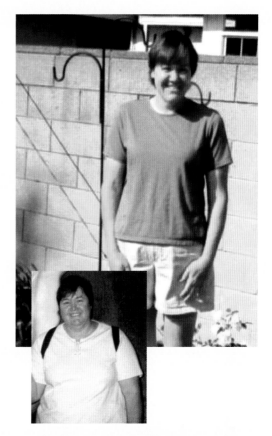

A mother of four, Cindy Bonsteel lost 50 kg and her family now practises new healthy habits.

the program and try to remember they're making changes that will become new habits. 'Before you know it, the weight will start coming off, and that really motivates you to keep sticking with it,' she says.

'I don't like to call this a diet, as everyone in the world has a "diet". You can have a junk-food diet or a healthy diet, and I choose to be healthy.'

Double-dig Gardeners know that the best soil is double-dug. So when you put in a new bed or turn over the soil in your vegetable patch in the spring, leave the power tiller in the shed and get out there with a sharp shovel. Dig each row twice – first to a single shovel's depth, then down one more shovel's worth. Refill the row by putting the first digging's soil in the bottom and the second's on top. You'll have fresh, more fertile soil on top and fluffy dirt down deep, so tender roots can grow strong, creating beautiful, healthy plants.

Plant bulbs Garden catalogues start advertising sales of autumn bulbs in midsummer. That's the time to think about daffodils, daylilies, tulips and a host of other gorgeous spring and summer flowers for next year. Order heaps and plant them over several cool autumn weekends. Your efforts will be rewarded with a stunning display once winter's gone.

Stop buying weed killer Be a friend to the earth and to your own muscles. Pull, dig out and cut back weeds yourself. Your arms and back will get a fantastic workout.

On the job: don't become desk-bound

It's easy to stay seated at work, jump up for lunch and then plonk down again until home time rolls around. Here's how to burn more kilojoules and add more energy to your day.

Get more 'face time' Instead of sending emails or calling co-workers, stop by their desks to ask a question or figure out a solution to a work issue. Doing this instead of sending just one email a day could save you 5 kilograms over 10 years!

Take energy breaks Every half an hour, walk around your office or down the hall for 5 minutes. Jump up and down in your office. Do push-ups with your hands resting against your desk. Do 10 leg lifts, then stand up and rise on your toes 10 times. Stretch your arms high 10 times, too.

Get a rolling chair Try sitting on a large exercise (Swiss) ball instead of a desk chair. You'll use your abdominal and back muscles all day to help you balance. You can buy exercise balls for a reasonable price at most sports shops.

Go the long way Walk right the way around your work building a few times before heading to lunch. Use the toilet or photocopier furthest away from your desk. Volunteer to help co-workers move boxes or carry files or books.

Take the stairs, of course *ChangeOne* recommends that you take the stairs at least twice a day. Just two flights daily could help you melt 3 kilograms in a year. Climbing stairs for just 2 minutes five days a week gives you the same kilojoule-burning, heart-rate-quickening results as a 36-minute walk!

Plan a walking meeting Need to schedule a small meeting? Suggest a walking meeting instead of getting together in an airless conference room. Take a small notebook and a pen. Chances are, you'll have better ideas and forge a better relationship with your fellow walkers.

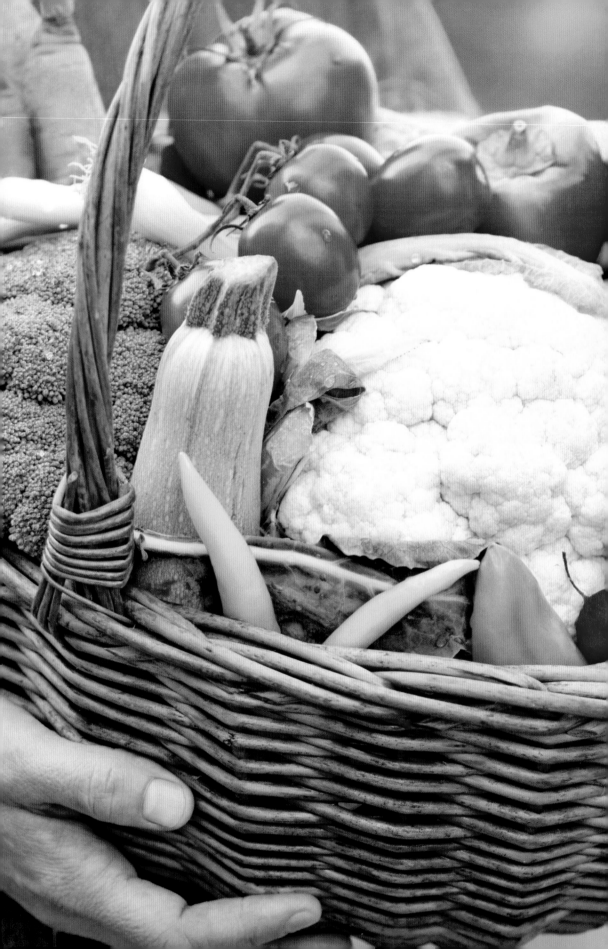

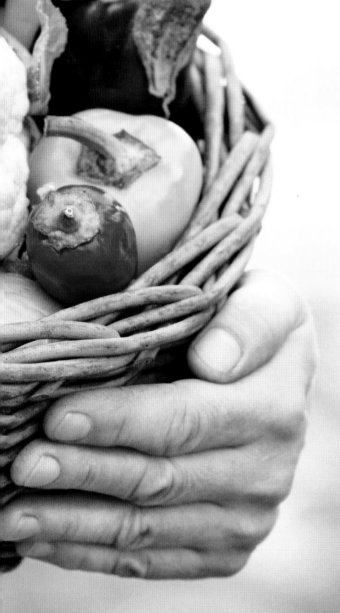

PART 3

RESOURCES

Meals
& recipes

We hope you've had a chance to try the recipes contained in the first 12 weeks of *ChangeOne*, and that you enjoyed them, because we have lots more for you.

In the following pages, you'll find a delicious mix of fresh ideas for breakfast, lunch, dinner and snacks.

You'll also discover tips, recipes, substitutions and the guidance you need to bring them to life in your own kitchen, with your own sense of style and taste.

Here is what you'll find.

- Quick breakfasts (pages 309 to 311)
- Smart lunches (pages 312 to 317)
- Delicious dinners (pages 318 to 325)
- Snacks & desserts (pages 326 to 330)

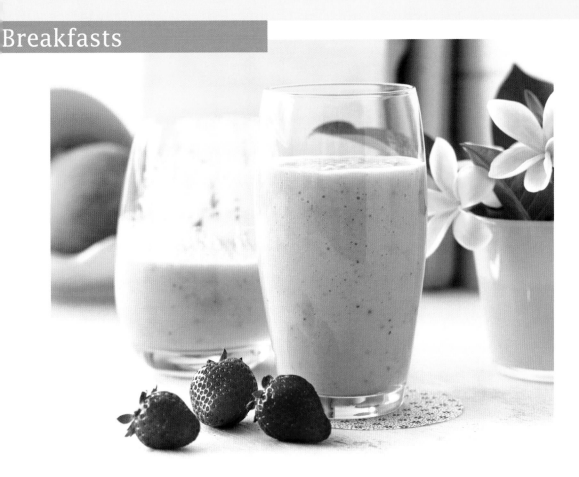

Smoothie breakfast

Shakes, smoothies – no matter what you call them, these frosty combinations of fruit and milk or yogurt refresh and nourish.

1 tropical smoothie (tall tumbler)

1 toasted English muffin half spread with 1 teaspoon (thumb tip) peanut butter

942 kJ, 225 kcal, 11 g protein, 5 g fat (<1 g sat fat), 5 mg cholesterol, 37 g carbohydrate (23 g sugars), 2 g fibre, 210 mg sodium

TROPICAL SMOOTHIE

Serves 2

1 cup (250 ml) low-fat milk
1 ripe banana or mango
¼ cup (40 g) fresh or frozen strawberries or blueberries
1 teaspoon honey, or to taste

1. Combine all the ingredients in a blender and blend until smooth.

2. Pour into glasses and serve.

HEALTH TIP

When buying a freshly made smoothie from a café, be sure to ask them to use low-fat natural yogurt or skim or reduced-fat milk.

The hearty frittata

This no-fuss Italian egg dish – really a thick, flat omelette – is cooked in a frying pan on the stove, then finished off under the grill.

12.5 cm wedge vegetable
  frittata (calculator)

½ cup (75 g) fresh blueberries
  (2 golf balls)

1 slice wholemeal toast

1284 kJ, 307 kcal, 20 g protein, 16 g fat (5 g sat fat),
246 mg cholesterol, 21 g carbohydrate (10 g sugars),
6 g fibre, 412 mg sodium

VEGETABLE FRITTATA

Serves 4
1 tablespoon olive oil
1 small onion, finely chopped
350 g small button mushrooms,
  quartered
250 g baby spinach leaves
5 eggs
2 tablespoons chopped fresh parsley
freshly ground black pepper
50 g grated cheddar or parmesan
8 tomatoes, sliced (optional)
1 small onion, thinly sliced (optional)

1. Heat the oil in a large frying pan. Fry the onion over medium heat, stirring occasionally, for 3–4 minutes, or until softened but not browned.

2. Add the mushrooms and fry, stirring frequently, for a further 3–4 minutes.

3. Add the spinach to the pan and cook over medium–high heat, stirring often, for 3–4 minutes, or until the leaves have wilted and excess liquid has evaporated. Reduce the heat to low.

4. Break the eggs into a bowl. Add 2 tablespoons cold water, the parsley and pepper, then beat together.

5. Pour the egg mixture over the spinach mixture and cook for 5 minutes, until the egg is set and golden. Preheat the grill to high.

6. Sprinkle the cheese over the top. Place under the grill and cook for 2–3 minutes, or until the frittata is set and the top is golden. Serve hot or cold, with a tomato and onion salad, if desired.

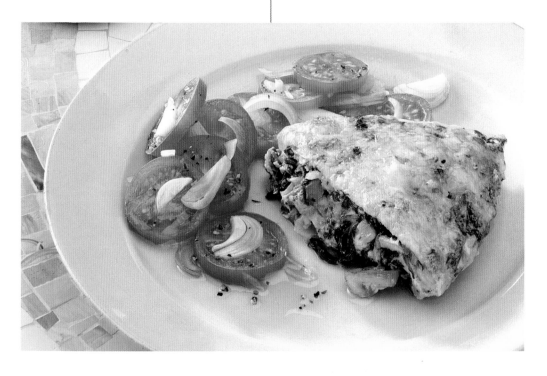

Fruit bread delight

Fruit breads, sometimes called 'quick breads', are a natural partner for a cup of tea, and with fresh fruit and a glass of milk they make a lovely breakfast.

1 thin slice peach and yogurt loaf
   (lip-balm thickness)

½ cup (60 g) fresh raspberries
   (2 golf balls)

1 cup (250 ml) skim milk or
   1 tub (150 g) low-fat yogurt

Cup of tea or coffee

1092 kJ, 261 kcal, 14 g protein, 4 g fat (<1 g sat fat),
21 mg cholesterol, 41 g carbohydrate (27 g sugars),
5 g fibre, 235 mg sodium

PEACH AND YOGURT LOAF

Serves 16
2 medium fresh peaches
1 ½ cups (210 g) plain flour
¾ cup (85 g) wholemeal plain flour
¼ cup (25 g) toasted wheat germ
¾ cup (150 g) caster sugar
1 teaspoon bicarbonate of soda
½ teaspoon salt
½ cup (125 g) natural yogurt
1 egg plus 2 egg whites
2 tablespoons sunflower or corn oil
1 teaspoon pure almond essence

1. Preheat the oven to 180ºC. Lightly spray a large loaf tin with cooking spray.

2. Blanch and peel the peaches, then remove the stones and chop flesh finely.

3. Combine the plain and wholemeal flours, wheat germ, sugar, bicarbonate of soda and salt in a large bowl.

4. In another bowl mix the yogurt, egg, eggwhites, oil and almond essence. Make a well in the dry ingredients and pour in the yogurt mixture. Stir until just combined. Do not overmix. Fold in the peaches.

5. Spoon the mixture into the tin and smooth the top. Bake for about 1 hour or until a skewer inserted in the centre comes out clean. Cool in the tin on a wire rack for 10 minutes, then turn out onto the rack to cool completely. One serve is one slice.

HEALTH TIP

When you order fruit bread like this at a coffee shop or café, your slice should be about the same thickness as a deck of cards. Save any extra for later.

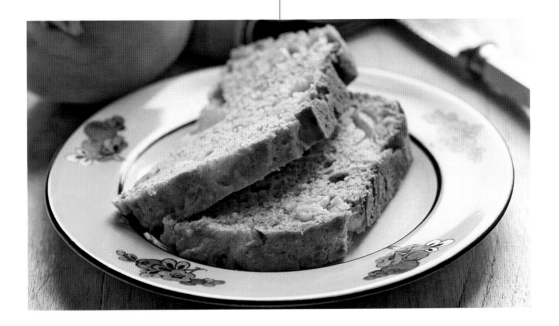

Soups

For a hearty, sustaining meal in the middle of the day, enjoy a mug of soup accompanied by a simple sandwich and a piece of fruit.

Soup and sandwich

Hearty split pea or cream of asparagus soup (coffee mug)

1 Bavarian sandwich

1 orange, apple or peach

1618 kJ, 387 kcal, 24 g protein, 11 g fat (5 g sat fat), 43 mg cholesterol, 47 g carbohydrate (16 g sugars), 11 g fibre, 351 mg sodium

HEARTY SPLIT PEA SOUP

Serves 8

1 teaspoon olive oil
1 tablespoon vegetable stock
1 large onion, finely chopped
3 cloves garlic, crushed
2 carrots, halved lengthwise and thinly sliced across
³⁄₄ cup (150 g) split peas
2 tablespoons tomato purée
250 g smoked chicken breast, diced
¹⁄₄ teaspoon salt
¹⁄₂ teaspoon freshly ground black pepper
¹⁄₂ teaspoon dried sage
4 cups (1 litre) water

¹⁄₃ cup (50 g) small pasta shapes
25 g parmesan, grated

1. Heat the oil and stock in a large non-stick saucepan over medium heat. Add the onion and garlic and cook, stirring frequently, for about 7 minutes or until the onion is golden brown. Add the carrots and cook for a further 5 minutes or until just tender.

2. Stir in the split peas, tomato purée, chicken breast, salt, pepper, sage and water. Bring to the boil. Reduce to a simmer, cover and cook for 30 minutes.

3. Uncover, add the pasta and cook for about 15 minutes or until the pasta and split peas are tender. Sprinkle each serve with some parmesan and serve hot. (Leftover soup will keep, refrigerated, for 3 to 4 days, or frozen, for 2 to 3 months.)

For a Bavarian sandwich

Spread 1 thin slice pumpernickel bread with honey mustard. Top with 15 g cheddar, shaved or grated, and lettuce or rocket. Add another slice of bread.

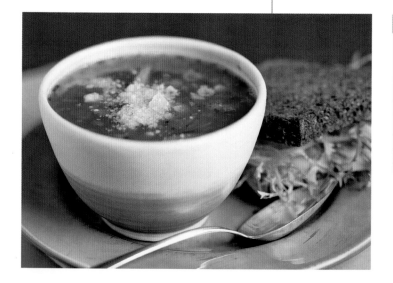

HEALTH TIP

At a restaurant or café, keep watch for high-kilojoule ingredients and ask how a soup is made. If necessary, skip the parmesan topping.

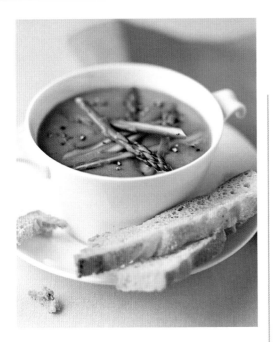

CREAM OF ASPARAGUS SOUP

Serves 4

625 g asparagus, tough ends trimmed
1½ teaspoons olive oil
4 spring onions (scallions), thinly sliced
250 g boiling potatoes, peeled and
   thinly sliced
400–450 ml water
1 teaspoon dried tarragon
¼ teaspoon salt
¼ teaspoon freshly ground black pepper
½ cup (125 ml) reduced-fat milk

1. Cut 10 thin asparagus spears into thirds
and reserve for the garnish. Chop the rest
of the asparagus into 1 cm lengths.

2. Heat the oil in a medium non-stick
saucepan over low heat. Add the spring
onions and cook, stirring frequently, for
about 2 minutes or until tender. Stir in
the potatoes and chopped asparagus.

3. Add the water, tarragon, salt and pepper,
and bring to the boil. Reduce to a simmer,
cover and cook for about 10 minutes or until
the potatoes and asparagus are tender.

4. Transfer to a food processor and blend
until smooth. Return to the saucepan and
stir in the milk and reserved asparagus.
Cook over low heat for 3 minutes, or until
the soup is heated through and the pieces
of asparagus are tender. Serve hot.

Instead of	Try
In split pea soup:	
Split peas	Lentils Canned beans
Smoked chicken	Smoked ham
In cream of asparagus soup:	
Asparagus	Broccoli
Asparagus and potatoes	Carrots and sweet potato

Caesar salads

Now hugely popular, Caesar salads are readily available with all sorts of toppings – grilled chicken breast, as shown here, or grilled fresh tuna or tiger prawns.

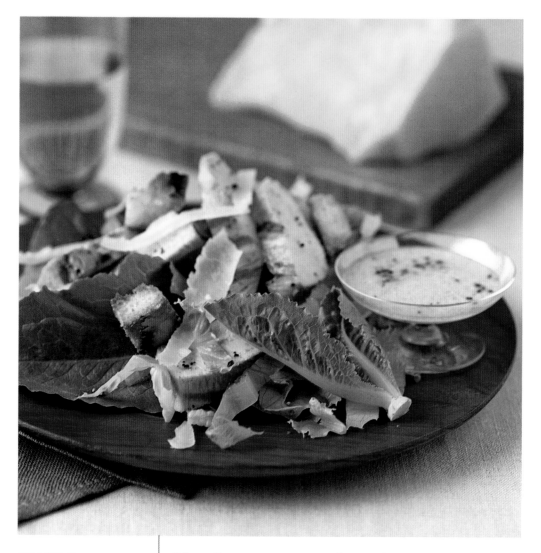

Time-saver
Wrap and refrigerate leftover grilled meat or fish for your next day's Caesar salad.

Chicken Caesar lunch

Grilled chicken Caesar salad (2 cricket balls)

½ cup (115 g) fresh fruit salad (2 golf balls)

1604 kJ, 383 kcal, 26 g protein, 21 g fat (6 g sat fat), 70 mg cholesterol, 22 g carbohydrate (13 g sugars), 6 g fibre, 470 mg sodium

GRILLED CHICKEN CAESAR SALAD

Serves 4

2 garlic cloves, peeled
3 tablespoons lemon juice
2 tablespoons low-fat natural yogurt
1 tablespoon olive oil
350 g boneless, skinless chicken breast
½ teaspoon freshly ground black pepper
1 large cos lettuce, torn into small pieces
100 g croutons (see right)
25 g parmesan

1. Preheat the grill or heat a ridged cast-iron grill pan. Finely crush the garlic cloves until paste-like. Put the garlic paste, lemon juice, yogurt and oil into a screwtop jar and shake until blended.

2. Sprinkle the chicken with the pepper and lightly coat with cooking spray. Grill for 4 to 5 minutes on each side or until cooked through. Cut across the grain into 1 cm slices.

3. Toss together the lettuce, croutons and chicken in a large bowl.

4. Shake the dressing to mix. Drizzle over the salad and toss lightly. Divide evenly among 4 plates. Using a vegetable peeler, shave strips of parmesan over the salads.

Instead of	Try
Grilled chicken	Grilled tuna
	Canned water-packed tuna, drained
	Grilled tofu cubes
	Grilled salmon
	Grilled steak
	Cooked peeled prawns

Prepare salad with 85 grams per serve for all these options.

ABOUT CAESAR SALAD

Legend has it that Caesar salad was invented by Caesar Cardini, a restaurant owner in Tijuana, Mexico, for a group of visiting movie stars. Then there are those who credit Caesar's brother, Alex, with the concoction. Whoever dreamed it up, the salad has become a classic. The original Caesar contained romaine (cos) lettuce, tossed at the table with a dressing of raw egg, lemon juice, garlic, olive oil and Worcestershire sauce, and was adorned with croutons and parmesan.

CROUTONS

■ To make croutons, cut 100 g day-old bread (crusty white bread, French bread, ciabatta, rye, etc) into small cubes and toss with 1½ tablespoons olive oil. Spread out on a baking sheet and bake at 200ºC for about 10 minutes, or until crisp and golden. Allow to cool slightly before using.

■ For garlic croutons, use savoury garlic-flavoured oil. For herb croutons, toss the hot, freshly baked croutons with finely chopped fresh herbs, such as parsley, basil and mint.

■ When buying croutons, compare brands and choose the one that is lowest in kilojoules.

HEALTH TIP

When you're eating out, ask for dressing to be served separately, if possible, so that you can control the amount on the salad. Classic Caesar dressing is made with lots of olive oil. As with all standard salad dressings, it contains a lot of kilojoules – about 420 – in each tablespoon. If the salad only comes ready-dressed, you may want to revise your choice.

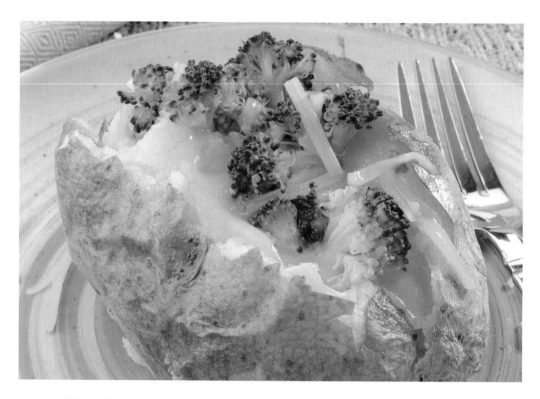

Well-dressed baked potato

With the right toppings, a baked potato makes a healthy and satisfying main dish.

1 medium baked potato, about
170 g (tennis ball), topped with:
steamed broccoli (unlimited)
¼ cup (30 g) cheddar, grated
(surface of palm)

Green salad (unlimited) with
1 tablespoon fat-free dressing
(1 salad dressing cap), or low-fat
dressing (adds about 125 kilojoules)

½ cup (75 g) berries in season
(2 golf balls)

1292 kJ, 309 kcal, 15 g protein, 11 g fat (6 g sat fat),
30 mg cholesterol, 35 g carbohydrate (10 g sugars),
11 g fibre, 502 mg sodium

Free toppings

The vegetable toppings for your potato
are 'free' – they carry few kilojoules, so
you can pile on as much as you wish.

Instead of	Try
Steamed broccoli	Diced tomatoes
	Chopped onions
	Steamed spinach
	Grilled mushrooms

Substitute toppings

You can swap the cheese for any of
these other toppings with about the
same number of kilojoules:

Instead of	Try
Grated cheddar	½ cup (85 g) canned beans (kidney, etc) or chilli con carne
	½ cup (125 g) low-fat cottage cheese

Wrap it up

Flour tortillas wrapped around a variety of fillings make a great alternative to a traditional bread sandwich as a hearty, diet-friendly lunch.

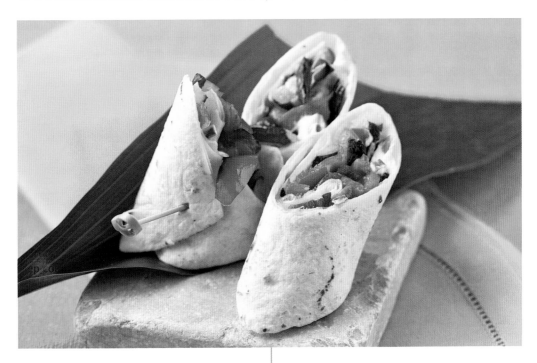

1 roasted vegetable wrap

Green salad (unlimited) with
1 tablespoon (1 salad dressing cap)
fat-free dressing

½ cup (115 g) diced honeydew melon
(2 golf balls), topped with a mint leaf

1068 kJ, 255 kcal, 9 g protein, 9 g fat (2 g sat fat),
4 mg cholesterol, 35 g carbohydrate (22 g sugars),
6 g fibre, 466 mg sodium

ROASTED VEGETABLE WRAPS WITH CHIVE SAUCE

Serves 4
- **1 tablespoon olive oil**
- **1 tablespoon rice vinegar**
- **1 teaspoon chopped fresh rosemary**
- **1 garlic clove, crushed**
- **2–3 zucchinis, 450 g total weight**
- **2 large red capsicums**
- **1 large red onion**
- **4 x 15 cm flour tortillas**
- **Yogurt cheese made from 1 cup (200 g) low-fat natural yogurt (see page 31)**
- **¼ teaspoon onion and chive seasoning**
- **1 tablespoon snipped fresh chives**

1. Preheat the oven to 230ºC. Lightly coat a baking tray with cooking spray. Whisk together the oil, vinegar, rosemary and garlic in a small bowl. Cut each zucchini across in half, then lengthwise into 5 mm slices. Cut each red capsicum into 8 strips. Cut the onion into 16 wedges.

2. Toss the vegetables and oil mixture in the baking tray. Roast, tossing frequently, for 30 minutes or until brown and tender. Sprinkle the tortillas with a little water, stack and wrap in foil, then heat in the oven with the vegetables for the last 5 minutes.

3. Combine the yogurt cheese and the onion and chive seasoning in a small bowl. Spread evenly on the tortillas and top with the vegetables. Fold in the sides of the tortillas and roll up. Cut each one into 3 pieces.

Chicken fillets

Chicken fillets (boneless, skinless chicken breasts) are the most convenient portion of chicken you can buy, and it's worth keeping a supply in your freezer. They can be sliced while frozen for stir-frying, or thawed to use whole, as they are, or pounded thin for escalopes. To keep this lean meat moist, pair it with a sauce.

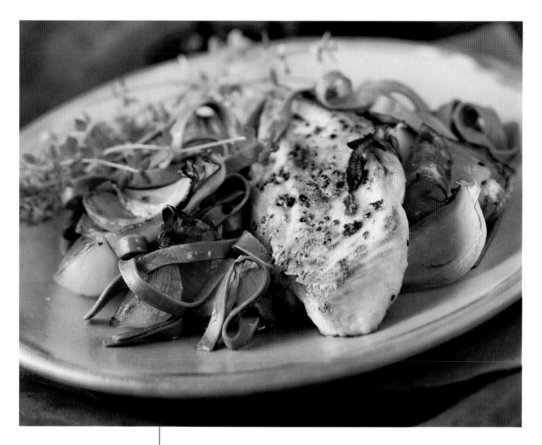

Chicken dinner

Chicken and caramelised onion stir-fry –
1 chicken fillet (palm size) **with onions** (2 golf balls)

Spinach fettuccine or tagliatelle (tennis ball)

Tossed salad (unlimited) – **mixed greens topped with tomato wedges, dressed with ½ teaspoon** (thumbnail) **olive oil, balsamic vinegar** (unlimited) **and freshly ground black pepper**

1973 kJ, 471 kcal, 34 g protein, 14 g fat (3 g sat fat), 74 mg cholesterol, 52 g carbohydrate (24 g sugars), 8 g fibre, 340 mg sodium

CHICKEN AND CARAMELISED ONION STIR-FRY

Serves 4

700 g red onions
4 skinless chicken fillets, 115 g to
  140 g each
¼ teaspoon salt
½ teaspoon freshly ground black pepper
4 teaspoons olive oil
2 tablespoons caster sugar
5 tablespoons chicken stock
1 teaspoon chopped fresh rosemary
1 teaspoon chopped fresh thyme
1 tablespoon red wine vinegar

1. Cut each onion into 6 wedges. Sprinkle the chicken with the salt and ¼ teaspoon freshly ground black pepper.

2. Coat a large non-stick frying pan with cooking spray. Add 2 teaspoons olive oil and heat over medium-high heat for about 30 seconds. Add the chicken and cook for about 3 minutes on each side or until browned. Transfer to a plate.

3. Reduce the heat to medium and add the remaining oil to the pan. Then add the onions and sprinkle with 1 tablespoon sugar and the remaining pepper. Cook for about 8 minutes or until the onions turn golden brown and caramelise. Stir frequently, breaking the onions apart as they cook. Add the stock and boil until it evaporates.

4. Stir in the rosemary, thyme and remaining sugar. Return the chicken to the pan and sprinkle with the vinegar. Cook, uncovered, for a further 4 minutes or until the chicken is cooked through (when a fillet is pierced the juices that run out should be clear).

Instead of	Try
Red onions	Leeks, spring onions (scallions) or golden (French) shallots

ABOUT CHICKEN AND OTHER POULTRY

Chicken is the most popular type of poultry and, like turkey, is endlessly versatile. Both chicken and turkey are very lean – turkey is the lower in fat and kilojoules – and most of their fat is in the skin. Lean duck, without skin and fat, has about the same amount of fat as lamb. Here is a kilojoule and fat comparison, based on an 85 g cooked serve, without skin and bone.

	Kilojoules	Fat (grams)
Turkey breast	480	0.6
Duck breast	500	2.1
Chicken breast	590	3.0
Duck leg meat	630	5.1
Turkey leg meat	640	6.1
Chicken leg meat	730	8.2
Goose	850	10.8

SKIN ON OR OFF?

It's best not to eat the skin of poultry – it can add almost a teaspoon of fat per 85 g serve – but it can be removed either before or after cooking.

Skin off: Skinless chicken fillets are great in simmered or stir-fried dishes where they are cooked with other moist ingredients or in a sauce.

Skin on: Chicken in its skin is perfect for roasting. The skin helps to keep the chicken moist, and a thin membrane between the skin and the flesh prevents the fat from getting into the meat.

ABOUT SPINACH PASTA

Pasta can be coloured and flavoured with a wide variety of vegetable purées and pastes, such as spinach (green), tomato or beetroot (red) and carrot (orange). There's not enough of the vegetable in it to make a nutritional difference, but it looks and tastes great.

Braised beef

Think of a succulent joint of beef simmering slowly with vegetables and wine, and your mouth waters – you can almost smell the savoury aromas. Make this on an afternoon when you have several hours spare for the beef to cook to perfection.

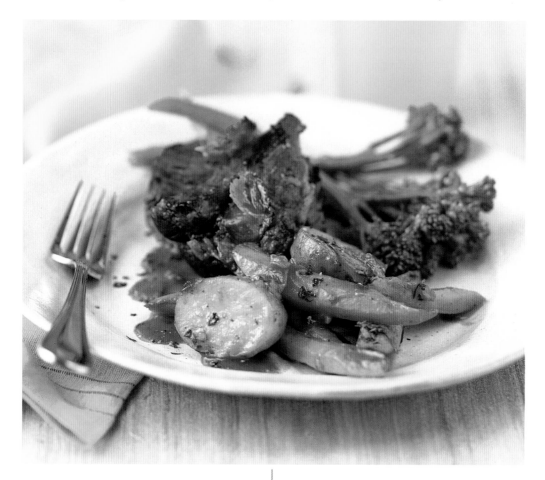

Braised beef dinner

85 g wine-braised beef (deck of cards) with vegetables (tennis ball)

Steamed broccoli (unlimited)

1 slice wholegrain bread (palm size)

832 kJ, 199 kcal, 26 g protein, 4 g fat (<1 g sat fat),
10 mg cholesterol, 12 g carbohydrate (3 g sugars),
18 g fibre, 200 mg sodium

WINE-BRAISED BEEF

Serves 12

1 boneless beef joint (e.g. chuck, topside), weighing about 1.5 kg, trimmed and tied into shape

1 teaspoon salt

1½ teaspoons freshly ground black pepper

8 large carrots, cut into 5 cm chunks

2 onions, coarsely chopped

4 garlic cloves, crushed

2 cans (about 400 g each) whole roma tomatoes

1 cup (55 g) fresh basil, chopped

2 cups dry red wine or beef stock
1 kg small new potatoes, scrubbed
2 teaspoons cornflour mixed with
   2 tablespoons water

1. Preheat the oven to 170ºC. Rub the beef with the salt and pepper. Put into a large flameproof casserole over medium-high heat and sear on all sides. Transfer to a plate.

2. Add the carrots, onions and garlic to the fat remaining in the casserole and cook for about 8 minutes or until the onions are browned. Stir in the tomatoes with their juice and half of the basil. Cook for 5 minutes, stirring and breaking up the tomatoes with a spoon.

3. Return the beef to the casserole. Add the wine or stock and enough water to bring the level of liquid up to 5 cm. Bring to the boil. Cover with foil and then with the lid to create a tight seal. Transfer to the oven and braise for 1 hour, turning the meat over once during cooking time.

4. Add the potatoes and remaining basil, plus additional water if needed to maintain liquid to a depth of 5 cm in the pot. Braise for a further 1 hour, or until the meat and vegetables are tender.

5. Cut the beef into small chunks and arrange on a platter with the vegetables. Strain the braising liquid into a saucepan and bring to a simmer. Whisk in the cornflour mixture and bring to the boil. Simmer for 1 minute, or until thickened. Ladle over the beef and vegetables, and serve.

6. Divide leftovers into individual serves. Cover and keep, refrigerated, for 1 to 2 days, or in the freezer for up to a month.

Serve bonus: Braise extra vegetables (except potatoes) with the beef to enhance the flavour and fill your plate.

TIPS FOR TENDER MEAT

- Keep the liquid in the casserole at the correct level.
- Cover the pot with foil and then the lid to create a tighter seal.
- Braise gently in a warm oven, or on top of the cooker on low heat.
- Allow enough time for cooking; never turn up the heat to hurry things along.
- Cook until the beef is 'fork tender': insert a large double-pronged fork into the thickest part of the joint. If the fork goes in easily and pulls out just as easily, the meat is done.

ABOUT BUYING BEEF FOR BRAISING

Lean muscular joints require long, moist cooking methods, as in this recipe, to make them tender and succulent. The best joints to use for braising are boned and rolled: blade and chuck, silverside and topside. Brisket is also excellent braised, but it is more fatty than the other braising joints.

TIPS FOR GREAT GRAVY

Meat cooked with moist heat creates delicious cooking juices that you can turn into gravy. After removing the joint and vegetables from the pot, pour the cooking juices into a gravy separator or measuring jug so that you can remove the fat. Or use a baster to suction off the liquid from under the thin layer of fat. Thicken by stirring in 2 teaspoons cornflour or 1 to 2 tablespoons plain flour, mixed to a paste with cold water, and gently simmering. Or serve the flavoursome juices just as they are.

Grilled fish

Fish is growing in popularity, and for good reason: it's low in saturated fat – the fat contained in oily fish is the heart-healthy type – and packed with vitamins and minerals. Nutritionists recommend that you eat fish at least twice a week.

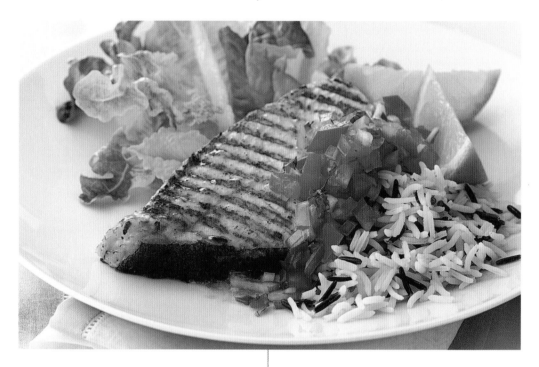

Fish from the grill

1 barbecued fish with salsa
(chequebook)

Wild and white rice (tennis ball)

Grilled mixed onions – 2 onion halves plus 2 spring onions (scallions)

2042 kJ, 488 kcal, 32 g protein, 16 g fat (3 g sat fat),
49 mg cholesterol, 53 g carbohydrate (13 g sugars),
5 g fibre, 131 mg sodium

BARBECUED FISH WITH SALSA

Serves 4
**4 firm white fish steaks (about 150 g each),
  such as swordfish or kingfish
2 tablespoons extra virgin olive oil
juice of 1 small orange
1 clove garlic, finely chopped or crushed
freshly ground black pepper
1 orange, cut into wedges to serve**

**Salsa
200 g roma tomatoes, diced
1/2 red capsicum, seeded and diced
1/2 red onion, finely chopped
juice of 1 small orange
1/2 cup (15 g) fresh basil, chopped
1 tablespoon balsamic vinegar
1 teaspoon caster sugar
freshly ground black pepper**

1. To prepare the fish steaks, place them in a shallow non-metallic dish. Whisk together the oil, orange juice, garlic and a little pepper to season. Spoon the marinade over the fish and turn to coat evenly. Set aside.

2. To make the salsa, combine the tomatoes, capsicum, onion, orange juice, basil, balsamic vinegar and sugar, and season with pepper. Spoon into a serving bowl.

3. Preheat a barbecue hotplate or grill rack to medium–high heat. Remove the fish from the marinade and cook on the hotplate or grill rack over direct heat, basting from time to time with the remaining marinade, for 4–5 minutes on each side, or until the fish is cooked through.

4. Transfer the fish to individual serving plates and grind over some additional black pepper. Garnish the fish with the salsa and serve with wedges of orange.

WILD AND WHITE RICE

Serves 4

225 g mixed basmati and wild rice
Pinch of salt

1. Bring a large saucepan of water to the boil. Add the rice and salt. Bring back to the boil and stir well, then lower the heat so the water is simmering. Cook for about 20 minutes or until the rice is tender.

2. Drain well, then allow to stand for 2 minutes before serving.

GRILLED MIXED ONIONS

Serves 4

4 small red onions
8 spring onions (scallions)

1. Slice the red onions in half lengthwise. Place the red and spring onions on a baking tray and spray all sides with cooking spray, or brush lightly with olive oil.

2. Cook under the grill (alongside the fish if there is room on the grill rack) until tender and browned, turning once.

TIPS FOR COOKING FISH

With the exception of grilled tuna, which is often served rare, most fish should be cooked until just done, with flaky but moist flesh, taking care not to overcook. The '10-minute rule' can help: cook fish for a total of 10 minutes for each 2.5 cm of thickness. Steaks and large fillets may take longer to cook, while thin fillets will cook in a matter of minutes. Here are a few guidelines.

Steaks: Grilling is good for fish steaks such as perch, salmon, shark, swordfish and tuna, which hold together well when you turn them.

Fillets: Higher-fat fish fillets like salmon and trout won't fall apart on the grill. Baking or pan-frying is best for thin fillets such as sole, bream, whiting and other varieties. They are more likely to fall apart on the grill.

Whole fish, large fillets: These can be grilled, steamed in a wok or fish steamer, baked or poached.

TIPS FOR ORDERING

When eating out, feel free to order any type of fish you fancy. Even though oily fish such as salmon are higher in kilojoules than white fish, they're also packed with heart-healthy omega-3 fatty acids – the health benefits are worth the extra kilojoules. Grilled and steamed fish are cooked with little or no extra fat, but baked or fried fish may be cooked with butter or served with a cheese-based or other high-fat sauce. So be sure to ask the waiter before ordering.

Super side dishes

The beauty of *ChangeOne* is its adaptability: you can mix and match main courses and side dishes for an infinite number of meal combinations.

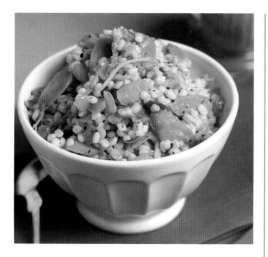

BARLEY PILAF WITH HERBS

Serves 4

1 ½ teaspoons olive oil
2 smoked poultry slices, coarsely chopped
1 onion, finely chopped
2 cloves garlic, crushed
2 carrots, thinly sliced
½ cup (100 g) pearl barley
¼ teaspoon salt
½ teaspoon dried sage
½ teaspoon dried thyme
2 ¼ cups (560 ml) water
½ teaspoon grated lemon zest
½ teaspoon freshly ground black pepper
¼ cup (50 g) grated parmesan

1. Heat the oil in a medium saucepan over medium heat. Add the chopped poultry and cook for 2 minutes. Add the onion and garlic and cook for a further 5 minutes, or until the onion is tender and golden brown.

2. Add the carrots and cook for 5 minutes, or until tender.

3. Add the barley, stirring to combine. Add the salt, sage, thyme and water, and bring to the boil. Reduce to a simmer and cook, stirring frequently, for about 45 minutes, or until the barley is tender.

4. Stir in the lemon zest, pepper and parmesan until evenly combined.

5. Divide into 4 serves. One serve is approximately the size of 1 tennis ball.

770 kJ, 184 kcal, 11 g protein, 7 g fat (3 g sat fat), 22 mg cholesterol, 19 g carbohydrate (3 g sugars), 4 g fibre, 362 mg sodium

SUMMER RATATOUILLE

Serves 4

1 eggplant, about 700 g
¼ teaspoon salt
1 small bulb fennel
2 teaspoons olive oil
2 small yellow zucchini, about 350 g total weight, chopped
1 small onion, cut into thin wedges
2 tablespoons chicken stock
2 large garlic cloves, crushed
1 can (about 400 g) whole roma tomatoes
1 tablespoon chopped fresh oregano
1 teaspoon chopped fresh rosemary, plus sprigs for garnish
1 green capsicum, chopped

1. Cut the eggplant across in slices. Sprinkle on both sides with salt and spread out on a double layer of kitchen paper. Leave to drain for 15 minutes, then rinse well and pat dry with kitchen paper. Cut into cubes. Trim and chop the fennel bulb.

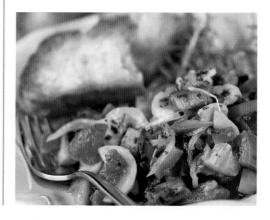

2. Heat 1 teaspoon oil in a large non-stick frying pan over medium-high heat. Cook the zucchini and onion for 5 minutes, or until the onion is softened. Transfer to a large bowl. Add ½ teaspoon oil and the stock to the pan. Stir in the eggplant and reduce the heat to medium. Cover and cook, stirring occasionally, for 12 minutes, or until the eggplant is tender. Add to the bowl.

3. Add the remaining oil and garlic to the pan and cook for 30 seconds. Stir in the tomatoes with their juice, the fennel, oregano and chopped rosemary, breaking up the tomatoes with a spoon. Cover and simmer for 5 minutes. Stir in the capsicum and simmer, covered, for a further 7 minutes. Return all the vegetables to the pan. Bring to the boil, and cook, uncovered, for 3 minutes, stirring occasionally.

4. Divide into 4 serves. One serve is about the size of 1 cricket ball. Serve warm or cool, garnished with rosemary.

449 kJ, 107 kcal, 5 g protein, 4 g fat (<1 g sat fat), 0 mg cholesterol, 14 g carbohydrate (12 g sugars), 10 g fibre, 271 mg sodium

ASPARAGUS WITH CONFETTI VINAIGRETTE

Serves 4
750 g asparagus
½ teaspoon salt
2 large red capsicums, finely chopped
2 large yellow capsicums, finely chopped
4 spring onions (scallions), thinly sliced
2 teaspoons fresh thyme or ½ teaspoon dried thyme
5 tablespoons reduced-salt chicken stock
3 tablespoons white wine vinegar
½ teaspoon freshly ground black pepper

1. Trim the asparagus. Bring 1 cm of water to a simmer in a large non-stick frying pan over medium-high heat. Add the asparagus and ¼ teaspoon salt. Simmer for 3–4 minutes, or until the asparagus is tender. Transfer to a plate. Keep warm.

2. Wipe the pan dry. Coat with cooking spray and set over medium-high heat. Cook the red and yellow capsicums for about 4 minutes or until tender. Stir in the spring onions and thyme, and cook for a further 1 minute.

3. Stir in the stock and vinegar and bring to a simmer. Sprinkle with the pepper and remaining salt, and pour over asparagus.

4. Divide into 4 serves. One serve equals approximately 5 spears.

275 kJ, 66 kcal, 7 g protein, <1 g fat (0 g sat fat), 0 mg cholesterol, 8 g carbohydrate (7 g sugars), 4 g fibre, 374 mg sodium

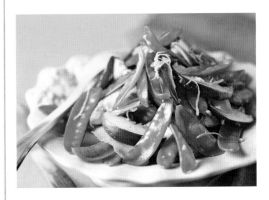

SNOWPEAS AND APPLES WITH GINGER

Serves 4
2 teaspoons olive oil
2 tablespoons peeled and finely chopped fresh ginger
3 cloves garlic, crushed
500 g snowpeas, strings removed
2 crisp red dessert apples, unpeeled, cut into thin wedges
¼ teaspoon salt

1. Heat the oil in a large non-stick frying pan over low heat. Add ginger and garlic, and cook for 2 minutes or until tender.

2. Add the snowpeas, apples and salt, and cook, stirring frequently, for about 7 minutes or until the snowpeas are tender but still crisp.

3. Divide into 4 serves. One serve is approximately the size of 1 tennis ball.

431 kJ, 103 kcal, 4 g protein, 3 g fat (<1 g sat fat), 0 mg cholesterol, 16 g carbohydrate (12 g sugars), 5 g fibre, 154 mg sodium

Snacks

As you know, smart snacking helps to hold off between-meal hunger. Here are a few more make-it-yourself snacks to try in addition to the snacks in Week 3. All but the roasted capsicum pinwheels will keep well in an airtight container, so you can have them on hand to enjoy each day. Each serve provides about 420 kilojoules.

CURRY-SPICED FRUITS, NUTS AND SEEDS

Makes 32 serves
1 tablespoon curry powder
2 teaspoons finely chopped fresh ginger
1 large eggwhite
¼ cup (25 g) quick-cook oats
1 cup (150 g) blanched almonds
1½ cups (150 g) pecan halves
1 cup (150 g) brazil nuts
⅓ cup (55 g) pumpkin seeds
⅓ cup (55 g) sunflower seeds
½ cup (75 g) sultanas
½ cup (75 g) dried cranberries

1. Preheat the oven to 130ºC. Mix together the curry powder, ginger, eggwhite and oats in a large bowl. Add all the nuts and seeds, and toss well to coat.

2. Transfer to a baking tin, spreading out evenly. Bake for about 1 hour, stirring occasionally, until lightly browned and crisp. Leave to cool in the tin.

3. Tip the nuts and seeds into a bowl. Add the sultanas and cranberries and mix well.

4. One serve is ⅓ cup (25 g). Store in an airtight container for up to 2 weeks.

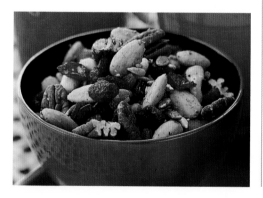

ROASTED CAPSICUM PINWHEELS

Makes 8 pieces
1 red capsicum, cut lengthwise into flat panels (about 4, depending on shape of the capsicum)
½ cup (55 g) canned chickpeas, rinsed and drained
1 tablespoon low-fat natural yogurt
½ teaspoon toasted sesame oil
½ teaspoon grated lemon peel
2 teaspoons lemon juice
2 teaspoons water
1 flour tortilla (20 cm in diameter), plain or flavoured
1 cup (100 g) mixed salad greens

1. Preheat the grill. Grill the capsicum pieces, skin side up, until charred. Transfer to a plate. When cool enough to handle, peel and cut into 1 cm-wide strips.

2. Combine the chickpeas, yogurt, sesame oil, lemon peel and juice, water and salt in a food processor and blend until smooth.

3. Spread the mixture evenly over one side of the tortilla, leaving a 1 cm border clear all round. Top with the salad greens and roasted capsicums. Roll up tortilla like a Swiss roll.

4. Wrap tightly in foil or cling wrap and chill for at least 1 hour, but no more than 4 hours. The roll will get softer and easier to slice as it sits in the refrigerator; if left longer than 4 hours it will become soggy. To serve, unwrap and cut across into 8 pieces (each 2.5 cm wide).

5. One serve equals 2 pieces. These pinwheels do not keep well and should be eaten the day they are made.

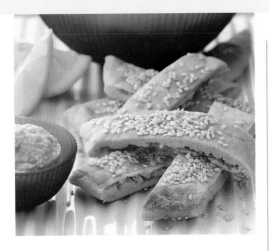

SESAME PITA CRISPS

Makes 36 pita crisps
6 pita breads
2 tablespoons olive oil
2 tablespoons sesame seeds

1. Preheat the grill to high. Spread the pitas on a baking tray. Using 1 tablespoon of the olive oil, brush the top side of each pita with oil. Sprinkle over half of the sesame seeds.

2. Grill for 1 minute or until the bread and the seeds are golden brown.

3. Turn the pitas over and brush with the remaining olive oil. Sprinkle over the rest of the sesame seeds. Grill for 1 minute or until bread and seeds are golden brown.

4. Using scissors, quickly cut the hot pitas across into 6 fingers. Leave to cool and become crisp.

5. One serve is 3 pita crisps. Can be stored in an airtight container for 1 to 2 days.

PARMESAN TWISTS

Makes 40 twists
1/2 cup (85 g) wholemeal plain flour
1/2 cup (85 g) white plain flour
50 g butter
50 g parmesan, grated
1 large egg
2 tablespoons reduced-fat milk
1 teaspoon paprika
1 tablespoon poppy seeds

1. Preheat the oven to 180°C. Sift the flours into a bowl, adding the bran from the sieve. Rub in the butter, then stir in the parmesan.

2. Whisk the egg and milk together. Reserve 1 teaspoon of the mixture and stir the rest into the flour mixture to make a firm dough. Knead briefly until smooth.

3. Sprinkle the paprika over a floured surface, then roll out the dough to a square just larger than 20 cm on all sides. Brush with the reserved egg mixture and sprinkle over the poppy seeds.

4. Cut the square of dough in half, then cut into 10 cm sticks that are about 1 cm wide. Twist the sticks and place on a baking tray lined with baking paper.

5. Bake for 15 minutes or until lightly browned and crisp. Cool on the baking tray for a few minutes, then transfer to a wire rack to cool completely.

6. One serve is 3 twists. Can be stored in an airtight container for up to 5 days.

TORTILLA CHIPS

Serves 8
8 corn tortillas, about 300 g
4 teaspoons canola oil
seasoning (e.g. ground cumin, or salt and freshly ground black pepper)

1. Preheat the oven to 170°C. Brush each tortilla with 1/2 teaspoon oil and sprinkle with seasoning.

2. Using kitchen scissors, cut each tortilla into wedges. Spread on a large baking tray.

3. Bake for 15 minutes or until crisp and firm. Transfer to a wire rack to cool. One serve equals chips from 1 tortilla.

4. Store in an airtight tin for 1 to 2 days.

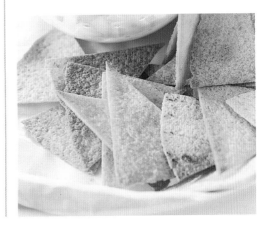

Fruit desserts

What could be more refreshing than a fruit-based dessert? Fruit adds colour and flavour to so many sweet dishes, together with weight-controlling fibre, vitamins and a whole host of other beneficial nutrients. Your family and friends will never know that you've lightened up the sweet course with these 420 kilojoule serves.

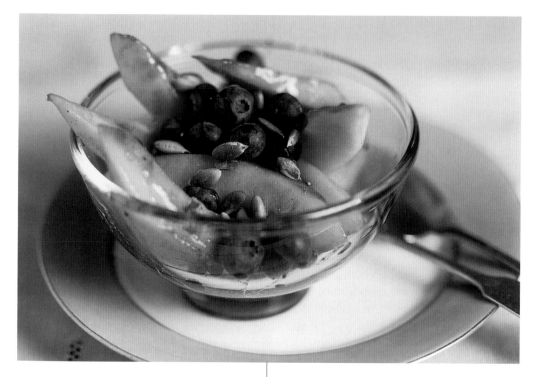

MELON SALAD WITH RASPBERRY VINAIGRETTE

Serves 4

- **1 tablespoon hulled pumpkin seeds**
- **4 tablespoons sugar-free seedless raspberry jam**
- **1 tablespoon balsamic vinegar**
- **2 teaspoons lemon juice**
- **¼ teaspoon ground cinnamon**
- **1 large rockmelon or other orange-fleshed melon, cut into 8 wedges**
- **1 cup (150 g) blueberries**

1. Toast the pumpkin seeds in a small, heavy frying pan over medium heat for about 5 minutes or until they begin to pop. Set aside to cool.

2. Whisk together the raspberry jam, vinegar, lemon juice and cinnamon in a large bowl.

Add the melon and blueberries and toss to combine. Sprinkle with the seeds.

3. One serve is 2 rockmelon wedges, a golf ball–sized serve of blueberries, and 1 teaspoon (thumb tip) of pumpkin seeds.

ABOUT MELONS

Melons – rockmelon, honeydew melon and watermelon – are among the lowest-kilojoule fruit because they have a high water content and less sugar than other fruit. Orange-fleshed melon especially is rich in vitamins C and A, two important nutrients that you get mainly from fruit and vegetables. A serve of melon cubes about the size of a fist contains between 200 and 250 kilojoules.

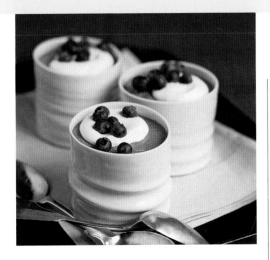

BLUEBERRY MOUSSE

Serves 4

½ cup (125 ml) reduced-fat milk
2 tablespoons dried skim milk
3 cups (450 g) blueberries
¼ cup (50 g) plus 1 teaspoon caster
sugar
½ cup (125 g) low-fat natural yogurt
1½ teaspoons powdered gelatine
2 tablespoons cold water

1. Combine the milk and dried milk in a small bowl and whisk until well blended. Place in the freezer for up to 30 minutes.

2. Reserve ½ cup (75 g) of the blueberries, and combine the rest with the ¼ cup (50 g) sugar in a medium saucepan over low heat. Bring to a simmer, stirring to dissolve the sugar, then cook for about 10 minutes or until the berries have broken up and the mixture has reduced to about 1 cup (250 ml). Cool to room temperature, then stir in three-quarters of the yogurt.

3. Sprinkle the gelatine over the cold water in a heatproof measuring jug. Soften for 5 minutes, then place jug in a saucepan of simmering water for 2 minutes or until the gelatine has dissolved completely. Cool.

4. Whisk the chilled milk until thick and soft peaks form. Whisk in the remaining teaspoon sugar and the gelatine mixture. Fold into the blueberry mixture.

5. Spoon into 4 dessert bowls or glasses. Chill for 2 hours or until set. Just before serving, top with the remaining yogurt and the reserved blueberries.

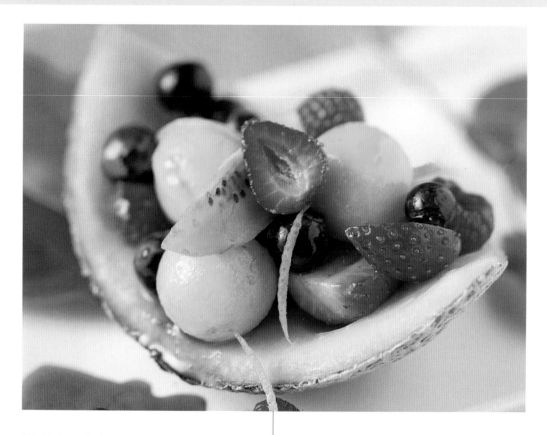

FRUIT BOATS WITH ORANGE AND BALSAMIC GLAZE

Serves 4

4 tablespoons balsamic vinegar
¼ teaspoon grated orange peel
2 tablespoons orange juice
2 teaspoons soft light brown sugar
1 large rockmelon or other melon
2 cups (350 g) strawberries, hulled and quartered
1 cup (150 g) blueberries
1 cup (150 g) raspberries
2 kiwifruit, peeled, halved and cut into thin wedges

1. To make the glaze, combine the vinegar, orange peel and juice, and brown sugar in a microwave-proof dish. Microwave on high for 2 to 3 minutes or until syrupy, or cook over medium-high heat in a small saucepan for 4 to 5 minutes. Set aside.

2. Cut the melon into quarters, discard seeds and scoop out balls of flesh, leaving a thin layer of flesh on the rind that you'll use as boats. Put the melon balls, strawberries, blueberries, raspberries and kiwifruit in a large bowl.

3. Drizzle over the glaze. Toss to coat the fruit evenly. Spoon into the 4 melon boats and serve immediately.

FRUIT AND HEALTH

Fruit and vegetables are extremely important to good health. This is reflected in the Dietitians Association of Australia's '7-a-day' recommendation – to eat at least 2 serves of fruit and 5 serves of vegetables every day. Fruit and vegetables offer a unique package of plant compounds, called phytochemicals, that are linked to lower risk of heart disease, high blood pressure, stroke, certain cancers and other long-term ailments. The evidence so far is that you get these benefits mainly from eating real fruit and vegetables, and much less so from taking vitamin and mineral supplements.

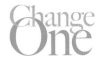

Meal plans & shopping guide

It's a vicious circle: if you don't know what you are going to be cooking in the week ahead, you can't shop for food effectively. And if you are not shopping effectively, it becomes very difficult to cook and eat well. As we've said a few times, eating well takes a little planning.

We're here to help. In this section, you'll find detailed weekly meal plans, plus strategies to buy and store food.

Following a rigid eating plan may seem unappealing, but give it a look. At worst, you'll get a quick overview of the *ChangeOne* program. And you may even stumble on a day or week that's worth a try.

Each day's meal plan comes very close to our target of 5500 kilojoules. For those in the 7000 Club, remember that you can double your starch or grain at breakfast, *or* double your protein at lunch or dinner, *or* add an extra serve of starch or grain at dinner.

And don't forget to check out the shopping strategies that follow the meal plans. You'll find tips and advice that will improve even the best-organised kitchen.

Week 1	Monday	Tuesday	Wednesday	
Breakfast	**Smoothie breakfast** (page 309) • Tropical smoothie • Toasted English muffin, half spread with peanut butter	**Bagel delight** (page 31) • Half bagel topped with cream cheese and jam • Yogurt with sliced ripe peach	**Breakfast on the go** (page 32) • Muesli bar • Yogurt topped with blueberries	
Lunch	**Chef's salad** (page 46) • Green salad topped with sliced chicken breast, ham and cheese • Crusty wholegrain roll • Diced melon	**Soup and sandwich** (page 312) • Hearty split pea soup • Bavarian sandwich • Seasonal fruit	**EATING OUT** **Friendly hamburger** (page 52) • Hamburger with lettuce, tomato and condiments • Tossed green salad	
Snack	Baked tortilla chips dipped in salsa	Cocoa made with skim milk	Baked apple (page 74)	
Dinner	**Fish from the grill** (page 322) • Barbecued fish with salsa, accompanied by grilled mixed onions • Wild and white rice	**Beef stew dinner** (page 94) • Beef stew • Egg noodles	**Thai noodle salad** (page 104) • Thai noodle salad	
Snack/ Dessert	Blueberry mousse (page 329)	Frozen yogurt	Yogurt smoothie	

Thursday	Friday	Saturday	Sunday
A perfect bowl of cereal (page 34) • Bran flakes topped with raisins and chopped nuts • Skim or reduced-fat milk	**Egg on a roll** (page 25) • Scrambled egg on a wholemeal roll • Fresh fruit salad • Skim or reduced-fat milk	**Pancakes with berries** (page 26) • Vanilla pancakes topped with maple syrup and sliced strawberries • Skim or reduced-fat milk	**Streusel cake** (page 231) • Skim or reduced-fat milk Brunch Hummus and pita Crudités platter (raw vegetables)
Pizza and salad (page 41) • Pita pizza • Green salad • Apple	**Soup and salad** (page 42) • Vegetable soup with breadsticks • Green salad topped with chicken • Green or red grapes	**Deli sandwich** (page 54) • Chicken and gruyère sandwich • Shredded vegetables • Melon salad	**The Sunday omelette** (page 134) • Vegetable cheese omelette • Chunky oven chips • Melon wedge • Orange juice
Frozen yogurt	Vita-Weat with low-fat cottage cheese	Tub of natural yogurt topped with fruit	
EATING OUT **Italian** (page 114) • Melon with prosciutto • Pasta arrabbiata with parmesan • Mixed salad • Fresh figs	**Pantry stew** (page 158) • Chickpea, sweet potato and carrot stew • Garlic bread	**EATING OUT** **Chinese** (page 116) • Hot-and-sour soup • Prawns stir-fried with ginger and spring onions (scallions) • Plain boiled rice • Fresh pineapple	**Fish parcels with Spanish rice** (page 102) • Baked salmon parcels with tomatoes • Spanish rice
Glazed bananas (page 74)	Latte made with skim or reduced-fat milk	Microwave popcorn	Apple

Week 2	Monday	Tuesday	Wednesday	
Breakfast	**Smoothie breakfast** (page 309) • Tropical smoothie • Toasted English muffin, half spread with peanut butter	**A perfect bowl of cereal** (page 34) • Bran flakes topped with sultanas and chopped nuts • Skim or reduced-fat milk	**Egg on a roll** (page 25) • Scrambled egg on a wholemeal roll • Fresh fruit salad • Skim or reduced-fat milk	
Lunch	**Tuna salad sandwich** (page 228) • Tuna salad sandwich • Carrot and celery sticks • Banana	**Chicken Caesar lunch** (page 314) • Grilled chicken Caesar salad • Fresh fruit salad	**Well-dressed baked potato** (page 316) • Baked potato stuffed with broccoli and cheese • Mixed green salad • Seasonal berries	
Snack	Mixed dried fruit	Parmesan twists (page 327)	Frozen yogurt	
Dinner	**Chicken dinner** (page 318) • Chicken and caramelised onion stir-fry • Spinach fettuccine • Tossed salad	**Braised beef dinner** (page 320) • Wine-braised beef with vegetables • Steamed broccoli • Crusty bread	**Pasta primavera dinner** (page 100) • Pasta primavera • Italian salad	
Snack/ Dessert	Fruit boats with orange and balsamic glaze (page 330)	Apple	Pineapple chunks	

Thursday	Friday	Saturday	Sunday
Bagel delight (page 31) • Half bagel topped with cream cheese and jam • Yogurt with sliced ripe peach	**Breakfast on the go** (page 32) • Muesli bar • Yogurt topped with blueberries	**Fruit bread delight** (page 311) • 1 slice peach and yogurt loaf • Fresh raspberries • Skim milk or low-fat yogurt	**Pancakes with berries** (page 26) • Vanilla pancakes topped with maple syrup and sliced strawberries • Skim or reduced-fat milk
Soup and sandwich (pages 312–313) • Cream of asparagus soup • Bavarian sandwich • Seasonal fruit	**Deli sandwich** (page 54) • Chicken and gruyère sandwich • Shredded vegetables • Melon salad	**Mexican wrap** (page 57) • Flour tortilla filled with chicken, beans and condiments • Orange	**Wrap it up** (page 317) • Roasted vegetable wraps with chive sauce • Green salad • Honeydew melon
Peanut butter on a rice cake	Strawberry smoothie	Rich tea biscuits with skim or reduced-fat milk	Pretzel sticks and reduced-fat cheddar
EATING OUT **Family restaurant** (page 122) • Tomato soup • Grilled chicken with potato wedges and tomato salsa • Large mixed salad with low-fat dressing • Ice-cream with strawberries	**Fish from the grill** (page 322) • Barbecued fish with salsa, accompanied by grilled mixed onions • Wild and white rice	**Barbecued chicken feast** (page 142) • Spicy barbecued chicken • Grilled summer vegetables • Warm potato salad with dijon vinaigrette • Sesame breadsticks	**Pantry stew** (page 158) • Chickpea, sweet potato and carrot stew • Garlic bread
Almond-flavoured milk	Sorbet	Frozen yogurt	Blueberry mousse (page 329)

Week 3	Monday	Tuesday	Wednesday	
Breakfast	**Fruit bread delight** (page 311) • 1 slice peach and yogurt loaf • Fresh raspberries • Skim milk or low-fat yogurt	**A perfect bowl of cereal** (page 34) • Bran flakes topped with sultanas and chopped nuts • Skim or reduced-fat milk	**Pancakes with berries** (page 26) • Vanilla pancakes topped with maple syrup and sliced strawberries • Skim or reduced-fat milk	
Lunch	**Soup and sandwich** (page 312) • Hearty split pea soup • Bavarian sandwich • Seasonal fruit	**Chicken Caesar lunch** (page 314) • Grilled chicken Caesar salad • Fresh fruit salad	**EATING OUT** **Friendly hamburger** (page 52) • Hamburger with lettuce, tomato and condiments • Tossed green salad	
Snack	Rice cake with peanut butter	Digestive biscuit and hot cocoa made with skim milk	Breadsticks with tomato salsa	
Dinner	**Fish parcels with Spanish rice** (page 102) • Baked salmon parcels with tomatoes • Spanish rice	**EATING OUT** **Indian** (page 120) • ½ vegetable samosa plus salad • Tandoori king prawns • Spicy lentil dhal • Fresh fruit salad	**Colourful stir-fry** (page 92) • Fried rice with tofu and vegetables	
Snack/ Dessert	Pineapple chunks		Frozen yogurt	

Thursday	Friday	Saturday	Sunday
Breakfast on the go (page 32) • Muesli bar • Yogurt topped with blueberries	**Bagel delight** (page 31) • Half bagel topped with cream cheese and jam • Yogurt with sliced ripe peach	**Hearty frittata** (page 310) • Vegetable frittata • 1 slice wholemeal toast • Fresh blueberries	**Quiche with fruit bread** (page 135) • Asparagus and cheddar quiche • 1 slice peach and yogurt loaf (page 311) • Orange juice
Pizza and salad (page 41) • Pita pizza • Green salad • Apple	**Deli sandwich** (page 54) • Chicken and gruyère sandwich • Shredded vegetables • Melon salad	**Soup and salad** (page 42) • Vegetable soup with breadsticks • Green salad topped with chicken • Green or red grapes	**Fishcake brunch** (page 132) • Crab cakes • Tossed salad • Crusty bread roll • Seasonal berries
Mixed dried fruit	Curry-spiced fruits, nuts and seeds (page 326)	Tub of low-fat yogurt	Mixed nuts
Chicken, beans and rice (page 161) • Quick beans and rice • Grilled chicken fillet • Green salad	**Thai noodle salad** (page 104) • Thai noodle salad	**Quick tuna pasta** (page 164) • Penne with tuna • Rocket salad	**EATING OUT** **Italian** (page 114) • Tomato bruschetta • Small serve of spaghetti with seafood • Granita
Frozen yogurt	Fresh fruit	Melon salad with raspberry vinaigrette (page 328)	Fresh fruit salad

Week 4	Monday	Tuesday	Wednesday	
Breakfast	**Egg on a roll** (page 25) • Scrambled egg on a wholemeal roll • Fresh fruit salad • Skim or reduced-fat milk	**Smoothie breakfast** (page 309) • Tropical smoothie • Toasted English muffin, half spread with peanut butter	**A perfect bowl of cereal** (page 34) • Bran flakes topped with sultanas and chopped nuts • Skim or reduced-fat milk	
Lunch	**Chicken Caesar lunch** (page 314) • Grilled chicken Caesar salad • Fresh fruit salad	**Mexican wrap** (page 57) • Flour tortilla filled with chicken, beans and condiments • Orange	**Chef's salad** (page 46) • Green salad topped with sliced chicken breast, ham and cheese • Crusty wholegrain roll • Diced melon	
Snack	Cocoa made with skim milk	Mixed nuts	Roasted capsicum pinwheels (page 326)	
Dinner	**Colourful stir-fry** (page 92) • Fried rice with tofu and vegetables	**Pasta primavera dinner** (page 100) • Pasta primavera • Italian salad	**EATING OUT** **Bistro and pub** (page 118) • Steamed mussels • Salmon fishcakes • Large mixed salad • Fresh berries	
Snack/ Dessert	Fruit boats with orange and balsamic glaze (page 336)	Fresh fruit salad		

Thursday	Friday	Saturday	Sunday
Breakfast on the go (page 32) • Muesli bar • Yogurt topped with blueberries	**Hearty frittata** (page 310) • Vegetable frittata • 1 slice wholemeal toast • Fresh blueberries	**Bagel delight** (page 31) • Half bagel topped with cream cheese and jam • Yogurt with sliced ripe peach	**The Sunday omelette** (page 134) • Vegetable cheese omelette • Chunky oven chips • Melon wedge • Orange juice
Pizza and salad (page 41) • Pita pizza • Green salad • Apple	**Well-dressed baked potato** (page 316) • Baked potato stuffed with broccoli and cheese • Mixed green salad • Seasonal berries	**Wrap it up** (page 317) • Roasted vegetable wraps with chive sauce • Green salad • Honeydew melon	**Soup and salad** (page 42) • Vegetable soup with breadsticks • Green salad topped with chicken • Green or red grapes
Mixed dried fruit	Tortilla chips (page 327)	Crudités	Sesame pita crisps (page 327)
Chicken dinner (page 318) • Chicken and caramelised onion stir-fry • Spinach fettuccine • Tossed salad	**Prawn kebab feast** (page 90) • Prawn and capsicum kebabs • Sesame broccoli • Wild and white rice	**Fish from the grill** (page 322) • Barbecued fish with salsa, accompanied by grilled mixed onions • Wild and white rice	**Braised beef dinner** (page 320) • Wine-braised beef with vegetables • Steamed broccoli • Crusty bread
Frozen yogurt	Sorbet	Blueberry mousse (page 329)	Seasonal fruit

Shopping strategies

Putting *ChangeOne* into action at the supermarket is easy with our guide to sensible shopping. Use it to make your own checklists to ensure you're never without the essentials.

Chances are, you already have many of the ingredients for the sample meals in our four-week plan. It is surprisingly easy to cook with flavour and richness when you have a good collection of condiments, herbs and spices, stocks, canned beans and baking supplies close by. They're part of the basic provisions – the pantry, refrigerator and freezer items to keep always on hand.

ChangeOne meals also call for lots of perishable foods such as fruit, vegetables, meats and dairy products. That's where a good checklist comes in handy. For your convenience, we've designed a *ChangeOne* shopping plan that takes care of these foods in two categories: long-life and short-life.

Supermarkets stock their produce separately from dairy, meats and seafood, so that's the way for you to set up efficient checklists for your *ChangeOne* shopping plan.

Long-life items such as apples, onions and other foodstuffs you can store in a cool place or in the refrigerator – they keep for a while and are good to have to hand all the time.

Fruit and vegetables
- Apples • Kiwifruit • Lemons and limes
- Melons (uncut) • Oranges • Cabbage
- Carrots • Celery • Garlic • Onions and spring onions (scallions) • Potatoes
- Pumpkin and other squash

Dairy products, meat and seafood
- Butter • Cheeses, hard and dry (e.g. parmesan) • Yogurt • Beef (in the freezer)
- Chicken joints (in the freezer) • Salami, hard Italian • Salmon (in the freezer)

Short-life items such as lettuce, milk and uncooked meats – these keep only a few days in the refrigerator and are best bought and used for a specific recipe.

Fruit and vegetables
- Berries in season • Grapes • Mangoes
- Peaches • Zucchini • Cucumbers
- Lettuce and salad greens • Capsicums, red and green • Tomatoes

Dairy products, meat and seafood
- Cheeses, medium (e.g. cheddar, mozzarella) • Cheeses, soft (e.g. ricotta, cottage) • Milk • Cooked deli meats
- Meats and seafood, uncooked

ChangeOne shopping plan

Monthly. At around the same time every month, check and replenish your kitchen staples.

Twice monthly. Replenish long-life fruit and vegetables, dairy products, meat and seafood as needed.

Weekly to twice weekly. Pick up short-life items for that week's meals. A few general tips can simplify your shopping even more.

- Plan a whole week's recipes and write your shopping list. Then check your pantry and refrigerator for items you will need that week.
- You can substitute just about any fruit or vegetable for another, so buy those that you like or those that are in season.

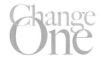

Personal tools

Throughout *ChangeOne*, we've asked you to write things down. How's the weight-loss progressing? What are your current goals? What did you eat today? What activities did you do?

But the truth is, few of us are in the habit of writing down such things. So we've tried to make it easier for you.

On the following pages are all the guides you need to progress through *ChangeOne.*

Each of these forms was conceived to be as simple to use as possible. They ask the tough questions, but in easily answerable ways. So give them a try. They take just a few minutes. You are free to make as many photocopies of each form as you need to track your progress.

Here's what you'll find.

- *ChangeOne* Contract
- Your healthy weight calculator
- Hunger profile
- Daily food diary
- Daily activity log
- Progress log

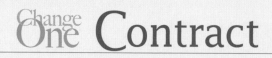

Contract

ChangeOne start date: _____

I VOW TO MYSELF that over the next three months I will learn and
practise the eating habits necessary to lose weight and improve my health.
I put forth the following goals:

Intermediate weight target: _____

Ultimate weight target: _____

HOW I EXPECT MY LIFE TO IMPROVE: _____

_____

_____

_____

HOW I EXPECT MY HEALTH TO IMPROVE: _____

_____

_____

_____

IN ADDITION to weekly weigh-ins on the scales, I will track my progress
by the two methods I will list below (for example, clothing size, appearance,
energy, notches in a belt, or self-confidence):

1. _____

2. _____

I HEREBY AFFIRM that the goals I have set meet the TRIM test. Each one is
Time-bound, Realistic, Inspiring and Measurable.

I agree to review my progress and re-evaluate my strategies for reaching my
goals every two weeks during the program.

I agree to keep this contract as a reminder of my commitment.

Signed: _____

Witnessed by (optional): _____

Your healthy weight calculator

What's your ideal weight? The answer depends on your body type. Researchers use a scale called Body Mass Index, or BMI, which assigns a number based on a combination of height and weight. Essentially, the number indicates whether you are carrying a healthy or unhealthy level of body fat.

To find your BMI on the chart below, locate your height in centimetres across the bottom of the chart. Then move your finger up the column to see if your weight falls into the healthy weight range. Finally, your BMI appears at the right of the chart.

You'll notice that a healthy weight range covers a range of BMIs. For example, the healthy weight range for someone who is 170 cm tall is between 54 kilograms and 72 kilograms, and the BMI is between 18.5 and 25. The reason for this is that people have different body types, some slender, some stocky, some small-boned, some large.

The BMI index isn't foolproof. It tends to overestimate body fat in athletes and people with very muscular builds. It tends to underestimate body fat in older people, who have usually lost muscle mass.

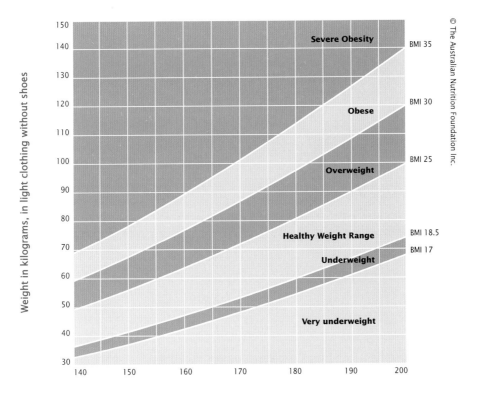

Height in centimetres, without shoes

Remember that losing even a few kilograms when you're overweight will improve your health, reducing your risk of heart disease and diabetes. Trying to bring your weight down to a normal BMI is a terrific goal. But if you have a long way to go to get there, set some milestones along the way. Reward yourself at each step, and don't get discouraged. Every little bit helps.

Date:

Hunger profile

Instructions: Make a copy of this form and carry it with you during the day. Every time you get hungry, record the time, how you felt (tired, bored, ravenous, stressed out, just plain hungry), what you ate or what you did instead of eating (took a walk, distracted yourself with work). This will help you to determine your eating habits – both good and bad – and make it easier to adjust your meal and snack times for healthy weight loss.

	TIME	HOW I FELT	WHAT I ATE	WHAT I DID
MORNING				
AFTERNOON				
EVENING				

Date:

Daily food diary

Instructions: First, write down what you eat. Next, estimate serves as carefully as you can, based on what you've learned throughout *ChangeOne*. For example, if one egg is the recommended serve at breakfast, and you eat two, then write in 'two serves'. Keep a copy of the form with you and fill it in as soon after a snack or meal as you can.

Adding up kilojoules is optional. We don't recommend that *ChangeOne* participants worry about kilojoules – managing serve sizes will take care of that. But if you really want to see how you are doing, here's how to find kilojoule information:
- For *ChangeOne* meals, use kilojoule counts that we provide;
- For *ChangeOne* snacks and desserts, estimate 420 kilojoules per serve;
- For other snacks and prepared foods, use their nutrition labels.

	WHAT I ATE	ESTIMATED SERVES	KILOJOULES
BREAKFAST			
LUNCH			
DINNER			
SNACKS			
	TOTAL KILOJOULES (optional):		

Date:

Daily activity log

Instructions: Use this form to track daily exercise. Include all activities of 5 minutes or more in duration and estimate their intensity. As general guidelines, light activities could include dusting, ironing, playing bowls. Moderate activities could include playing golf, raking the lawn, walking, washing the car or dancing. Strenuous activities could include aerobic dance, jogging, bicycling, swimming, hiking with a backpack and playing tennis. When you're done, add up the number of minutes you spent doing light, moderate and strenuous activities.

	WHAT I DID	TIME SPENT IN MINUTES PER INTENSITY		
AM		Light	Moderate	Strenuous
6:00				
7:00				
8:00				
9:00				
10:00				
11:00				
PM				
12:00				
1:00				
2:00				
3:00				
4:00				
5:00				
6:00				
7:00				
8:00				
9:00				
10:00				
11:00				
AM				
12:00				
1:00				
2:00				
3:00				
4:00				
5:00				
	TOTAL MINUTES:			

Progress log

Instructions: Once a week, record your weight and estimate how much time you spend being active. Jot down notes on any problems or issues you're facing. Try to weigh yourself and fill in the form at the same time each week.

Week of: _____ Weight: _____

AVERAGE DAILY ACTIVITY
❏ 45 minutes or more
❏ 30 minutes
❏ Less than 30 minutes

HOW I'M FEELING
❏ Great
❏ Okay
❏ Stressed out
❏ Discouraged
❏ _____

NOTES
_____
_____
_____
_____
_____

Week of: _____ Weight: _____

AVERAGE DAILY ACTIVITY
❏ 45 minutes or more
❏ 30 minutes
❏ Less than 30 minutes

HOW I'M FEELING
❏ Great
❏ Okay
❏ Stressed out
❏ Discouraged
❏ _____

NOTES
_____
_____
_____
_____
_____

Week of: _____ Weight: _____

AVERAGE DAILY ACTIVITY
❏ 45 minutes or more
❏ 30 minutes
❏ Less than 30 minutes

HOW I'M FEELING
❏ Great
❏ Okay
❏ Stressed out
❏ Discouraged
❏ _____

NOTES
_____
_____
_____
_____
_____

Week of: _____ Weight: _____

AVERAGE DAILY ACTIVITY
❏ 45 minutes or more
❏ 30 minutes
❏ Less than 30 minutes

HOW I'M FEELING
❏ Great
❏ Okay
❏ Stressed out
❏ Discouraged
❏ _____

NOTES
_____
_____
_____
_____
_____

		WEEK 1	WEEK 2	WEEK 3	WEEK 4
At the end of the month, plot a graph to chart weight changes during the month.	+3.5 kg				
	+2.5 kg				
	+1.5 kg				
	+1 kg				
_____ STARTING WEIGHT					
	−1 kg				
	−1.5 kg				
	−2.5 kg				
	−3.5 kg				

Index

Entries in *italics* refer to recipes

FOR READER'S DIGEST AUSTRALIA

Senior Editor
Barbara McClenahan

Designer Avril Makula

Nutritional Analysis
Toni Gumley

Food photography
Elizabeth Watt and John Freeman

Exercise photography
Cara Howe/StudioW26

Portion guide photographs
Christine Bronco

Portraits George Kamper

Success Story portraits provided
and reproduced by permission
of the participants

Senior Production Controller
Monique Tesoriero

READER'S DIGEST GENERAL BOOKS
Editorial Director Lynn Lewis

Managing Editor
Rosemary McDonald

Art Director Carole Orbell

Credits
All images © Reader's Digest,
except the following: cover,
1, 2–3, 4–5, 7 *br*, 10–11,
199, 201, 202, 204, 207,
210, 226, 234–5, 306–7, 316
(Shutterstock)

ChangeOne, the diet and fitness plan is published by
Reader's Digest (Australia) Pty Limited, 80 Bay Street,
Ultimo, NSW 2007
www.readersdigest.com.au, www.readersdigest.co.nz,
www.rdasia.com

First Australian and New Zealand edition 2006
Reprinted 2007 (paperback)
Revised and updated edition 2014

This book was originated by the editorial teams of The Reader's
Digest Association, Inc., USA, and The Reader's Digest Association
Limited, London.

National Library of Australia Cataloguing-in-Publication data:

Title: ChangeOne: the diet and fitness plan: the 12-week program
that will change your life forever.

Edition: Revised and updated edition.

ISBN: 978-1-922085-23-8 (paperback)
Notes: Includes index.
Subjects: Reducing diets. Reducing diets – Recipes. Reducing diets –
Menus. Reducing exercises.
Other Authors/Contributors: Reader's Digest (Australia)
Dewey Number: 613.25

Prepress by Colourpedia, Sydney
Printed and bound by Leo Paper, China

We are interested in receiving your comments on the content
of this book. Write to:
The Editor, General Books Editorial, Reader's Digest (Australia)
Pty Limited, GPO Box 4353, Sydney, NSW 2001
or e-mail us at bookeditors.au@readersdigest.com

To order additional copies of *ChangeOne, the diet and fitness plan*,
please contact us as follows:
www.readersdigest.com.au, 1300 300 030 (Australia);
www.readersdigest.co.nz, 0800 400 060 (New Zealand);
or e-mail us at customerservice@readersdigest.com.au

Product Code 041-5269
Concept Code US9100/IC

2–3 CDs
About 55–85 grams
**Use for sandwich meats,
sliced cheese**

Serve guide

These shapes will help you visualise
serve sizes in *ChangeOne* meals.

CHEQUEBOOK
About 165 grams
**Use for serves of
chicken breast fillet,
light-fleshed fish**